The Ultimate Breastfeeding
Book of Answers

The *The* Ultimate Breastfeeding Book of Answers

REVISED AND UPDATED

The Most Comprehensive

Problem-Solving Guide to

Breastfeeding from the Foremost

Expert in North America

Jack Newman, M.D., *and* Teresa Pitman

 Three Rivers Press • New York

To Adele, Daniel, Elise, and David Marc,
without whom I would never have understood any of this.
J.N.

To Matthew, Lisa, Daniel, and Jeremy, who taught me
that breastfeeding is about more than just giving milk.
T.P.

Library of Congress Cataloging-in-Publication Data

Newman, Jack, 1946–
The ultimate breastfeeding book of answers :
the most comprehensive problem-solving guide
to breastfeeding from the foremost expert in North America /
Jack Newman and Teresa Pitman.—Rev. and updated.
p. cm.
Includes index.
1. Breastfeeding. 2. Infants (Newborn)—Nutrition.
3. Infants (Newborn)—Care. 4. Lactation.
I. Pitman, Teresa. II. Title.
RJ216.N49 2006
649'.33—dc22   2006018606

ISBN-10: 0-307-34558-0
ISBN-13: 978-0-307-34558-5

Printed in the United States of America

10 9 8 7 6 5 4 3

First United States Edition

Contents

Introduction

Why is this breastfeeding book unique? Surely there are enough books and information pamphlets on breastfeeding available that another is not necessary! Or is it?

Women have, of course, managed to breastfeed throughout the human race's time on earth without the benefit of "breastfeeding experts" (though women's experience and knowledge used to be transmitted from generation to generation in a way they aren't for many women today), and have managed to do so using techniques and ways of holding babies that might seem impossibly inefficient to some. Many women still use such techniques, and succeed just fine.

In fact, there are women who do things very differently from what most lactation experts would recommend. Their babies are not latched on well, they stick to scheduled feedings, they hold the baby in awkward positions. And yet, they manage to breastfeed.

For many women, though, this isn't the case. With a little practical help, they will be able to succeed at breastfeeding; without it, they may not. The information they need is still hard to find. They hear conflicting advice from their doctors, the hospital nurses, their mothers and their friends, and the books they read tell them something else again. It can be hard to separate myth from reality.

The Ultimate Breastfeeding Book of Answers will help you do so.

This book is based on my understanding of breastfeeding and breastfeeding issues. And this understanding is based on the experience of my own family, much learning from others interested in lactation, and almost 20 years of helping mothers with breastfeeding problems. The knowledge I have gained over the years is what I hope to share with the reader of this book—knowledge that has helped many women breastfeed successfully, despite some challenges and difficulties along the way.

I will readily admit that I do not always do things as others might. I differ from many lactation specialists, for example, in my disdain for the use of measurements as the approach to understanding what is going on with a particular mother and baby. I don't find it helpful to weigh babies frequently or to wake them every three hours, for example, because I believe that a baby who is breastfeeding well doesn't need to be woken up—he'll let you know when he is hungry. And if the baby is not feeding well, his going to the breast more often won't help—drinking nothing *eight* times a day is no better than drinking nothing *six* times a day. The issue for me is whether the baby is feeding well or not.

My approach is based on observing mothers and babies, and giving them help, support, and information. Even with such aid, a very few mothers will not be able to breastfeed. But for the majority of women, these factors can make the difference between breastfeeding well—or having to give up.

When I speak at conferences about breastfeeding, I am almost always asked how I became interested in this field. I think the question itself speaks volumes about how we see roles in our society. Breastfeeding, obviously, is done by mothers and babies. The fact that a male pediatrician is interested in breastfeeding seems unusual to many people—a downright bizarre career choice.

In the past, some physicians took an interest in breastfeeding only in order to find alternatives to it. They looked for some way of feeding infants whose mothers had died, for example. Wet-nurses often fed these babies, but it was not always possible to find one. So infant formula was developed, and, through trial and error, improved so that babies usually survived with it, and even thrived. But physicians were rarely concerned about the science and art of breastfeeding.

So how did I end up specializing in helping women breastfeed?

I had the same medical education as the other students who attended medical school with me, and that training included nothing about breastfeeding. I remember quite well the only lecture we had on infant feeding. It lasted an hour. Breastfeeding was not even mentioned. We were taught, in 1969, that to make formula, you took one part cow's milk, two parts water, and one tablespoon of corn syrup, and then . . . Actually, I couldn't remember what then, and maybe that's why I was so receptive to the idea of breastfeeding—when I found out that it existed.

That happened when I was doing my fourth-year rotation of obstetrics and gynecology. One day, at the six-week postpartum clinic, I was asked by the resident to examine a woman—ask her how she was doing, if she had any symptoms, examine her uterus and her breasts. When I examined her breasts, milk shot out at least a yard. I was amazed. What was going on here? What was that? I am not kidding you—I had no idea such a thing was possible, and I wasn't sure what this all meant. They hadn't prepared me for this in medical school. Surely they should have mentioned something about this secretion that occurs in the breast after birth?

I also knew it was not possible for the mother to have milk, because I knew that the routine orders on the maternity floor were to give the mothers an injection to *dry up* their milk. As far as I could see, this was done with everyone, and as far as I could determine, nobody ever asked the mothers if they wanted the injection. Perhaps the mothers were asked before they delivered whether they were going to breastfeed, but they certainly were not asked again if they were sure before receiving the injection.

That was it for a while. That's all I ever got in medical school about breastfeeding. And, of course, breastfeeding was so unimportant in the curriculum that there was not a single question about it on the final exams.

I remember, a few years later, I saw a woman breastfeeding in the market in San Cristóbal de las Casas, Mexico. It was such an unusual sight for me that I actually took a photo of her. Quaint, right? How Third World of her! Good *National Geographic* photo.

Then my wife and I had our first baby in 1976. I cannot tell you why neither Adele nor I ever considered anything for our son except breastfeeding. It was not even in our minds to feed formula, and I'm not at all sure why. We learned that breastfeeding may be natural, but that it is not always easy. But it worked well enough, and our baby was breastfed exclusively, except for a few bottles of sugar water here and there when he seemed to want to nurse all the time (and no, I would not recommend that today). Since I was working as the only doctor in the small town where we lived at the time, and my wife was the only nurse, we didn't have anyone to ask. We muddled through. Daniel breastfed until he was almost four years old.

Because I was now the father of a breastfed baby, I became a bit more interested in the topic. I began to notice news reports about babies in Africa and other countries who were dying because they were not breastfed. I realized that most of the pediatricians I was working with knew very little about breastfeeding—not even the little I had learned watching Adele and Daniel nursing together. In my first year of pediatrics, breastfeeding did not come up at all as a topic of discussion. I remember that neither staff nor residents ever asked women if they were breastfeeding or not. I remember we did not ask mothers of babies in the special care unit to bring in milk. All babies were fed formula by bottle. By today's standards, this formula was completely inappropriate for premature babies, much less appropriate than breastmilk would have been. Yet the notion of using breastmilk for the premature babies was never a priority or even discussed. That was in one hospital where I trained.

Then I moved to the Hospital for Sick Children in Toronto. I thought things would be different. They were, a little. Breastfeeding was mentioned more, mostly in the context of how it was getting in the way of measuring the amount of fluids a baby was getting. One older staff pediatrician mentioned that his children were breastfed and implied that he felt it was important. That impressed me. But generally, formula was used without a thought. In the intensive care unit, we wrote orders for formula, often without even asking if the mothers were providing milk. (The mothers were always elsewhere, since the Hospital for Sick Children did not have babies born there.)

When I finished my residency in pediatrics, I went to work in Africa in 1981, and what I saw there confirmed what I had heard about the horrors of bottle-feeding in those circumstances. Every day, babies died because they were not breastfed—or even if they were partially breastfed—because they were getting extra formula. The water used to prepare the formula was often contaminated, and these babies weren't getting the vital antibodies from breastmilk that would have helped them fight off infections. The mothers often didn't have enough money to buy sufficient formula, so they watered down the small amounts they had. Starving babies and children were admitted every day to the hospital, babies and children who shouldn't have been starving.

I realized that if we could institute three fairly simple public health measures—two of which were taken for granted in Canada—we could be sitting around twiddling our thumbs much of the day instead of running around hopelessly trying to catch up with all the sick children.

- All children would be immunized. Every day children died of measles, in particular. Polio was common, tetanus frequent. Whooping cough seemed uncommon, but devastating when it did occur.
- All the tuberculosis contacts would be followed up and treated. Tuberculosis was epidemic.
- All babies would be breastfed exclusively to about six months, and would continue to breastfeed for two years and beyond.

Obviously, I couldn't do everything, so I concentrated on helping mothers breastfeed. This seemed to me to be easier and less expensive to accomplish than tackling the other issues. Little did I know how much resistance the formula companies and other physicians, especially some of the physicians in the private hospital (in Africa!), could put up.

In fact, I did get lots of support from most colleagues and co-workers. The nurses who worked in the hospital were incredible. They could get babies breastfeeding who had been off the breast for weeks, and they managed to get milk supplies to increase. I know now that I should have paid much more attention to what the nurses were doing, but I didn't. At the time, I thought there wasn't much to know about breastfeeding. You just put the baby to the breast, right? I'd figured out that you don't give bottles or time feedings, but that was it.

When I returned to Canada, I went to work in the Hospital for Sick Children emergency department as a staff pediatrician. Every day, I saw mothers and babies suffering with breastfeeding problems. Some mothers knew their frustrations were related to breastfeeding; some did not. What was striking, however, was how lousy the information was that they were getting about breastfeeding. Not only was the advice bad, but it sometimes defied logic and common sense. And I heard this same bad advice quoted by many different mothers, so I knew it was widespread. I did what I could to help the women, but I didn't know how to solve many of the larger issues surrounding breastfeeding.

One day, our chief of emergency came to a staff meeting and suggested that we should take four hours a week out of our schedules to do something other than emergency—to prevent burnout. I did not want to do what most of the others were doing—a general clinic, which involved dealing with children with behavior and learning problems and other chronic issues. I was an emergency pediatrician; long-term issues were not my thing. So I decided to start a breastfeeding clinic. My experiences in the emergency department had shown me that there was a definite need.

During the first full year of the clinic at the Hospital for Sick Children, 1985, only 70 mothers and their babies came. Many Monday mornings there were no mothers and babies at all. But slowly, the clinic got busier. Some of the mothers who came succeeded brilliantly (probably not because of anything I did, because I still knew very little). But their success encouraged me, and I was learning all the time. The word started to spread. I am now seeing, personally, 1,200 or more mothers and their babies each year.

The success of the clinic created its own momentum. I began to attend seminars on breastfeeding and to learn from the mothers I worked with and other breastfeeding experts. Soon I realized that the breastfeeding issues that most of the mothers were coming to see me with should not have been issues at all. Their problems were caused by the ignorance of the nurses and doctors in the postpartum areas about breastfeeding and about how to help mothers with breastfeeding. More than 90 percent of the difficulties women have with breastfeeding could be—and should be—prevented.

When I saw these situations, I believed that the hospitals, doctors, and nurses would want to know how their policies and advice were causing breastfeeding difficulties for the women they worked with. I started writing letters to these people, explaining what the problems were. The response wasn't what I expected. I got angry letters back insisting that the mothers I had seen had not told me the truth about their experiences in the hospital. Sometimes I would simply be told to mind my own business. Sometimes they would write to the Chief of Pediatrics to complain about me.

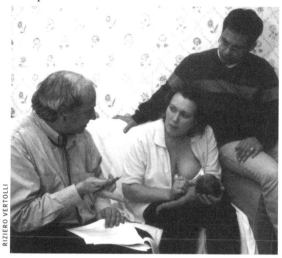

Consultations with the whole family . . .

But I couldn't stop being concerned about the babies who cried and suffered because they weren't getting enough milk, the mothers who struggled with agonizingly sore nipples and painful breasts, and the many other problems caused by breastfeeding mismanagement.

So when the Hospital for Sick Children decided to close the breastfeeding clinic there, I began seeing women at other hospitals around the city of Toronto. Now, I usually see between 10 and 20 mothers and babies each day.

And I have not stopped writing letters, speaking at conferences and workshops, and trying to prevent breastfeeding problems. Once one takes up a cause, it becomes more and more difficult to ignore the real issues. I began to see how the formula companies aggressively and, to my mind, unethically marketed their products. I began to see how the whole health system

collaborated, quite willingly, with the formula companies. I began to see that infant feeding was not a question of the mother making an informed choice between breastfeeding and bottle-feeding. Not at all.

Once I started examining it, I realized the whole system works against mothers and babies breastfeeding. We have stacks of research to show that breastfeeding is important for the health and optimal development of babies, and yet it is too often seen as expendable and unimportant. In my efforts to support breastfeeding, I sometimes found myself in conflict with obstetricians, pediatricians, and hospital nurses—not to mention dietitians who were concerned because they couldn't measure everything, radiologists who told mothers they couldn't breastfeed after MRI (Magnetic Resonance Imaging) scans, anesthetists who told mothers they couldn't breastfeed after a general anesthetic, and many other health professionals who seemed to recom-

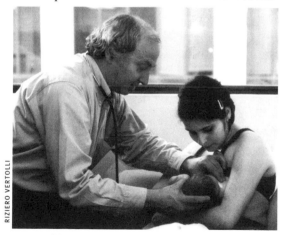

. . . and hands-on work with a mother and her baby

mend weaning in almost any situation. I found myself in opposition to child protection services that believe separation of breastfeeding mothers and babies is not an issue, and judges in family court who believe fathers deserve to have alternate weeks with their children even if it means destroying the breastfeeding relationship.

Breastfeeding should *never* be expendable. Only under extraordinary circumstances should breastfeeding be interrupted. It is too important to the physical and mental health of the child and the mother for them to give it up the way one might give up ice cream.

The purpose of this book is to empower women. Their right to breastfeed, and their babies' right to be breastfed, should be paramount. It is more important than the comfort of the person sitting near them in the restaurant who is offended by seeing a baby breastfeed. It is more important than the physician's desire to recommend a particular drug for the mother without bothering to find something compatible with breastfeeding. It is more important than the other hospital routines and paperwork that take up the time of the postpartum nurses.

My hope is that this book will help mothers and fathers understand how breastfeeding works, how it can be accomplished, and how it is being undermined. In these pages, you will find information about getting breastfeeding off to a good start, dealing with challenging situations, and handling breastfeeding in special circumstances. I also hope to counteract many of the widely held myths about breastfeeding—myths that can become obstacles to the new mother.

Breastfeeding is important. It is worth making the effort to overcome challenges such as sore nipples or a premature baby's weak sucking reflex so that breastfeeding can succeed. And it is equally important to make the changes needed in our medical system and our society so that breastfeeding becomes easier and more acceptable.

It's been a slow process, but we're getting there. Each mother who has a happy, successful breastfeeding experience brings us one step closer to a society where breastfeeding is, once again, the norm.

I

The Normal Way
to Feed a Baby

1

Why Breastfeeding
Is Important

Myth: Infant formulas are pretty much the same as breastmilk, so it doesn't make much difference which you choose.

Fact: The risks to feeding a baby with anything other than the milk nature designed for him are real, and are a concern even in societies where medical care and treatment for the problems caused by these formulas are readily available. In some parts of the world, the use of breastmilk substitutes means many babies will very probably not survive. While the vast majority of bottle-fed babies in North America will survive, that doesn't mean the health problems and risks are not real and potentially serious for both the individuals affected and the larger society that must help to care for them.

Health care providers, childbirth educators, and others often talk about the "advantages" of breastfeeding. But to describe the differences between breastfeeding and artificial feeding this way includes the underlying assumption that artificial feeding is what is normal and acceptable, even though there may be some "fringe benefits" to breastfeeding.

The warning messages on packages of cigarettes don't say, "Non-smokers may have lower rates of heart disease or lung cancer," they say, "Smoking increases your risk of heart disease and lung cancer." That's because we know that

breathing in smoke-filled air is not normal or good for the human lungs.

The different way we express this information is even clearer when we present statistics and percentages from research. If women who were breastfed as infants show (as they did in a recent study) a decrease of 25 percent in breast cancer rates when compared to women fed formula as infants, this can—more accurately—be restated this way: Women who were fed formula as infants had a 33.3 percent increase in breast cancer rates. Looks more significant, doesn't it?

It is *breastfeeding* that is the normal way to feed a baby. Breastfeeding is what the baby's body and developing systems are designed to expect, and there are many factors involved in breastfeeding that are not yet fully understood. The important difference between the two methods of infant feeding is that there are risks to artificial feeding.

One area of risk is in the manufacturer's preparation of these breastmilk substitutes. As with any manufactured food item, there are sometimes mistakes in the composition of the food; contamination with bacteria and other material; and errors in the processing. There is a long history of formula recalls for various reasons—important ingredients left out, bacteria or other contaminants found in some cans, incorrect labeling and more.

While these can happen with any food product,

9

infant formulas are different because they are the only food the baby gets for several months. If an important ingredient is missing (as has happened in the past), the effect on the baby can be serious. Babies have suffered brain damage and permanent developmental delays because of chloride-deficient formulas; babies have become ill with diseases such as meningitis from contaminated formulas. A recent study of several brands of formulas found that some cans contained more than four times the amount of Vitamin D listed on the label—and Vitamin D in excess is toxic. Choosing to use these substitutes for breastmilk means relying on a manufacturer's assembly line, which will inevitably produce some errors and problems, and parents simply have to hope that their baby isn't unlucky enough to get that batch of formula, and that they notice when a particular lot number is recalled.

We often assume that if breastfeeding is not possible—a rare situation—formula is the second-best solution for feeding the baby. The World Health Organization (WHO), though, makes it very clear that infant formulas are not second best to breastfeeding. Second best would be the mother's own milk, pumped or expressed, and fed to her baby (perhaps with a cup or tube). This is only second best because the value of breastfeeding includes such benefits as the development of the baby's jaw and facial muscles as he nurses at the breast, and the transfer of germs back and forth between the mother and the baby, which helps protect the baby against infection and allergies, is more likely to occur when the mother and baby are together, touching, skin to skin and mouth to breast. Expressed milk won't provide those important factors, but it is the next best thing to breastfeeding. If pumping or expressing is impossible, the third feeding suggestion on WHO's list is

donated milk from a breastmilk bank. Only if that is also unavailable would artificial baby-milk feedings be used—the fourth-best solution.

But even the most complete, best prepared formula of any brand has significant risks when compared to "the real thing"—breastmilk.

Let's look at some of the areas that have been researched and consider the risks to babies fed artificially.

Intelligence and Cognitive Development

We know that the human baby's brain is not yet fully developed at birth, and that it continues to grow and make important connections between the cells of the brain for about three years after birth. Once that process is completed, brain cells may die but no new ones can be added. Breastmilk, because it is designed for human babies, contains all the nutrients a baby's brain needs to reach its maximum potential.

Breastmilk substitutes (formulas), however, don't have all these components. In fact, we don't really know what all of them are.

Researchers have known from early on that children who breastfed as infants scored, on average, higher on tests of intelligence and development, but researchers tended to attribute this to other factors. Perhaps mothers who chose to breastfeed were more motivated to do good things for their children, and this led to their being more involved in teaching their children as they grew up. Or perhaps the extra holding and skin-to-skin contact involved in breastfeeding was the reason these children were brighter, and mothers using breastmilk substitutes could achieve the same results by simply holding their babies more.

Holding babies more and teaching them more are both good things. But a 1992 study tried to eliminate these factors by looking at premature babies who were being fed through a tube. Some of these babies were given their mothers' milk, and some were given breastmilk substitutes—and the results were significant. When they reached school age, the children who had received breastmilk scored higher on tests of intelligence. The milk itself makes a difference.

Other researchers have studied babies who were breastfed for varying lengths of time, and found that intelligence scores were higher (on average) for babies who were breastfed longer.

It may be that the increased skin-to-skin contact and holding is also a factor. While mothers who are giving their babies formula will usually hold them during feedings when the babies are very small, once the baby is old enough to hold his own bottle, he is often set down in an infant seat to feed himself. As he gets older still, he's likely to be given his bottle while sitting in a high chair or while walking around. A breastfeeding mother, on the other hand, always sits or lies down with her baby, to hold him on her lap or cuddle him beside her. This contact is undoubtedly beneficial to both of them.

Diabetes

Diabetes is a serious disease that is becoming increasingly common. Type I is the type seen in children, and there is clearly a genetic component that makes some children vulnerable to this illness. While the evidence is not conclusive, studies have shown that when formula or cow's milk is not introduced to the baby's diet until he is older (some have recommended waiting at least one year), the baby is less likely to develop diabetes.

SIDS

SIDS stands for Sudden Infant Death Syndrome—situations in which a baby dies, usually while asleep. This is also known as crib death or cot death. No cause for this syndrome has been discovered, and there are probably several factors involved. (After many years of advising parents always to put the baby to bed lying on his stomach, for example, doctors are now recommending that babies sleep on their backs to reduce the incidence of SIDS.) Researchers have found that feeding a baby with formula does increase the risk of the baby dying from SIDS.

Respiratory Illnesses

If you've noticed the steadily increasing numbers of children with asthma, you're not alone. There are multiple causes of this problem, too (one being the increasing amount of air pollution in our cities, and another, the larger numbers of children in day care situations, where they are exposed to more viruses at an earlier age).

Once again, though, feeding the baby with formula is a risk factor for developing asthma. Babies fed formula instead of breastmilk are also at a higher risk of other respiratory illnesses, including respiratory syncytial virus (RSV). They also take longer to recover from these illnesses than do breastfed babies.

Ear Infections

Since ear infections are quite common in infants and young children, this area has been frequently researched, and formula-feeding has been repeatedly shown to be a risk factor in developing otitis media (ear infection). Ear infections are often very painful for the baby, and can lead to further complications—fluid can stay in the ear for a period of time after the infection has been treated, affecting the baby's hearing and speech development.

Childhood Cancer

At least three studies have found that formula-feeding increases the risk of developing cancer during childhood. These studies are not conclusive, but there are good theoretical reasons why the conclusions may be correct.

Gastrointestinal Infections and Diseases

It seems logical that the baby's gastrointestinal system would be affected by the choice of infant feeding method—and it is. Formula significantly increases the baby's risk of diarrhea caused by various infections, and babies who are fed artificially also take longer to recover from these illnesses. This is in part because they often have to be taken off their formula and given only clear fluids while they are sick—meaning that they get fewer nutrients—while a breastfed baby can, and should, continue nursing and receiving high-quality nutrition plus antibodies to kill off the germs that are causing the illness.

Breastfed babies are much less likely to become constipated. In fact, their bowel movements are usually very loose, even if they become infrequent. Formula is much more likely to cause constipation and painful bowel movements.

Effectiveness of Vaccines

Artificial feeding reduces the effectiveness of vaccinations by diminishing the baby's response and production of the necessary antibodies. Breastfed babies have a better response to vaccinations, and produce more antibodies.

Normal Development of Jaw and Facial Muscles

Anyone who has carefully observed a baby suck on a bottle and compared it to the way a baby suckles at the breast knows that these are two very different techniques. Naturally, they lead to different development of muscles in the baby's cheeks, jaw, and tongue. Some people claim they can recognize a breastfed baby on sight, just by looking for the rounded, well-developed cheeks! The importance of this becomes clear as the child gets older—children who were artificially fed as babies are more likely to need orthodontic work. Long-term breastfeeding, in particular, seems to promote the development of a well-shaped jaw and straight teeth.

Other Conditions

Artificial feeding increases the baby's risk of many other problems as well. Several recent studies found that artificially fed babies are much more likely to become obese as children and teens. They are at greater risk of colitis, meningitis, Crohn's disease, necrotizing enterocolitis, eczema, certain types of heart disease, and allergies, among others.

Risks to the Mother

Breastfeeding helps new mothers to recover from giving birth by encouraging the uterus to contract normally and by reducing the amount of blood loss.

It also reduces the risk of developing breast cancer. Some early studies didn't reveal this benefit; they tended to lump together women who had breastfed for only a few days with those who had breastfed for several years. Since then, more careful research has shown that the length of breastfeeding is important—the greater the total number of months of breastfeeding, the lower the risk of developing breast cancer.

Myth: Breastfeeding is too difficult and time-consuming for today's mother.

Fact: Breastfeeding is convenient, easy once you get the hang of it, and an enjoyable experience for most women.

The topic of the first meeting in the standard La Leche League series of four meetings is Advantages of Breastfeeding. (Yes, they should probably change it to Risks of Artificial Feeding if they want

ready, always at the right temperature. It takes just a second to lift up a shirt or undo a button and offer the breast to the baby. They find breastfeeding easy when they're traveling to places where it might be hard to store formula at the right temperature or find a place to heat it. They love being able to just roll over in bed and feed the baby when he fusses with hunger in the night. And they appreciate not having to spend time preparing or cleaning bottles, because it means extra time with the baby.

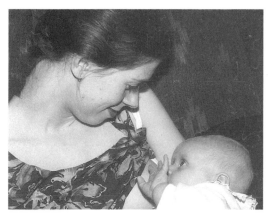

Breastfeeding is about more than just giving milk. Mothers *and* babies benefit from the special closeness of the breastfeeding relationship.

to discuss the medical issues.) Often the leader of the group invites each mother to share the reason she thinks breastfeeding is important or valuable, and the discussion then flows around the room.

Some mothers talk about how breastfeeding reduces allergies or ear infections. Some talk about the studies they've seen reported on how breastfed babies who are in day care stay healthier because of the extra antibodies, so the mothers will have to miss less work. Some might mention they hope to reduce their own risk of breast cancer.

But they're the minority. Most mothers talk about the emotional side of breastfeeding and how it makes mothering a baby, toddler, or young child easier and more enjoyable.

They like the convenience: the milk is always

Mothers often say it takes them a few weeks to really understand that breastfeeding is more than just another way of getting food into the baby. At first, they are focused on the mechanics of getting the baby to latch on properly and figuring out how much he is eating. But once those techniques are mastered, some of the other important aspects of breastfeeding become apparent.

Breastfeeding is a great comfort to a baby who has been hurt or scared or upset for some other reason. It soothes a baby who has to be given a vaccination, and calms a baby who has been startled by a dog suddenly barking, or is stressed by being separated from his mother. It reminds the baby of being in the womb: "Ah, yes, there's that familiar heartbeat, and that voice I've always heard, and that familiar smell, and I'm warm and comfortable," and makes the transition to the outside world a little easier.

Breastfeeding is a good thing for new mothers, too. Mothers at the meetings talk about how breastfeeding forces them to slow down in a busy world and spend time with their babies. You can't prop up a breast and leave the baby to eat while you finish washing the dishes. Breastfeeding guarantees that you and baby will be skin to skin, relaxing together, several times a day. And those restful feeding times can be helpful in recovering from pregnancy and birth.

They love the smell of the breastfed baby—that clean smell that doesn't come from any soap or talcum powder. Even the baby's bowel movements don't smell unpleasant—they give off that faint yeasty odor that warns you right before it all runs out of the diaper and down the baby's leg.

They talk about how breastfeeding tunes them in to their baby's signals. Mothers tell stories about how they couldn't consciously recognize their baby's crying, but their breasts did, and started to leak milk at the sound of his voice. They talk about how often they wake up just a minute or so before the baby does. Some tell stories about how they knew their baby was ill because of a small change in the way he suckled or behaved at the breast.

Mothers talk about how they learned, through the ongoing experience of breastfeeding, to understand the baby's sometimes subtle cues. One mother was nursing her baby while chatting with a public health nurse. At some point during the conversation, the mother moved the baby to the other breast. The nurse stopped what she was saying and asked, "Why did you change breasts?" The mother, surprised, said, "He was finished that side, and he wanted the other one." The nurse insisted that she hadn't seen any signals from the baby. But the mother had felt the baby preparing to let go of the nipple, and without even thinking about it, moved the baby to offer the other breast. These kinds of interaction become unconscious after a while. Experienced nursing mothers can tend to other children, prepare meals, talk with friends and still be aware of the baby's suckling so that they know when to adjust the baby's latch, when to change breasts, and when the feeding is over and the baby wants to be moved to another position.

They will talk about the sheer pleasure of being skin to skin with their baby, and of seeing him drift off to sleep at the breast with a trickle of milk running down his chin. As the baby gets older, and breastfeeding doesn't take all the baby's energy and concentration, he'll begin to play at the breast, letting go to smile up at Mom, patting Mom's cheek or investigating her dental work, making happy noises as he nurses. These are all part of the joy of parenting.

> "Taking a little one to nurse, watching him grow to manhood, that's what love is."
> Carol Shields, *The Stone Diaries*

Mothers who work outside the home talk about how much they appreciate that bond. It's hard to leave your baby in someone else's care, but being able to put the baby to the breast when you get home at the end of the day can re-establish the connection, and be relaxing for both mother and baby. These mothers like having something special between them and their babies—something the babysitter can't do.

These experiences are difficult to measure in a scientific way, but they are very real to mothers, and they are important considerations in deciding whether to breastfeed or bottle-feed.

Yes, It's Worth Solving the Problems

Twenty years ago, almost any difficulty encountered by a breastfeeding mother had a single solution: wean the baby. Sore nipples? *Stop nursing.* Breast infection? *Wean immediately.* Baby isn't gaining weight well? *Quit nursing.* This probably seemed pretty easy and straightforward to the doctor giving out the advice, but it was often devastating to the mother who really wanted to breastfeed.

If the baby was premature or smaller than average in size, even if born full term, the mother was usually advised not to even try breastfeeding, because suckling would be too hard for the baby, and breastmilk wouldn't have enough calories to help him gain weight. If a baby was bigger than average, mothers were often told that their breastmilk wouldn't be enough to sustain him, and that giving formula would be better. If either baby or mother had any health issues, breastfeeding would be stopped.

Now mothers are more likely to be aware of the benefits and importance of breastfeeding, but may still have difficulty getting the help they need to make breastfeeding work.

MOTHERS' STORIES
LESLEY

Lesley's labor was induced a week before her due date because her blood pressure was high, and her doctor was concerned. After a short but intense labor, her daughter was born weighing just over seven pounds (3 kg). She seemed very sleepy, and Lesley wasn't able to get her to nurse right away. The nurse expressed concerns about the baby's breathing, and took the infant to the nursery for observation.

When Lesley went home a day later, the baby had nursed a couple of times but not well, and Lesley's nipples were getting sore. By the time the baby was three days old, Lesley's nipples were unbearably painful, and the engorgement she was experiencing made it even harder to get the baby on the breast. When she took the baby to the doctor, he recommended supplementing with a bottle of formula after each feeding, and suggested she take painkillers before she nursed, to make the feedings more comfortable.

Dissatisfied with that, Lesley called the public health department, and a nurse made a home visit. The nurse watched Lesley try to breastfeed her baby and examined her nipples—which were cracked and beginning to bleed. Her advice: "Put the baby on a bottle. This isn't working." Lesley wanted to breastfeed, not wean. She found a book in the library that explained how sore nipples could be caused by the baby not being well latched on, but it took several more calls before she found someone who could help her get the baby correctly latched on. Her sore nipples healed.

Lesley was well aware of the reasons breastfeeding her baby was important, but she needed more than that—she needed some practical help. It is only when more people become informed about the importance of breastfeeding for babies that more help will be available to nursing mothers.

Breastfeeding and Guilt

One reason that the many significant differences between breastfeeding and formula-feeding have been downplayed is that people are concerned about making mothers who do not breastfeed feel guilty.

But this concern about guilt is, in reality, just a ploy. It is an argument that deflects attention from the lack of knowledge and understanding of many health professionals about breastfeeding.

This allows *them* not to feel guilty for their ignorance regarding how to help women overcome difficulties with breastfeeding (many of which could be prevented in the first place). This argument also allows formula companies and health professionals to pass out formula company literature and free samples of formula to pregnant women without any guilt pangs, even though it has been clearly demonstrated that this literature and the free samples decrease the frequency and duration of breastfeeding. There are often deliberate attempts to make the two methods of feeding seem equivalent—for example, lists of "pros and cons" of breastfeeding and formula mention things such as "baby's bowel movements smell better" as a reason for breastfeeding—an unimportant benefit that is easily canceled out by one of the listed "benefits" of formula-feeding, such as "father can feed baby, too." The list may be rigged to come out with the same number of benefits to both types of feeding—but only if dozens of significant advantages to breastfeeding are completely ignored.

This is not how health professionals discuss other decisions with their patients when there are health implications. If a pregnant woman went to her physician and admitted she smoked a pack of cigarettes, is there not a strong chance that she would leave the office feeling guilty about endangering her developing baby? If she admitted to drinking a couple of beers every so often, surely she would leave the office feeling guilty?

How about if she went to the doctor's office with her one-week-old baby and told the physician that she was feeding her baby homogenized milk? What would the physician's reaction be? Most would practically collapse and have a fit. And they would have no problem at all making that mother feel guilty for feeding her baby cow's milk, and then pressuring her to feed the baby formula instead (not pressuring her to breastfeed, of course, because they wouldn't want to make her feel guilty about not breastfeeding).

Why is there such indulgence for formula? The reason, of course, is that the formula companies have succeeded so brilliantly with their advertising in convincing most of the world that formula-feeding is just about as good as breastfeeding, and that there is therefore no need to make a big deal about women not breastfeeding. It is also reassuring for the many health professionals who themselves did not breastfeed, or whose wives did not breastfeed.

While a doctor would not hesitate to press for a mother to use formula rather than plain cow's milk, the truth is that while formula is theoretically more appropriate for a baby than cow's milk, there are no long-term clinical studies showing any difference. Not one. The differences between cow's milk and formula are much smaller than the differences between formula and breastmilk. Furthermore, we have a wealth of clinical data to show how much better off the breastfed child is, and almost every day there are new studies showing additional health benefits.

So how should breastfeeding be supported? All pregnant women and their families need to know the risks of formula-feeding. It does matter. All should be encouraged to breastfeed, and all should get the best support available to start breastfeeding once the baby arrives. This support is critical. It is no use telling women how breastfeeding will benefit their babies, and then making it difficult for them to breastfeed—thanks to unhelpful hospital routines or bad advice from health professionals.

If mothers get the information about the risks of formula-feeding, and have a good source of support and help, and still decide to formula-feed, they will have made an informed decision. Their information about feeding should not come from the formula companies, however, as it so often does. The formula company pamphlets give some advantages of breastfeeding, but then go on to imply that their formula is just as good. If mothers get good help with breastfeeding but still find it is not for them, they can decide to switch to bottle-feeding, if they choose. It is not difficult to go from breastfeeding to bottle-feeding; it is much more difficult to switch from bottle-feeding to breastfeeding.

While You're Pregnant

You can begin to prepare for breastfeeding while you are pregnant—not by "toughening up your nipples" as mothers were at one time advised to do, but by planning for your baby's birth and getting the information you need. Some ideas:

- Attend at least one meeting of a breastfeeding support group like La Leche League while you are pregnant. You will get to see babies breastfeeding, and meet people who can provide you with information and support once the baby arrives.

- If you will be giving birth in a hospital, ask about the hospital policies. Make it clear that you want your baby to be with you from birth on, unless there is a medical problem.

- Discuss with your partner and your doctor or midwife what you can do to get breastfeeding initiated if there are problems such as a cesarean birth, premature baby, or if either you or the baby is ill.

- Arrange for support and practical help once you go home from the hospital, so you can concentrate on learning to breastfeed.

2

Finding
Good Breastfeeding Help

Myth: Health professionals know more about breastfeeding than other people do.

Fact: All health professionals—nurses, midwives, physicians—say they are supportive of breastfeeding. It would be difficult for them not to, as the evidence of the superiority of breastfeeding increases on a daily basis, and all the major professional organizations (such as the Canadian Paediatric Society and the American Academy of Pediatrics) have made statements about its importance. But the claims to support breastfeeding are sometimes only on the surface, and professionals' ability to provide real, practical help to breastfeeding mothers may be seriously inadequate.

This inability to help may come from their own experiences as parents. It is difficult to provide a lot of support and encouragement for mothers around breastfeeding when your own breastfeeding experience (or that of your wife) involved a lot of pain, a fussy baby, and early weaning to formula. It's also difficult when your medical training did not actually include much information on breastfeeding techniques, getting things off to a good start, or solving any problems that come up. Once medical school is over, it doesn't get any better. Instead of being supplied with good information about breastfeeding, the doctor's office is deluged with advertising from formula companies and invita-

tions to seminars on infant nutrition—sponsored, of course, by a formula company.

Many health professionals are supportive only when breastfeeding is going well and easily. Some are not supportive even then. As soon as there are any difficulties with breastfeeding, or the baby is not fitting precisely into the growth charts, or the life of the new mother is not perfect, too many health care professionals advise weaning the baby or supplementing breastfeeding with formula. This is almost always unnecessary, or could be avoided with proper help.

How can you know if the person you are relying on for your medical care is *not* supportive of breastfeeding? Here are some clues:

He or she gives you formula samples or literature from one or more formula companies when you are pregnant or soon after you have had your baby.

What is the purpose of these formula samples and information? Why do formula companies give them out and urge doctors to distribute them? There is only one purpose: to advertise and market infant formulas. The brochures, videos, and samples of formula are given to you to encourage you to use the formula, to wean your baby early or supplement unnecessarily, so that you will eventually depend on a formula company for your baby's food. The brochures and videos usually contain a mix of accurate and subtly misleading information that undermines breastfeeding, and the handy can of formula is a powerful suggestion to the mother that her milk will not be enough—that at some point she will need this formula. They are not innocent gifts or harmless samples.

And we know that it works. The research results are clear: mothers who are given these samples of formula wean their babies earlier than mothers who are not. The effectiveness of

is also true that not all breastfed babies grow up to be healthy and secure. But this does not mean that it doesn't make any difference how you feed your baby.

Breastmilk is very different in composition from formula. Not only does it contain antibodies and living white blood cells to protect babies from illness, but it changes from day to day and month to month as the baby's needs

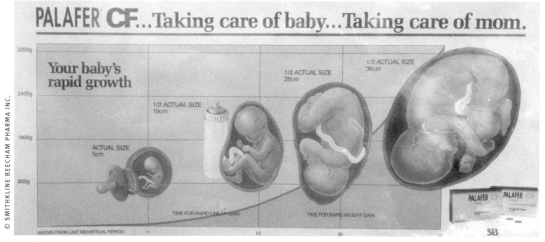

An ad for iron tablets for pregnant women in a women's health clinic. The company does not make formula or bottles, but the poster shows well the pervasive nature of bottles and pacifiers as symbols for babyhood in our society. This "bottle-feeding" mentality interferes with our understanding of how breastfeeding works, and often is at the root of health professionals' advising that mothers stop breastfeeding, *almost always* unnecessarily.

this approach is further demonstrated by the determination shown by formula companies in getting these samples into the hands of pregnant women and new mothers. If it didn't work, they wouldn't invest so much time, money, and effort into this form of advertising.

Ask yourself why your health professional is marketing infant formula. And ask yourself why he or she is not marketing breastfeeding.

She or he tells you that breastfeeding and bottle-feeding are essentially the same.

It is true that most bottle-fed babies grow up to be physically healthy and emotionally secure. It

change. It even changes from the beginning of the feeding to the end. It is easily digested, and the nutrients are readily absorbed.

Formula, on the other hand, is just a rough approximation of what we knew several years ago about what goes into breastmilk, and it is based on the milk of an entirely different species. There are many things in breastmilk that can't be duplicated in formula, and formula can't change to meet the baby's changing needs.

Breastfeeding is also not the same as bottle-feeding. It is a different kind of relationship. The breastfed baby is guaranteed a certain amount of holding and skin-to-skin contact as long as he continues nursing. This doesn't mean that bottle-feeding parents can't give their babies lots of holding and skin-to-skin contact. It just takes more effort and thought.

Health professionals often describe breast-feeding and bottle-feeding as being more or less equivalent because they are concerned that mothers who are not able to breastfeed will feel guilty or disappointed. If you are not able to breastfeed, it is unfortunate. To pretend that it is unimportant or insignificant is patronizing and medically inaccurate. A baby does not have to be breastfed in order to grow up healthy and secure, but breastfeeding is clearly beneficial to both mother and baby, and it is natural to be disappointed if you are, for whatever reason, unable to breastfeed.

He or she tells you that a particular brand of formula is the best.

There is no evidence that one brand of formula is better than any other brand for the normal, healthy baby. Some babies do seem to tolerate one better than another, but this is very individual. When a health professional recommends one over another, it may be because that formula representative has most recently dropped by with more information. Or it may mean that his or her own children tolerated that brand of formula the best.

Either way, this should tell you that the health professional is making recommendations based on something other than research. This should concern you, because the doctor is not strongly supporting and encouraging breastfeeding.

She or he tells you that it is not necessary to breastfeed the baby immediately after birth, since you will be too tired and the baby is often not interested anyway.

While breastfeeding in the first hour or two after birth may not be necessary in terms of the baby's survival at that time, it is helpful in getting breastfeeding well established. While you may be tired after labor, you will also be excited about meeting your new baby and eager to connect with him. This is a time when both you and your baby are most ready to begin breastfeeding.

The baby can nurse even if you have to lie flat after giving birth. Some babies are not interested in taking the breast immediately after birth, but most will latch on within an hour or two, and if they are kept close to their mothers they will begin to search for the nipple when they are ready. If they are taken away from their mothers, many will go into a deep sleep and not show any interest in nursing for many hours. Early breastfeeding has been shown in many research studies to be helpful in getting breastfeeding established, and the colostrum that your breasts produce in the first few days after the baby is born is valuable for the baby.

Often it seems as though hospital routines—weighing the baby, taking footprints, giving eyedrops and Vitamin K injections—all take priority over keeping mother and baby together and getting breastfeeding established. There is no reason why any of these things can't wait for a couple of hours, while mother and baby begin nursing. When these other tasks are given a higher priority, breastfeeding is made to seem unimportant, and again this calls into question the health professional's commitment to breastfeeding.

He or she tells you there is no such thing as nipple confusion, and that you should start giving bottles early to your baby to make sure he will accept the bottle nipple.

The health professional who assumes that an artificial nipple is harmless is looking at the world as if bottle-feeding, not breastfeeding, is the normal method of infant feeding. Why would anyone stress the importance of getting a baby used to an artificial nipple, when there are so many other ways to supplement a baby's food intake, should that become necessary?

The artificial nipple has not been proven harmless to breastfeeding. Just because there are some—or even many—babies who are given bottles and pacifiers from time to time and who continue to breastfeed without apparent problems, that does not mean that other babies do not develop problems. We have no way of predicting in advance which babies will be able to cope with both, and which will not. And often there is a combination of factors—one of which is the use of artificial nipples—which together add up to breastfeeding difficulties and, often, early weaning.

And if there is no problem with confusion or switching back and forth between bottles and breasts, then why the emphasis on starting a baby on a bottle early, to be sure he will accept it? There is an underlying assumption here, that at some point you will need to give your baby bottles, even though many breastfed babies *never* get bottles and end up, eventually, weaning from the breast and drinking out of a cup. Health professionals should be supporting breastfeeding without setting up the idea that before too long the baby will be on a bottle.

She or he tells you that you must stop breastfeeding because you are ill, or your baby is ill, or you need medication or medical tests.

There are some rare situations in which illness in the mother or baby means that breastfeeding cannot continue. Too often, though, health professionals recommend weaning the baby without any further investigation, and almost always it is not necessary. A health professional who is truly supportive of breastfeeding will make every effort to find ways to continue breastfeeding even while coping with medical conditions.

A few years ago, most doctors recommended that women with breast infections should immediately wean their babies. In some cases, this made the situation worse and led to a breast abscess. Now most understand that nursing through a breast infection is not only quite safe for the baby, but will help the mother heal more quickly and with fewer complications.

Mothers with illnesses such as the flu or gastrointestinal ailments are often advised to wean their babies and are warned that they risk dehydration if they continue to nurse. However, most find it easier to continue breastfeeding than to deal with a miserable baby and engorged breasts. Taking small, frequent drinks of juice or flat ginger ale will help to keep the mother hydrated, and she can nurse her baby while lying in bed if she's not feeling well. She doesn't need to worry about passing the infection on to the baby, because the baby was already exposed to the virus before the mother had any symptoms. Now the baby will benefit from the antibodies his mother's body is producing and passing on in the milk.

What about more serious illnesses, for which the mother needs medication? In most cases, the mother will be able to continue breastfeeding because the medication will not affect her baby. In situations where the drug is not safe during breastfeeding, there is almost always an alternative drug that can be used. It is extremely uncommon for there to be only one medication for a particular condition. The Compendium of Pharmaceuticals and Specialties (CPS) is not a good resource for this, because drug manufacturers tend to say all drugs are contraindicated for breastfeeding mothers, in order to protect themselves from legal liability. See Chapter 11, Breastfeeding While on Medication, for more information and for some good resources.

If your health professional's first suggestion is a medication that requires you to stop breastfeeding, you have a right to be concerned that not enough attention is being paid to the importance of breastfeeding.

He or she is surprised to learn that your six-month-old is still breastfeeding.

One public health nurse—who often stressed how much she supported breastfeeding—had a call about another question from the mother of a seven-month-old baby. The nurse asked the mother what the baby was eating, and the mother said, "Oh, he's breastfeeding." The nurse asked what the mother gave the baby when she gave him bottles: "Are you giving him formula or straight cow's milk in his bottle?" The mother repeated, "No, he's breastfeeding. No bottles, no solid foods." The nurse paused for a moment and said, "Well, you're brave."

The nurse's expression of surprise that a seven-month-old baby would still be nursing, and her expectation that this baby would be getting bottles even though the mother had clearly stated that he was breastfed, were both unsupportive of breastfeeding. She was suggesting that there was something abnormal or strange about a baby breastfeeding at this age, and that he should have been getting at least some bottles.

In fact, in most of the world, breastfeeding for at least two or three years or longer is common, normal, and recognized as a desirable thing. Research by anthropologist Kathy Dettwyler suggests that the natural age of weaning for

humans is somewhere between 2½ years and 7 years. Breastfeeding for this length of time seems to promote optimum brain development, and good development of the baby's teeth and jaw, and to reduce the incidence and severity of many illnesses and allergies.

It is not unusual to see a North American three-year-old carrying around a bottle or using a pacifier. Even more children this age have a bottle or pacifier at bedtime or naptime, even if they don't use them the rest of the time. Both of these are substitutes for being at the breast, yet we often consider them to be more acceptable than breastfeeding—the real thing.

The same professionals who think it is strange to continue breastfeeding after six months usually recommend giving babies formula until they are at least nine or 12 months old. Many recommend special follow-up formulas designed for babies who are eating solid foods. But remember that these formulas are only imitations of breastmilk—modifications of cow's milk (or soy milk) intended to make them more digestible and closer to breastmilk. Why should the imitation be considered better than the original?

He or she tells you that there is no value in breastmilk after the baby reaches a certain age—six months, 12 months, or whatever.

This is simply not true. Even if it were true, even if breastmilk suddenly turned to water at a certain age, there would still be value in *breastfeeding*. The closeness of mother and child, the ability to comfort and soothe at the breast, the interaction between two people in love, would all be just as important even without the milk.

But breastmilk, at whatever age and stage the baby has reached, is still milk. It still has all the calcium, fats, protein, vitamins, and minerals that it always did, and these are all readily absorbed and used by the child's body. It is a milk uniquely designed for humans. If there is value in a young child drinking cow's milk—which, while it contains important nutrients, is harder for the child's body to digest and absorb—surely there is far more value for that child in having breastmilk.

In addition, the concentration of some immune factors in breastmilk actually increases as the child grows older, providing even more protection against illnesses such as gastroenteritis, respiratory infections, ear infections, etc. This protection is important, because older babies and toddlers are much more likely to eat cookies off the floor, kiss (or bite) other children, and otherwise be exposed to a wider range of germs. If your child is in day care or around large numbers of children, these protective antibodies will be very important.

He or she tells you that you must never allow your baby to fall asleep at the breast.

Why not? It is fine and sometimes convenient if a baby can also fall asleep without nursing, but one of the great advantages of breastfeeding is that you have a handy way of putting a tired baby to sleep. Nothing calms a baby or toddler like breastfeeding. Even a child who has become overtired or overexcited by the busy activities around him will usually calm down, relax, and fall asleep at the breast.

For mothers who are told not to let their babies fall asleep at the breast, breastfeeding is more difficult. What is a mother supposed to do if her baby is both tired and hungry, and she knows that he's likely to fall asleep nursing? If she doesn't feed him, he may fall asleep on his own but wake up after a short time because he's so hungry. If she tries to keep him awake while he nurses by tickling his feet or stimulating him in other ways, he's

likely to get annoyed and may even bite, refuse the breast, or end up crying. She may stop the feeding before the baby has really had all he wants, in order to prevent him from falling asleep—and that means he'll wake up sooner than he would have otherwise, because he's hungry again. The feeding becomes a tense experience instead of being relaxed and happy. Sometimes mothers who are told not to let their babies sleep at the breast end up resorting to using pacifiers to put the baby to sleep, even though pacifier use may interfere with breastfeeding, especially if there are already breastfeeding difficulties.

She or he tells you not to stay in the hospital to breastfeed your sick child because it is important for you to rest at home.

Babies who are ill do not need breastfeeding less than healthy babies, they need it *more*. Your doctor and your hospital should be making every effort to create an environment where you can get the rest you need while staying with—and breastfeeding—your baby. When your baby is ill, it is *not* the time to introduce formula to his system. This is the time when he needs your milk the most, with its perfect nutrition and active disease-fighting components. How much rest would you really get, anyway, if you went home? You'd be awake worrying about your baby.

If your medical advisor makes these statements, don't accept them at face value. Ask for more information. Ask for a second opinion—and look for someone with expertise in breastfeeding.

So How Do You Find Good Breastfeeding Help?

When you are choosing a family doctor or a pediatrician, ask about breastfeeding. Of course, your doctor supports breastfeeding. But ask more questions: *What percentage of your patients breastfeed? At three months? At six months? At a year? Two years? In what situations would you recommend weaning from the breast?* If the list is a long one, be careful. *What books or videos about breastfeeding would you recommend?* (If they are all distributed by formula companies, that's a bad sign.)

If you are planning a hospital birth, look for a hospital that has earned the **Baby Friendly** designation. There are currently three Baby Friendly hospitals in Canada and 52 in the United States.

To become a Baby Friendly hospital, the policies and routines must match the steps I describe in Chapter 4, Getting Off to the Best Start (plus a few more). If none of the hospitals available to you are officially Baby Friendly, you can certainly ask questions to see how close they come to meeting the requirements. Do mothers and babies stay together after birth, or is there a standard "observation period" during which the baby is kept in the nursery? If breastfeeding needs to be supplemented, how is that supplement given? You will probably be going on a hospital tour or two anyway, to see what it is like to give birth there, so this is a great opportunity to ask questions about breastfeeding.

La Leche League (LLL) groups hold monthly meetings in most parts of North America, and they encourage mothers to begin attending meetings while they are still pregnant. Find out, before your baby is born, about such support groups in your community. La Leche League is a volunteer organization that for almost 50 years has provided mother-to-mother help for women interested in breastfeeding. Every La Leche League leader has breastfed at least one child, but she draws on far more than her own personal experience in sharing information and support. She has access to a considerable network of breastfeeding research and knowledge.

At LLL meetings you will meet other mothers, many with new babies and some with older babies. If you haven't been around babies much, it will be helpful for you to watch these infants as they latch on to the breast, change sides, fall asleep at the breast, and nurse in different positions. Just being around other new mothers and hearing their stories can be encouraging.

La Leche League leaders may also be a good resource if you run into problems. Each individual leader's experience will vary, of course, but if your situation is more challenging, the leader can probably put you in touch with someone who can help you.

In some communities, other breastfeeding support groups have been initiated by the public health department or have sprung up informally. These can be helpful, too, although you may have to look elsewhere if you run into any significant difficulties.

Lactation consultants are a new type of health care professional. At the moment, the use of this title is not regulated, so anyone can call themselves a lactation consultant. In some hospitals, this is simply the title of the nurse who is expected to deal with breastfeeding problems, even if she hasn't done any additional training in breastfeeding. However, to be an International Board Certified Lactation Consultant and use the letters IBCLC after their names, applicants must have considerable experience in working with breastfeeding mothers and babies, and must pass a stringent examination on breastfeeding. So an IBCLC—and there are many in private practice, as well as many working with hospitals, clinics, or doctor's offices—would, in general, be a good source of breastfeeding help.

Breastfeeding clinics have sprouted up around the country, and vary in their level of knowledge and helpfulness. Some are connected with hospitals or with public health units, while others are run independently by physicians or lactation consultants. At one hospital clinic, for example, the only lactation consultant on staff worked in the clinic part-time. The rest of the time other nurses—some with only minimal interest in breastfeeding—rotated through. The quality of help a breastfeeding mother would receive depended a lot on what day she showed up at the clinic. But clinics often have experienced, knowledgeable, and interested staff, and can be a good resource.

Good breastfeeding help is sometimes hard to find. Keep looking; keep asking. If you are told that you need to wean your baby, make sure you get a second or third opinion. Talk to other breastfeeding mothers about the doctors, clinics, or other resources they find helpful. Don't be discouraged—information about breastfeeding is spreading, and the resources available for new mothers continue to grow in number and improve in quality.

Some signs that your doctor or midwife is supportive of breastfeeding

• No formula company marketing materials are on display or in use around the office. The weight conversion guide near the scales for weighing the baby, for example, does not include a formula company logo.

• Schedules for La Leche League meetings, or meetings of other breastfeeding support groups in your community, are posted and lists of the phone numbers to call are readily available.

• You are not given any brochures or videos about breastfeeding that have been created by formula companies. When you ask for information about breastfeeding, you are referred to La Leche League, a lactation consultant in your community, or books and other materials written by people who are not paid by formula companies.

• There are no "gift packs" with formula samples to be given out.

• Before you give birth, you and your doctor discuss ways to help you get breastfeeding off to a good start, by nursing as soon as possible after birth and keeping the baby with you so you can nurse according to the baby's cues. Your doctor explains how to know if the baby is latched on well and drinking milk. You also discuss strategies in case there are complications, such as a premature birth or a cesarean section.

• In the waiting room, you see other mothers breastfeeding. There may be pictures or posters of breastfeeding on the walls.

3

The Sale and Promotion of Infant Formula

Myth: Companies have the right to use any marketing methods they like to get consumers to buy their products.

Fact: Not true. There are many restraints put on companies to make sure their products are marketed in such a way that the consumer is protected. For example, false claims cannot be made about what a product might do. Many products cannot be advertised to children. And where health is an issue, some products are available only by prescription, or are required to carry warning labels.

What does this have to do with breastfeeding? Many breastfeeding advocates feel that the inappropriate marketing of formula is one of women's biggest barriers to successfully breastfeeding.

Third World Deaths

The hazards of formula first attracted worldwide attention in the 1970s, when newspapers published photos of emaciated and dying babies in developing countries. The pictures were shocking, and people demanded to know the reasons for this tragedy.

The cause, it was revealed, was the marketing of baby formula to women who could not afford to pay for it, who could not be assured of clean water to prepare formula, who did not have the resources to boil water, and who did not realize how the use of formula would interfere with breastfeeding. Babies were undernourished because of the high cost of formula; mothers often diluted it to make it last. Babies did not have the protection of breastfeeding—or at least not the full protection—since they were not breastfeeding exclusively, and so often developed diarrhea or respiratory infections. Many died.

Hearings were held in the U.S. Senate in 1978, where the world was able to listen as a representative of Nestlé was asked if he felt any responsibility to find out the extent to which formula was being used with impure water, or being diluted to a dangerous extent. He stated that the company could not have that responsibility. Nestlé promotes and sells the most formula in developing countries and has the largest market share in the world.

Groups of concerned consumers organized a boycott of Nestlé products in response to this, stopping in 1984 only when Nestlé finally seemed to give in and promise to market formula according to certain guidelines. However, the boycott has been restarted in recent years as more evidence has accumulated of Nestlé's continuing direct-marketing practices.

The International Code on the Marketing of Breastmilk Substitutes (1981)

Shocked by the unnecessary, tragic deaths of so many babies, nongovernmental organizations, the World Health Organization, UNICEF, scientific bodies, and the formula companies themselves hammered out a code of ethics on the marketing of infant formula, bottles and teats (artificial nipples), and any food or drink that could replace breastmilk in a child's diet.

The final code was a compromise and included the following provisions:

- No marketing of any products (formula, bottles and teats, or other foods) should directly or indirectly target the consumer. This included no company representatives giving information to pregnant women, new mothers, or their families. Formula companies at one time sent special representatives to hospital maternity wards to give out information and free samples of formula, often dressing in white coats and passing themselves off as nurses or dietitians.
- No free samples or reduced price samples of formula should be given to pregnant women, new mothers, or their families.
- Only scientific information about formulas should be given to health care providers. Much marketing is aimed at health care providers such as doctors and nurses. It works particularly well because many health care providers do not believe they are influenced by advertising.
- Literature on infant feeding must be provided not by formula companies, but by government.
- All donations of money or equipment by formula companies to health care facilities must be done openly, and no special benefits should be granted the companies because of these donations.

It is important to remember that representatives of the formula companies were present and had input into the final form of the code. In 1981, all countries of the world, with the notable exception of the United States, voted to adopt the code. The United States has since come on board.

Unfortunately, from the very first, the formula companies disregarded the code completely and continued to market their products in ways they had just agreed to avoid. How was this justified? Representatives of formula companies told governments and health professionals the following:

- *The code was designed for Third World countries only.* This is untrue. Both the World Health Organization and UNICEF made it clear from the beginning that the code of marketing was meant for every country of the world. Actually, the code is, in many ways, more necessary in so-called First World countries, because knowledge of breastfeeding and the art of breastfeeding have essentially been lost, and women in industrialized countries are thus far more susceptible to misinformation propagated by the formula companies.
- *The code is too strong for industrialized countries.* This is not at all what the designers of the code intended. In fact, the code was intended to define a minimum standard that would be strengthened, not weakened, depending on each country's particular needs.
- *The code bans the use of formula, and is therefore too extreme.* The code does *not* ban formulas—indeed, there are provisions in the code designed to protect babies who must be fed artificial baby milk. For example, outdated formula was often being sold in developing countries. The code requires that an expiry date be clearly visible on all tins of formula.

Another problem was that instructions for making up formula were often not written in the language of the people to whom it was being sold. The code requires that instructions on preparing formula be written in the language of the target market.

Canada signed on to the code in 1981, but since then has essentially ignored the flagrant violations of the formula companies. While the code is not law, and violations are not punishable as crimes, these companies were not even given a little tap on the wrist! No "Tsk, tsk, you should try to be a little less obvious, you know."

At that time, and into the early 1990s, the majority of the formula sold in Canada was made by three companies: Mead Johnson (Enfalac), Ross (Similac), and Wyeth (SMA). A small Canadian company that made a product called Unilac was also in the picture, but has since gone under, unable to fight competition from the big players.

The big three do much of their marketing through the health system, even though this is forbidden by the World Health Organization (WHO) code. These companies vie for exclusive contracts with hospitals so that their product will be the only one used in a particular facility. Studies have shown that 93 percent of women start off using the same formula for their babies as is used in the hospital in which the baby was born. (One mother commented that mothers in the Ontario town where she lived would ask each other, "Are you breastfeeding or using Enfalac?" When she moved to another town, the question was, "Are you breastfeeding or using SMA?" Each town had one hospital, and the formula given out in its maternity ward became a generic word in that community.)

These exclusive contracts often last five to 10

years. The company gives cash, plus money for equipment, money for continuing medical education, free formula for the hospital nurseries, maternity wards and pediatric departments, and such little things as tape measures (with advertising), growth charts (with advertising), pads of paper (with advertising), pens (with advertising), coffee cups (with advertising), and myriad other useful little items that show up in every office and staff room.

The contract with the hospital often includes the provision of a "discharge" package for all mothers, whether they are breastfeeding or bottlefeeding. These giftpacks include samples of formula, as well as literature on breastfeeding and, of course, formula-feeding.

Neither the hospitals nor the formula companies were unhappy with this situation. (Breastfeeding mothers and babies may not have been happy, but since nobody makes any money from breastfeeding, this wasn't a huge concern.) But in 1989, Nestlé moved into the North American market and upset the applecart.

Already the largest food company in the world, Nestlé bought Carnation and started marketing directly to the consumer, sending free formula and literature to mothers at their homes. The other companies were outraged. How could Nestlé market directly to mothers in violation of the WHO code? (They ignored the fact that in giving free samples and brochures to mothers at the hospital, they were also marketing directly to them.)

In 1989, Ross placed the following ad in pediatric and pediatric nursing journals:

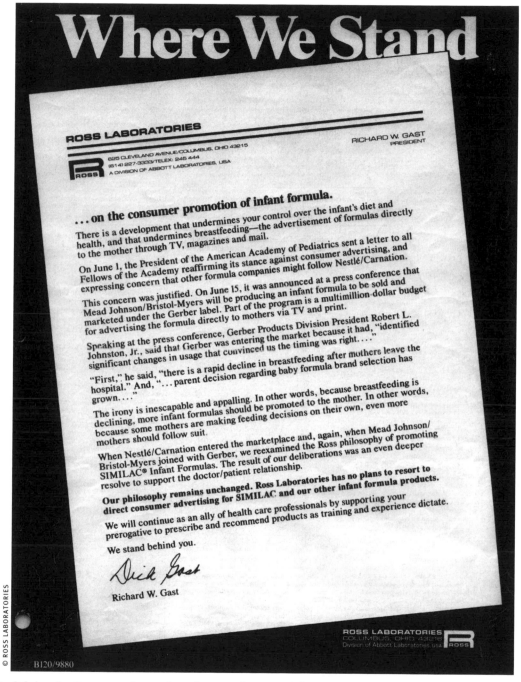

Where We Stand

ROSS LABORATORIES

RICHARD W. GAST
PRESIDENT

625 CLEVELAND AVENUE/COLUMBUS, OHIO 43215
(614) 227-3333/TELEX: 245 444
A DIVISION OF ABBOTT LABORATORIES, USA

... on the consumer promotion of infant formula.

There is a development that undermines your control over the infant's diet and health, and that undermines breastfeeding—the advertisement of formulas directly to the mother through TV, magazines and mail.

On June 1, the President of the American Academy of Pediatrics sent a letter to all Fellows of the Academy reaffirming its stance against consumer advertising, and expressing concern that other formula companies might follow Nestlé/Carnation.

This concern was justified. On June 15, it was announced at a press conference that Mead Johnson/Bristol-Myers will be producing an infant formula to be sold and marketed under the Gerber label. Part of the program is a multimillion-dollar budget for advertising the formula directly to mothers via TV and print.

Speaking at the press conference, Gerber Products Division President Robert L. Johnston, Jr., said that Gerber was entering the market because it had, "identified significant changes in usage that convinced us the timing was right...."

"First," he said, "there is a rapid decline in breastfeeding after mothers leave the hospital." And, "...parent decision regarding baby formula brand selection has grown...."

The irony is inescapable and appalling. In other words, because breastfeeding is declining, more infant formulas should be promoted to the mother. In other words, because some mothers are making feeding decisions on their own, even more mothers should follow suit.

When Nestlé/Carnation entered the marketplace and, again, when Mead Johnson/Bristol-Myers joined with Gerber, we reexamined the Ross philosophy of promoting SIMILAC® Infant Formulas. The result of our deliberations was an even deeper resolve to support the doctor/patient relationship.

Our philosophy remains unchanged. Ross Laboratories has no plans to resort to direct consumer advertising for SIMILAC and our other infant formula products.

We will continue as an ally of health care professionals by supporting your prerogative to prescribe and recommend products as training and experience dictate.

We stand behind you.

Dick Gast

Richard W. Gast

ROSS LABORATORIES
COLUMBUS, OHIO 43216
Division of Abbott Laboratories, USA

© ROSS LABORATORIES

B120/9880

It didn't take Ross very long, though, to realize that nobody really cared if direct advertising undermined breastfeeding and the health professional's "control over the infant's diet." So within a short time Ross was also marketing directly to the mother, in spite of the philosophy so firmly stated in its ad.

It is interesting that Ross's advertisement states

that the health professional should control the infant's diet. Surely the role of the health professional is to advise, not to control, and choices and decisions are up to the parents. I was also fascinated by Ross's exhortation about "prescribing and recommending products as training and experience dictate." What is the training of health professionals on breastfeeding? Very little. Their training about formula comes mostly from the formula companies. And, of course, the experience of most Canadian health care providers at that time would have been with Ross infant formulas, because Ross had the largest market share. So "as training and experience dictate" would mean, most of the time, recommending Ross formulas.

Nestlé, of course, deserves more than a slap across the wrist for initiating direct mail advertising and magazine advertising for formula in North America, but the other companies jumped on the bandwagon pretty quickly. In fact, it is now Mead Johnson, at least in Canada, that most aggressively markets to new mothers and pregnant women. I know this because I ask women who come to my clinic for help with breastfeeding if they have received any free samples of formula. The majority tell me yes, and often it has arrived in the mail even before the baby is born.

It does not matter that many mothers filled in forms asking for the formula because, according to the WHO code, the company is still not supposed to *send* the formula. In many cases, the mothers do not know they are filling in forms for formula. Maternity shops will ask mothers to fill in forms to get "free gifts"—and, of course, the gift pack includes formula. Newspapers send gift packs to mothers when they place a birth announcement and—guess what—it includes formula. Mothers can also end up on the mailing list of a formula company by entering contests.

The formula companies have managed to involve many other companies and organizations in their marketing efforts.

Why do companies give out all these free samples? Because they work.

Sending samples directly to pregnant women and new mothers isn't the only way formula is marketed. Mead Johnson, for example, offers nutrition seminars for pregnant women, at which breastfeeding is briefly discussed, and then formula is presented as a wonderful alternative, and free samples are handed out.

It's clear that the WHO code is being violated. But what's really wrong with this? Why shouldn't formula be marketed in these ways?

The problem is that infant formula is not like diapers. If a mother decides, because of a free sample she received in the hospital, that she will use a particular brand of diaper, she has been influenced by the free sample. After trying it for a while, though, the mother may find that the diaper gives her baby a rash or doesn't fit properly. Or she may decide to use another brand because it is cheaper, or looks more attractive. No problem. Next time she goes to the store, she switches brands. She can even go from disposable to cloth, or vice versa, without any difficulty.

However, let's look at the situation when an expectant mother gets a free sample of formula in the mail, reads the brochure that comes with it, and decides to give her baby that brand when it is born. When the baby is a few days old, the mother realizes that her baby seems to have a lot of digestive problems, the formula is very expensive and her breasts are aching with milk. She wants to switch to breastfeeding.

Some mothers will be able to make the switch. But for many, it will be impossible or at least very difficult. We know that what happens in the first few days after birth can have a significant effect on whether breastfeeding is successful. The mother who has given her baby formula for several days is likely to have trouble building up a good supply of her own milk, and her baby may not nurse well after several days of bottles. The mother may find she has no choice but to continue with bottlefeeding. That's what makes the marketing of formula different.

The formula companies argue that they are only competing with other brands of formula, but the fact is that they are competing with breastfeeding, too. And since the majority of new mothers begin by breastfeeding, *that* has become the strongest competitor.

I believe the companies are aware of this because I see strong—but subtle—anti-breastfeeding messages in the pamphlets they distribute to mothers. They don't say "our formula is as good as or better than breastmilk." They acknowledge that breastmilk is better, then proceed to make breastfeeding sound tiring,

restrictive, painful, and difficult—and explain how formula can help your baby grow and thrive.

The photos on this page and the next page, from a booklet created and distributed by a major formula company, demonstrate the approach I am describing. I call it "breastfeeding mother as brazen harlot, formula-feeding mother as convent girl."

Women in Western countries still feel that one of the problems of breastfeeding is that it "ties you down." After all, you can't go out with your baby and nurse him because you will be exposing yourself. Of course, this isn't true; you *can* breastfeed discreetly. (I will add that I am an advocate of "indiscreet" breastfeeding—the more people see babies at the breast, the more "normal" and accepted it will be.)

The photos in the brochure play on this fear of exposure. The breastfeeding mother is very exposed. In one of the photos, even the breast she is not using to feed the baby is completely exposed. The photo of her expressing her milk is

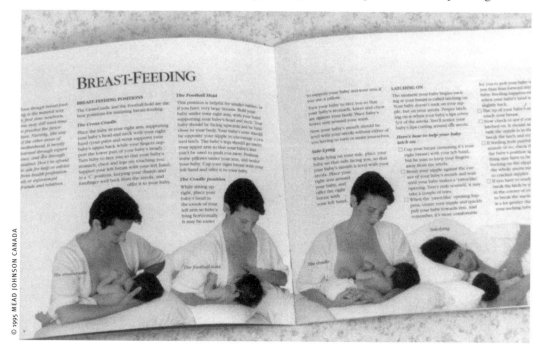

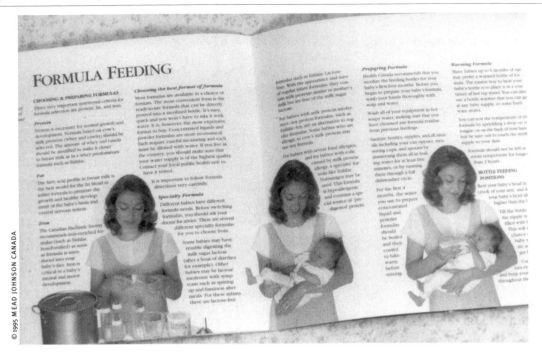

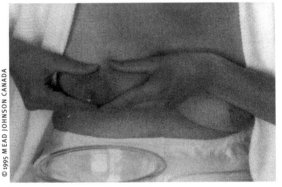

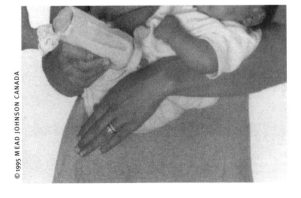

not very useful as information, but might make the pregnant woman who sees it feel uncomfortable about the idea of handling her breast in this way.

The formula-feeding mother, on the other hand, is dressed very modestly. She exudes a feeling of innocence that is really very touching. Now look at the picture of the breastfeeding mother where her left hand is exposed. And the one where the formula-feeding mother is showing off her left hand. Difference? One has a wedding ring and the other, not. Accidental? What do you think?

These two pictures are included to show that it is not just one company doing this. Look at these photos from a formula-company booklet, which is written (or at least signed) by a prominent pediatrician, and which, ostensibly, deals with the baby's developing senses. But marketing formula has not been forgotten.

Note that in the first picture, the breastfeeding family is stiff and the baby could be a doll, for all the life he shows. You can't see the baby's face, and you cannot even be sure that he is breastfeeding. The father is awkward and appears disconnected from the mother and baby.

Now look at the bottle-feeding family. They are better-looking, they are relaxed, they are cuddling. They are unbelievably lovey-dovey. The baby is seen prominently and is playing with Dad, who is obviously not cut out (as the other picture implies). Coincidence? What do you think?

Incidentally, the Canadian Paediatric Society teamed up with one of these companies to send out a booklet on infants that included infant feeding information. The booklet was accompanied by formula-company information and samples of formula. After protests, the package, which was given to pediatricians and family doctors as a "first visit pack," was withdrawn. However, the fact that this organization, which says it represents Canadian pediatricians, would collaborate in such a way with a formula company speaks volumes about its commitment to breastfeeding and its lack of understanding of the issues.

All this might not be so terrible if, at least, there was an equal amount of marketing for breastfeeding. Is there? Of course not. Who makes money on breastfeeding? I do. A few lactation consultants do, but most would make a lot more selling hot dogs on the street. Some lose money. Pump manufacturers do pretty

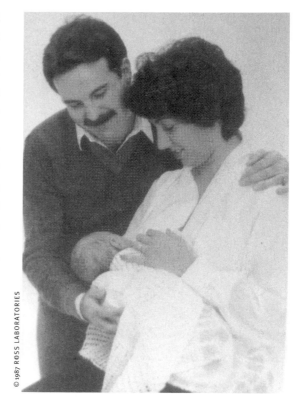

© 1987 ROSS LABORATORIES

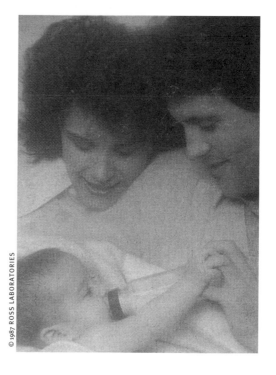

© 1987 ROSS LABORATORIES

well, and those who rent pumps sometimes make some money, but essentially, there is very little money out there to promote breastfeeding. The Canadian government has given a risible amount to promote breastfeeding. Many provincial governments do even less. And the Canadian Paediatric Society does more to help the formula companies than it does to help those who advocate breastfeeding.

Formula Contamination

Infant formulas, like all manufactured products, may become contaminated during the manufacturing process or may have ingredients accidentally left out. This is more serious when it happens to formula, because it is the only source of food for the baby, and bottle-fed babies don't have the immunities to protect them from bacterial infections. Parents who feed their babies formula should always keep track of the lot numbers of the formula they purchase and watch for announcements of recalls.

A few recent formula recalls, taken from the U.S. Food and Drug Administration, reports:

2001: Carnation (Nestlé)—excessive magnesium in ready-to-feed formula.

2001: Nutramigen (Mead Johnson)—incorrect preparation instructions on the label.

2003: Enfacre Lipil (Mead Johnson)—formula for premature babies contaminated with *E. sakazaki* bacteria.

2006: Gentlease (Mead Johnson)—contained metal particles as large as 2.7 ml.

Other recalls in the past included formula with nutrients accidentally left out or added in insufficient quantities; concentrated formula that was mislabeled with the instructions "do not add water"; formula with glass particles in it; and formula contaminated with various bacteria.

What about parenting magazines? Some actually are not that bad with regard to their information about breastfeeding. But most, with very few exceptions, also have ads for infant formula. And unfortunately, advertising is often more effective than articles, which take time to read.

Many parenting magazines have terribly inaccurate information about breastfeeding in their articles. Sometimes this is because the magazine's staff "doesn't want to make mothers feel guilty for not breastfeeding." This makes no more sense than saying we should not discuss why vaginal birth is, in fact, better for the mother and baby, because to do so will make mothers who have cesarean sections feel guilty. It is a statement often made by people who do not understand why breastfeeding is so important for both mother and baby.

How about health professionals—the doctors and nurses and others who work with pregnant women and new babies? Surely these are the people to help and advise women, and counteract the marketing efforts of the formula companies?

The reality, as I have discussed elsewhere, is that many health professionals learn very little about breastfeeding during their training. Even if they learn something about the benefits, they get no instruction on how to help mothers solve problems. On the other hand, they get lots of information about formula—most of it straight from the formula companies themselves.

The result is that while most health care professionals support breastfeeding in theory, many don't know how to help mothers get off to a good start, and their only advice in response to problems is "Give the baby formula."

While there is justifiable concern about marketing directed at new parents, physicians probably get targeted more than any other group. Brochures arrive at their offices, ads are in all the medical journals, formula company booths are set up at every medical conference. The formula company may provide a free lunch for all the doctors attending a conference—complete with a speaker to introduce a new formula and let everyone know how good it is. Though the WHO code states that all advertising to health professionals should contain scientific information only, this article of the code, like the rest, is widely disregarded.

Physicians, in particular, are very susceptible to this advertising, particularly because many think they are too intelligent and sophisticated to be affected by it. But we know it works. If it didn't, the formula companies would have stopped doing it.

For a few pennies, the formula companies supply the health professional, particularly the physician, with pens, tape measures, growth charts, pocket savers, notepads—all with formula advertising. And, of course, they encourage the health professional to give out free samples of their formula.

But the companies don't only target physicians. Dietitians, nutritionists, nurses, in fact all health professionals who could have anything to do with new mothers and their infants, are getting the flood of information about formula.

So here are the barriers pregnant women face when they are making decisions about how to feed their babies:

- They are living in a society where bottle-feeding is seen as the normal way to feed a baby.
- Breastfeeding is acknowledged as being "better," but formula is really "just as good," and, besides, breastfeeding is very difficult.
- The art of breastfeeding has largely been lost,

and the new mother may have no close relatives who have breastfed and could share their expertise with her.
- Health professionals share the society's attitudes and in addition have been taught that formula-feeding and bottle-feeding are solutions for breastfeeding problems.
- Government agencies do not understand the importance of breastfeeding, and why government money and support should be given to breastfeeding.
- Media get money from formula-company advertising, and editors and writers, having generally grown up in this bottle-feeding society, cannot understand what all the fuss is about. They are terribly indulgent about the abuses of formula companies in a way they would never be if the abuses were by, for example, automobile manufacturers.
- Formula companies have spent huge sums of money to market aggressively—and in my opinion, unethically—since they were involved in the drafting of the WHO code on the marketing of breastmilk substitutes.
- There is a general agreement among all parties that we should not make mothers feel guilty for *not* breastfeeding.

I think this question of guilt is an important one. We *shouldn't* be making mothers feel guilty for not breastfeeding, should we? We shouldn't make mothers feel guilty for anything, actually. Most mothers are doing the best they can, sometimes under very difficult circumstances. We all make mistakes. We all sometimes say the wrong thing, do the wrong thing, choose the wrong approach—some of us more than others. But generally parents try hard to do the best they can.

But we certainly make mothers feel bad about their choices in many other situations. If you are a smoker and your child has asthma, it is probable that you will leave your physician's office feeling guilty. If you are pregnant, and you drink alcohol, even small amounts, you will probably leave your doctor's office with stern warnings ringing in your ears and guilt in your heart. Tell the doctor you aren't planning to use a car seat when you take your baby out in the car, and you'll get another dose of guilt. Why would the physician do that? Because he or she really believes that your continuing to smoke or drink alcohol may harm the baby.

Obviously, the physician who says that we should not make mothers feel guilty for not breastfeeding doesn't believe that breastfeeding makes a difference. But there is lots of evidence that it does—for the mother, for the baby, and for society.

We have a double standard for breastfeeding and for infant formula. For example, consider the following:

Formulas are getting better than they used to be and they are, in theory, much better for infants than whole cow's milk. For example, the amount of protein is less, which is better; the amount of salt is less, which is better; the amount of iron is greater, which is good, because humans absorb iron poorly from animal milks and formulas. Despite being "better" in theory, however, there is little scientific evidence that it makes a difference in the long term or even short term whether you feed a baby formula or straight cow's milk. In fact, a couple of generations ago, many babies were fed straight cow's milk, or simple homemade formulas based on cow's milk.

Breastmilk has far more theoretical advantages over formula than formula has over straight cow's milk. For example, breastmilk contains (and formula does not) many, many immune factors, growth factors that stimulate the gut and nerves to develop, fats that help the brain and retina to develop appropriately, less aluminum and other metals. In addition, there are lots of scientific studies showing that there are not only theoretical advantages, but real differences between breastfed and artificially fed babies. (This has been discussed elsewhere, particularly in the section on drugs and breastfeeding.)

I can assure you that even if only one percent of the number of studies showing that breastfeeding is better than formula-feeding were to prove that formula from camel's milk was better than formula from cow's milk, there would be camel farms all over North America, and physicians would be urging mothers to use camel's milk formulas instead of cow's milk formulas!

Despite this, what happens if you go to the doctor and tell him that you are feeding your one-week-old baby straight cow's milk? Your doctor will have a fit. You will be told that this food is not appropriate for babies and that you are putting your baby at risk. You will be ordered to put the baby on formula (and you will probably be feeling pretty guilty at this point), and if you seem uncooperative, the doctor might even report you to the Children's Aid Society.

On the other hand, if you tell the physician that you are formula-feeding your one-week-old baby, what will you hear? Perhaps "That's fine, make sure it's iron-enriched." It's unlikely that the doctor will even ask why you are not breastfeeding. Maybe you were given wrong information (for example, were told that you could not breastfeed while taking a certain medication) and really *want* to breastfeed. It might not be too late, one week postpartum, to get your baby back to the breast. But your doctor won't ask you that question, because she doesn't want to make you feel *guilty*.

It is a false and absurd argument, yet it disarms even some breastfeeding advocates. It prevents physicians from talking to pregnant women about breastfeeding during the pregnancy. Many physicians ask about smoking, alcohol consumption, and diet, and offer suggestions and comments about what they believe is important for the baby. If they ask about feeding at all, they will not say to a woman who says she plans to formula-feed, "But have you considered breastfeeding? It's so much better for you and your baby." The pregnant woman might believe, as some women do, that she can't breastfeed because her breasts are too small or too large, or because her mother wasn't able to, or because she takes asthma medication, or any number of other myths that discourage women from breastfeeding. By not even asking the mother-to-be about her feeding plans, the doctor sends a message that breastfeeding isn't important.

Women should get the information they need to make an informed choice about breastfeeding. And this information must not come from formula companies. The aim of these companies is not to help with breastfeeding, but to make sure you use their product. Women should be told that there is good evidence that their baby will be smarter if they breastfeed, and that the baby will have less risk of developing diabetes, respiratory illnesses, gut infections, and ear infections. Women should be told they may decrease their own and the baby's risk, if the baby is a girl, of breast cancer, as well as their own risk of developing osteoporosis and perhaps ovarian cancer. If the mother then decides she will formula-feed, that is her informed choice.

Even then, it can be difficult to make a really informed choice. A pregnant woman who has seen very few babies nursing may find it difficult to imagine what it will be like to have a baby suckling at her breast. But she's probably seen lots of babies bottle-feeding. How can you choose what you don't know, what you have never tried? It seems to me that the best way for a mother to make an informed choice is to start breastfeeding, get good help to establish breastfeeding, and then, if she decides it's not for her . . . Well, who is going to say she did the wrong thing?

We sometimes hear that advocates of breastfeeding "force" women to breastfeed. You cannot *force* a woman to breastfeed; that is absurd. But let me ask this: has any woman in North America who has decided to bottle-feed been told in hospital that she *must* put the baby to the breast? I doubt it very much. Has any woman who wanted to breastfeed been told in hospital that she *must* give the baby formula? Oh, yes, this happens every day, in almost every hospital in North America. Who is forcing whom? In the majority of such cases, the formula is not only unnecessary, but is going to make breastfeeding success less likely. If a baby in the first few days goes to the breast and spits up, is it not sometimes recommended that the mother not breastfeed because the baby is not tolerating her milk? Oh, yes, even today, even after all we know about breastfeeding. If a baby in the first few days is formula-fed and spits up, is the mother ever told that she should try breastfeeding? Sometimes, but not often. The usual approach is, "Let's try another formula."

The real problem is the lack of knowledge among altogether too many health professionals with regard to breastfeeding, especially its practical aspects. For this reason, about 10 years ago, UNICEF announced the Baby Friendly Hospital Initiative.

The idea of the initiative is to make labor and birth and the immediate period after the birth of the baby conducive to establishing breastfeeding. To qualify, a hospital has to abide by 10 steps, none of them especially demanding. However, maternity ward routines in most North American hospitals are so unhelpful when it comes to breastfeeding that few come close to meeting the guidelines. Here are the 10 steps, each followed by my comment.

1. The hospital should have a breastfeeding policy that is consistent, covers the 10 points, and is communicated to all staff.

What could be more reasonable? Yet many hospitals that have policies for even the most trivial of procedures do not consider breastfeeding important enough to warrant a policy. This often leads to new mothers getting different advice from each nurse, doctor, and dietitian who speaks to her.

2. All staff dealing with pregnant women and new mothers should be trained to put into practice the breastfeeding policy.

No sense in having a policy if you can't carry it out. This is the most difficult of all the steps, because it costs money to train staff. Physicians also are included here. Typically, physicians are not interested in attending seminars on breastfeeding. The biggest problem is one of changing attitudes. Unfortunately, many staff still believe the best thing would be that every mother formula-feed, since this saves them lots of work and trouble. Others are reluctant to believe that the information they have been giving out and the way they have been dealing with breastfeeding for many years has actually done more harm than good.

3. Inform all pregnant women of the advantages of breastfeeding and teach them the basics of breast-feeding management.

This allows women to make an informed choice. No formula company samples and no formula company "teaching" materials are to be given out or made available. No group classes should be held to teach formula-feeding.

4. Help mothers initiate breastfeeding within 30 minutes of birth, or at least have the mother and baby together skin to skin within a half-hour.

Actually having the baby nursing is not always possible, but close early contact increases the probability of later success. This is quite reasonable for most mothers and babies, and should not be a problem to implement, except when the mother or baby is too sick. Too many false reasons are used to separate mothers and babies. Back to staff training and attitudes.

5. Help the mother initiate lactation and teach her how to maintain her milk supply if she and her baby must be separated.

If the mother is separated from her baby, she should get help as soon as is reasonable to start expressing her milk for her baby. This is often not done. The focus may be on the baby's illness, and breastfeeding may be seen as unimportant. But if the baby is sick, the mother's milk is more important than ever! Back to staff training and attitudes.

6. No supplements of any kind should be given to breastfed babies, except when there is a medical reason.

Unfortunately, medical and nursing staff knowledge of the practice of breastfeeding is often so meager, that supplements are given for no reason at all. Often, when there seems to be a problem that requires supplementation, it can be solved if the staff help the mother with breast-feeding technique. More training issues.

7. The mother and baby should room in together.

Rooming in means 24 hours a day. The staff are not doing the mother or baby a favor by separating them at night in order to "let the mother sleep." Keeping them together helps them get "in sync" with each other, helps the mother learn to recognize her baby's signals, and reduces the risk of engorgement and later milk supply problems.

8. Encourage breastfeeding as the baby needs it.

Babies should be fed according to their needs, not according to some schedule. Babies rarely do well on a schedule. Furthermore, note that the word used is *breastfeeding*, not simply "being at the breast." The staff need to be able to *show* the mother how to know a baby is well latched on, and how to know the baby is getting milk. Yes, more training.

9. Give no artificial nipples to breastfed babies.

Even if supplements are required, which they rarely are, it is hardly ever necessary to use a bottle. Supplements can be given by lactation aid (the preferred method), cup, finger-feeding, and a host of other methods, without using a bottle. The pacifier is almost never necessary if the baby breastfeeds well.

10. Encourage the establishment of support groups outside the hospital and ensure that new mothers get referred to them on discharge.

Since we have lost a whole generation or more of experienced nursing grandmothers who used to advise their daughters on breastfeeding, other support needs to be available. La Leche League, doulas, and public health nurses can all do the job, but information has to be consistent, and every mother needs close and early follow-up. It is sad that often the least qualified to provide this support and follow-up is the physician—although there are exceptions.

All this information should be expected from a hospital where babies are born. Nothing radical here. Except that very few hospitals manage it.

In 1999, after 10 years, Canada got its first Baby Friendly hospital. Sweden, on the other hand, has many. In fact, every hospital with a maternity ward in Sweden had Baby Friendly designation within the first few years of the launch of the initiative. And there are more than 14,000 Baby Friendly hospitals around the world.

In North America, staff training issues present a big stumbling block. But training is crucial to implementing the 10 steps. Even more important is the question of attitude. If a physician doesn't believe that helping mothers breastfeed is an important part of his or her job, he won't be bothered, no matter how many hours of training he is compelled to attend. If the physician thinks that every baby needs a 4- (or 6- or 8- or 12- or 24-) hour "observation period" in the nursery after birth—no matter how useless such a period of observation is, no matter how much it interferes with breastfeeding—nothing will change. If the administration cannot understand why the hospital should not accept free formula from formula companies, nothing will change.

And why shouldn't hospitals accept free formula from formula companies? With so many funding cutbacks hitting hospitals, surely they need to save all the money they can? I think the more important question is, How much is integrity worth? The research tells us that when a hospital accepts free formula, fewer babies are breastfed exclusively, and fewer babies leave hospital breastfeeding. These babies are then subject to all the risks and increased health problems caused by formula-feeding.

Why does this happen? When the maternity ward has lots of formula on hand—and free formula, at that—it becomes the quick and easy solution to any problem. *The mother is tired, so we'll give the baby a bottle and let her sleep. The baby isn't latching on well, so we'll supplement with a little formula.* The message the mother gets is: if you have a problem—any problem—formula is probably the answer. And she's already had some formula sent to her home, and will get another free sample when she leaves the hospital, so when breastfeeding isn't going smoothly, she opens the can and fills up the bottle . . . Before she really knows what has happened, the baby is weaned.

I hope this chapter will encourage you to read with a more critical eye any breastfeeding information or booklets you are given. I hope you will be more aware, as you look around your doctor's office, of the subtle and not-so-subtle advertising for formula. When you see it, tell your doctor, who may not even be aware of the items the formula company representative has dropped off and which are being displayed or even handed out to patients by the receptionist.

And I hope you will put pressure on your local hospital to become Baby Friendly, and will urge your government to enforce the WHO code. These are small steps, but they are necessary if we are going to give women real, truly informed choices about feeding their babies. In the long run, the only thing that will prompt change is pressure from parents.

II

An Ounce
of Prevention

4

Getting Off
to the Best Start

For breastfeeding to get going properly, there is a right way to start off, which can be crucial—although it is also true that some mothers and babies manage to get breastfeeding established even when many of the principles mentioned below are ignored. It is a remarkable testimony to the adaptability of human beings that breastfeeding often works in spite of everything that is done to undermine it.

A mother's experience of breastfeeding can be profoundly affected by what happens during the first hours after her baby's birth. A good beginning can help her find breastfeeding easy and painless; a bad beginning can make it painful and difficult.

The important steps to getting breastfeeding established are aimed at getting the baby well latched on to the breast. They are as follows:

1. If possible, have a natural childbirth.

If you want to help get breastfeeding off to a good start, plan to give birth with as few interventions as possible. We know that all medications and other interventions used in labor affect the baby and may create breastfeeding problems.

If your labor is induced with pitocin, the fluids given to you by IV may increase the amount of engorgement you experience and result in the baby having more difficulty latching on. A poor latch leads to poor feeding, and often, a lethargic baby who is jaundiced because of poor intake of milk. In some hospitals, where they don't understand that the poor feeding is the problem, instead of helping the mother with the breastfeeding, the baby may be separated from her for "treatment." The best treatment, though, is getting the baby breastfeeding well, not separation and even stopping breastfeeding, the latter being completely inappropriate.

If you have Demerol or other painkilling medications close to the time of the baby's birth, your baby will be sleepy and will have trouble coordinating his sucking motions. These medications may affect your baby for more than two weeks after the birth—a crucial time for getting breastfeeding established.

Epidurals are currently the most popular form of pain relief during labor in North America, but they can also make it harder for mothers to establish breastfeeding. A 1999 study by Jan Riordan had knowledgeable lactation consultants evaluate babies' ability to latch on and suck well. The babies who had not been exposed to epidural medication scored an average of 11.1 (out of 12) in suckling ability; the average score for the epidural babies was only 8.5.

Another study was done in Sweden, where newborn babies are usually allowed to self-attach at the breast. In this study, all the unmedicated babies found the mother's breast, self-attached, and began to suckle within an hour after birth. Of those exposed to the epidural, only 25 percent were able to attach and suckle, and some of these had to be helped by the mother or were found to be latched on incorrectly. The epidural babies also cried substantially more often and for longer periods of time.

The other interventions and side effects associated with epidurals can have their own effects on breastfeeding. When you have an epidural, you will also be given intravenous fluids, which may increase engorgement after the baby is born and may make it harder for the baby to latch on. You are more likely to need forceps or a vacuum extractor to help deliver the baby, and both of these can cause the baby to have a headache that may make nursing uncomfortable and difficult.

Women who have doulas with them during labor and birth are less likely to need medication and other interventions. Having a midwife to provide your care may also be helpful, if midwives are available in your community.

2. The baby is put to the breast immediately after delivery.

There is no reason why the majority of newborns cannot be put to the breast within 30 minutes of birth. Babies usually experience a time of quiet alertness in the first hour or two after birth. They are awake but not crying, and seem to be primed to take in new experiences—such as learning to breastfeed.

The mother is also usually emotionally ready to begin making this breastfeeding connection with her baby. Even if the labor has been long, hard, and exhausting, she usually finds holding the baby in her arms or on her body to be the perfect reward. The tired mother may need to have someone who can sit with her and wait patiently for breastfeeding to be initiated by the baby. She might need some help in getting herself into a comfortable position, but even if she must lie flat, the baby can still be brought to the breast.

When the baby is first put to the breast, he will often simply lick or nuzzle the nipple. This is fine, and it isn't necessary to aggressively force the baby to latch on to the breast. In fact, continued pushing of the baby into the breast when the baby won't latch on, as many inexperienced nurses and lactation consultants do when the baby refuses to feed, probably accounts for many babies' developing a resistance to going to the breast. If the mother can have relaxed, unhurried time with her baby, he will soon indicate his readiness to nurse. This may be 10 minutes, 15 minutes, or an hour after birth, but it is important that mother and baby stay together during this time, with skin-to-skin contact, so that the process can happen naturally. It might be necessary for the mother and baby to be moved, together, to a warmer room if they are in a chilly delivery room, or to be provided with a radiant heater over the mother's bed. It would be helpful if delivery rooms were not kept so cold. In many hospitals, babies are born in the same room where mother and baby will be for their entire hospital stay, and these rooms are often kept at a more comfortable temperature.

This initial time of quite alertness seems to be a special window of opportunity for establishing breastfeeding. Some babies, if they are taken from their mothers before this first feeding, seem to "shut down." They become sleepy and are hard to wake up later to feed. The longer they go without feeding, the harder it may be to get them interested in taking the breast.

Even worse is the situation in which the baby does not get a chance to nurse—perhaps because medical staff are concerned that the mother is too tired—and is instead given a bottle of formula or sugar water. This often has a very negative effect on the baby's suckling. Here he is, primed to learn to breastfeed, and he is given a rigid bottle nipple and expected to form his lips and tongue to manage its rapid flow. Because the baby is so sensitive at this stage, even one feeding from a bottle can create long-lasting problems. True, one bottle does not always cause problems, and may not cause a problem in the majority of cases. And yes, most problems can be fixed. But why create them in the first place? It does neither the mother nor the baby any favor to separate them. If the baby needs to be fed, he should be breastfeeding. How tiring is it, really, for a mother to lie in bed with her baby beside her, sucking at her breast?

> "The benefits to the mother of immediate breastfeeding are innumerable, not the least of which after the weariness of labor and birth is the emotional gratification, the feeling of strength, composure, and the sense of fulfillment that comes with the handling and suckling of the baby."
>
> —Ashley Montagu, *Touching*

Most—but not all—mothers and babies will learn to breastfeed even if the baby doesn't go to the breast immediately. But it is better to start early, because it is impossible to predict which baby will have difficulties stemming from a delayed start.

Researchers have filmed newborn babies crawling up the mother's abdomen—with no help or assistance from the mother or medical personnel—and finding and latching on to the breast. In fact, any "help" often hinders the baby from moving up to the breast and latching on. This doesn't mean we should never help the baby latch on after birth, but it is a powerful demonstration of the instincts and abilities that babies are born with, and what they can do if given the opportunity. They know how to find

the breast and they know what to do when they get there—if we don't mess it up. The researchers also found that narcotics given during labor can interfere with the baby's ability to crawl up to his mother's breast, locate the nipple, and latch on to the breast by himself.

Incidentally, have you ever wondered why the nipple and areola are a different color than the rest of the breast? Could the color difference be a visual cue for the baby to direct him to the right place? Researchers have also found that if one breast is washed and the other isn't, the baby tends to latch on to the unwashed nipple rather than the cleaned one. Good hygiene is important, but maybe we are a little obsessed by it and thus unwittingly interfere with natural processes.

Newborn babies don't necessarily crawl to the breast and latch on in five or ten minutes. The whole process may take an hour or more, and even when medication hasn't been given during labor some babies will not "self-attach." But there is no harm in allowing the mother and baby this time together, even if the baby only nuzzles at the breast. The benefits are real.

Remember, too, that every baby is an individual. Some babies will latch on right away, all by themselves. Some will need a little gentle urging from the mother. Some mothers and babies will benefit from a little help from a knowledgeable nurse, midwife, or other caregiver. And some babies will take a few hours to decide they are ready to nurse. It is no use forcing a baby to take the breast when he doesn't want to—forcing will only make him angry or upset, or he will simply go to sleep. As long as mother and baby are together, there is no rush. They can cuddle together, and the mother will be ready to respond when the baby does show interest in breastfeeding.

Some babies who have been heavily suctioned fight being put to the breast right after birth. It is routine in many hospitals to suction mucus from the baby's mouth, nose, and throat right after birth, but deeper suctioning—if meconium was present in the amniotic fluid—may interfere with the baby's latching on. It is not necessary for a full-term, healthy baby who is having no problems after birth to be suctioned. Even suctioning meconium has not been shown to be useful, although most obstetricians and pediatricians will do it, because it is traditional.

If you are expecting a baby, plan well before your baby's birth to have this time together. The baby can be examined while lying on the mother's body, and the mother can be examined while she is holding her baby. Even if you have had a cesarean section, your baby can be helped to breastfeed soon after the birth. Since your arms will probably be taken up with intravenous lines, you will need someone to help you bring the baby to your breast. The baby's father is an obvious choice, in many cases.

What if your nipples are flat or inverted? Nipples come in a variety of shapes and sizes. Some are large, some are small, some are flat or actually seem to sink into the breast, and some are protruding. Often mothers are told that their nipples are flat or inverted when they are not. Breasts and nipples change in the first few days after the birth of a baby, and nipples that seem flat or inverted on day one may no longer be so on day two or day six. At any rate, this should not be a concern. All these nipples can be made to work. They are all good for breastfeeding. Some may be more difficult to latch on to, at least at first, but most of the time it will work out.

The baby at birth does not have a particular expectation of what a breast and nipple should look like or feel like. It is true that a nipple that protudes and is firmer makes it a bit easier to stimulate the baby's sucking reflexes (as the nipple touches the roof of the baby's mouth), but this type of nipple is certainly not necessary for successful breastfeeding. When the baby is properly latched on, he takes a good mouthful of the breast as well as the nipple, and uses his gums and tongue to compress the milk ducts. This works just as well when the nipple is flat or inverted as when it is large and protruding.

But when the mother has flat or inverted nipples, it is particularly important to avoid giving the baby a bottle or pacifier. If the baby becomes used to a hard nipple that fills his mouth and stimulates him to suck, he will be looking for that nipple when he is put to the breast, and will be frustrated and confused when he can't find it. This doesn't mean he can't learn to breastfeed—he can. But giving the baby an artificial nipple to suck on will make it more difficult.

3. The baby and the mother should room in together.

There is *absolutely no medical reason for healthy mothers and babies to be separated after birth*. Rooming in should mean 24 hours a day, not only daylight hours.

Sometimes people encourage mothers to send the baby to the nursery at night because they think the mother will get more rest if she is separated from the baby. But this isn't so. Mothers and babies who are together will get "in sync" as they sleep and wake at the same time.

Women will often describe how they wake up at night and see that their babies are just starting to wake up. What happens is this: the baby who is deeply asleep begins to feel hungry and starts to move to a less-deep level of sleep. His breathing changes, becoming more rapid. The mother, who is attuned to her baby from birth, will respond in her sleep to these subtle changes in her still-sleeping baby's breathing. Her milk will begin to let down, and she will also begin, gradually, to wake up. By the time the baby has progressed from the change in breathing to moving around or perhaps trying to suck on his fingers or making quiet noises, his mother will be awake and ready to feed him. Because he isn't ravenously hungry, he can be patient if getting latched on well takes a couple of tries, or if the mother needs to arrange some pillows or her clothes to prepare for feeding. He will take the food he needs and fall asleep again, and his mother can sleep as well.

This is very different from the scenario when the baby is in a separate nursery. When his breathing changes to the "I'm getting hungry and waking up soon" type of breathing, the nursery staff are unlikely to notice. They have several other babies to watch as well. His mother, too far away to pick up on these subtle signals, is in a deep sleep. When the baby finally starts to cry loudly, because nobody has come to feed him, the nurse may have paperwork to finish or another baby to tend to before she can take him to his mother. Finally, she brings him to the room and wakes the mother from a sound sleep. The baby continues to cry, and his mother, groggy from being woken up and struggling to deal with a frantic baby, will start to feed him. But her milk hasn't let down, and even when the very hungry baby latches on, he doesn't at first get anything to drink. He gets more upset, and in his frustration may even refuse to take the breast.

Although hospital stays today tend to be short, they can be a good time for mother and baby to stay together and become accustomed to each other, while someone else is providing their meals and helping to take care of them. But for this to work, the mother and baby need to be together so that the mother can learn her baby's signals.

4. Artificial nipples must not be given to the baby.

You only need to watch babies suck on a bottle nipple and suckle at the breast to see that these are two very different processes. The baby at the breast must use his mouth and tongue quite differently from a baby sucking on a rubber bottle nipple or even a pacifier.

During the first few days after giving birth, mothers produce only a small amount of a special kind of milk, called colostrum. This milk is very high in antibodies and is a laxative, helping to prepare the baby's intestines—which were not used to digesting food before birth—to handle the milk that the breasts will soon be producing. The breasts of a new mother are fairly soft as well. This makes it easier for the new baby to learn to latch on.

So the baby's initial feedings at the breast do not yield large volumes of milk. This is how nature intended it to be while the baby is learning to breastfeed. But if the baby is given a bottle of formula, or even of expressed breastmilk, he learns a very different style of sucking. The bottle nipple is rigid and can be forced into the baby's mouth.

It is true that some babies learn to drink from a bottle as well as from the breast, but many do not, and it is difficult to know in advance which babies will have problems. A baby who is already having some problems with latching on, or is reluctant to take the breast, will almost certainly have even more difficulties if given bottles or pacifiers. And even babies who are doing fine at the breast can be confused or have their breast-feeding technique disrupted if they are given bottles. Even one bottle can create problems, especially if it is given early on.

Actually, the babies are not *confused*. They know exactly what they want. If they go to the breast and don't get much milk because they are not latched on well, and are then given a bottle and get a fast flow of milk, they will develop a preference for the bottle. Babies don't have to be potential rocket scientists to figure it out.

For this reason, many will describe this situation as "nipple preference" rather than "nipple confusion." This term can be pretty upsetting to the mother, however, who may already be feeling emotional about the problems she is having breastfeeding her baby, and now is told that the baby "prefers" the bottle to her breasts. It may feel like the baby is rejecting her. "Nipple confusion" suggests that the baby really does want to breastfeed but is temporarily confused.

The solution here is to fix the latch so that the baby is able to get milk just as readily at the breast.

Even when babies seem to be able to do some feedings at the breast and some from a bottle, this is often the first step to early weaning. The baby's suckling technique, which may be "good enough" in the early weeks when the mother's milk supply is very plentiful, may deteriorate as time goes by, and then the mother's breasts don't get enough stimulation to keep up her milk production. As it gets harder for the baby to get milk from his mother's breasts, he begins to prefer the bottle. Recognizing that her milk supply is down, his mother gives him additional bottles, and her milk supply decreases further. Before long, the baby shows a definite preference for the bottle—and ends up weaning.

A range of problems may result from the early introduction of rubber nipples, which causes the baby to latch on poorly. These include breast refusal, poor weight gain, high bilirubin levels, sore nipples, colic, and breast infections.

It is surprising that some people deny the existence of "nipple confusion." These individuals have probably seen one of the babies who seem to manage both breast and bottle. These same people would certainly agree that a baby may prefer one sort of rubber nipple over another; that a baby may take both breasts but prefer one side over the other; that a baby might prefer the mother's protruding nipple over her other flatter nipple. Almost every mother's nipples are flat compared to a bottle nipple, so it's not surprising that babies might learn to prefer the bottle nipple to the breast, or to at least be confused about the sucking technique they should use.

It's also interesting that many of the people who say there is no such thing as nipple confusion are the same ones who urge parents to give their babies a bottle early on so that the baby will be willing to take one. They warn parents that if they delay introducing a bottle, the baby may always resist being given a bottle. In other words, their concern is that the baby will have a persistent preference for the breast. What they forget to mention is that a bottle is not the only way to supplement a breastfed baby, should that become necessary (see Chapter 5, Not Enough Milk).

5. There should be no restriction on length of feedings or frequency of feedings.

One book on breastfeeding given to new mothers 25 years ago said that the most important piece of equipment needed for successful breastfeeding was a reliable watch or clock. An emphasis on timing of feedings is an unfortunate legacy from a decade when babies' lives were rigidly scheduled, even though those schedules frequently led to breastfeeding failure.

From the beginning of human existence, mothers have breastfed their babies without the benefit of clocks, watches, or schedules. In many parts of the world this is still true, and these mothers almost universally succeed at breastfeeding.

Unrestricted feedings encourage the mother to learn her baby's cues. If she isn't watching the clock, she will be watching her baby and learning how he indicates that he's getting hungry—perhaps by moving around in a restless way, perhaps by making sucking motions with his lips and tongue, perhaps by trying to raise his hands to his mouth. If he doesn't feed well at one feeding, it isn't a big deal—he'll be able to feed again as soon as he needs to, and that feeding may well go better.

In traditional societies, it is common for babies to nurse frequently for short periods of time. Anthropologist Kathy Dettwyler describes babies in Mali nursing for a few minutes at a time, several times an hour, with some longer stretches between feedings when the baby is in a deeper sleep. The shorter, more frequent feeding pattern also leads to the production of milk with a higher fat content; when there is a longer time between feedings, the milk has a higher water content. These babies are undoubtedly "snacking" at the breast, drinking only small amounts at each feeding, so they want to return to the breast frequently. There is nothing wrong with this. It is important, however, to remember that a baby who is not feeding well, and not really getting milk, will also want to come to the breast frequently. Mothers need to be sure that the baby is well latched on and drinking at each feeding.

Restricting the length and frequency of feedings was at one time thought to be a way of preventing sore nipples. The idea was that if the mother started by nursing only for short periods of time, her nipples would gradually "toughen up." But research has shown that this does not prevent sore nipples—getting the baby properly latched on is the key to pain-free breastfeeding. In fact, limiting and scheduling feedings can actually increase the risk of sore nipples. If the baby is ravenously hungry when he comes to the breast,

he may grab at the nipple and not be patient enough to wait until his mother gets him properly positioned. His frustration when the milk doesn't flow quickly enough may make him pull at the breast, often coming off it and relatching poorly, causing more pain. If the mother gives him bottles or a pacifier to help him wait until the next scheduled feeding time, his latch and the way he sucks may get even worse, and the mother will be even more likely to have nipple pain.

What about the baby who is at the breast for hours? Most often, this means the baby is not properly latched on and is not really getting much milk. He is at the breast, but he is not actually breastfeeding. These babies usually use a rapid, fluttering kind of suck that may stimulate some milk to let down, so they are able to drink a little bit; however, they don't do the slow suckling with distinct pauses that indicates a good flow of milk. Once the baby is latched on well, his sucking usually changes dramatically, his tummy gets filled up, and he no longer spends hours at the breast.

There are babies who seem to want to spend more time at the breast than others, even if they are getting plenty of milk. Some seem to need the extra comfort that breastfeeding gives them. Some are just "high need." These babies can become upset even if their mothers have lots of milk—they want to suckle more than they want to eat! It's important to watch the baby at the breast to figure out what is really going on.

> "Never again, never in the future that dawned later on, were we so sated. We were suckled and suckled. Always superabundance was flowing into us. Never any question of enough is enough or let's not overdo it. Never were we given a pacifier and told to be reasonable. It was always suckling time."
>
> —Günter Grass, *The Flounder*

6. Supplements of water, sugar water, and/or formula are rarely required.

Many hospitals used to routinely supplement all breastfed babies' feedings with water or sugar water, at least for the first few days. This is now not supposed to be routine for all babies, yet many babies receive these supplements for a variety of reasons—most of which are not valid—because many health professionals are not confident about breastfeeding working well.

There are very few medical reasons for giving supplements to babies. If there is a true medical issue and the baby needs a supplement, it should be given by a lactation aid or supplemental nurser while the baby is at the breast. If the mother and baby have to be separated (and again, there are rarely good medical reasons for this), then the baby could receive his supplement from a cup or by finger-feeding (see Chapter 5, Not Enough Milk).

In most cases, though, the best way to provide extra milk for the baby is to get the baby well latched on. That way he is getting the maximum amount of milk possible from his own mother.

7. Free samples of formula must not be given to pregnant women, new mothers, or their families.

The World Health Organization (WHO) has specifically advised against this, for good reason. These "gifts" are gifts only for the formula companies. The free samples undermine breastfeeding, and have been shown to decrease the amount and duration of breastfeeding because they undermine the mother's confidence. They are also too easy to use when problems crop up, so the mother gives formula instead of seeking out help with breastfeeding.

8. Proper positioning and latching on are crucial to success.

For most mothers and babies, this is the most important step. "Latching on" refers to the way the baby takes the breast into his mouth. A good latch means pain-free breastfeeding; it also means that the baby will get the milk he needs and you will be on your way to a successful breastfeeding experience.

We have many things in our society conspiring against getting a baby well latched on. Most women have seen many more bottle-fed babies than breastfed babies, and the images imprinted on their brains of "how babies are fed" include babies lying on their backs, turned away from their mothers, with a rubber nipple pushed into their mouths. Very often you see new mothers attempt to breastfeed their babies in a bottle-feeding position. Or the new mother may try to hold her breast and insert the nipple into the baby's mouth, just as she would a bottle. This is exactly the wrong way of getting a baby onto the breast. (Of course, even the wrong way of getting the baby onto the breast will work for some mothers.)

The hospital staff who are trying to help the mother breastfeed may not be experienced and may not have the skills needed to recognize a good latch or correct a bad one. While some nurses have taken courses in breastfeeding or have developed the ability to deal with stumbling blocks, many have not. However, the nurse's feelings about breastfeeding are probably more important than the number of courses she has taken. If her own children were bottle-fed, and she feels breastfeeding is not important, she is not likely to be very helpful to a new mother.

It can be hard for these nurses to accept that they may have been teaching new mothers incorrect breastfeeding techniques for many years. Many insist that breastfeeding is inevitably

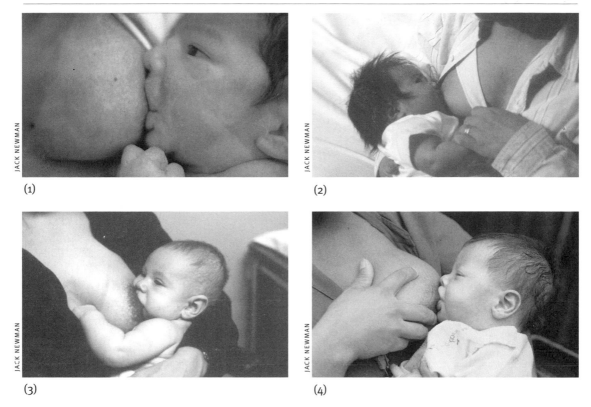

(1)   (2)

(3)   (4)

A series of bad latches. (1) The baby's mouth is puckered up, and he is not latched on at all; he falls off the breast when moved away from the mother. (2) Baby is nipple-feeding only. He is gaining well because of formula supplementation. (3) The baby's head is too far above the breast; his lower gums cannot compress the milk sinuses. The baby depends on the letdown reflex to get any milk at all. (4) Again, the baby is attached to the nipple only. His growth is good because the mother has an abundance of milk.

painful, and don't recognize that they are contributing to that painful experience by not helping the mother and baby to get breastfeeding well established.

The exact technique of getting the baby on the breast is not always as simple as "Apply Part A to Part B." Babies are individuals, and every breast is a little different—even breasts on the same mother! Sometimes mothers find the baby takes one breast easily, but not the other. Sometimes mothers use a cradle hold for one breast, and switch to the football hold for the other. Some women find it easier to get breastfeeding going if they are lying down instead of sitting up.

Blanket rules, such as "The baby should take the whole areola into his mouth as well as the nipple," don't hold true in most cases. Some women have small areolas, and if the baby takes only the areola, he won't have enough of the breast tissue in his mouth. Other women have very large areolas that cover most of their breasts, and it simply isn't possible for the baby to take the entire areola into his mouth when he is nursing. Some women also have very large nipples that fill the baby's mouth and limit the amount of additional breast tissue that he can take in.

Babies are different, too. Some are eager nursers from the very first day, others are calmer, while others take a day or two before they really figure out what's what. Some are sleepy because of narcotics their mothers received in labor. Some have a tight frenulum that can make it difficult to get their tongue forward. (The frenulum is the thin piece of flesh that attaches the tongue to the bottom of the mouth. In some babies, the frenulum is so tight that it restricts movement of the tongue.)

People who help mothers with breastfeeding need to be aware of these differences, and of how to manage them.

For these reasons, it can be difficult for a new mother to get good help with breastfeeding. If you are feeling real pain when the baby is breastfeeding, the baby is probably not latched on well, no matter what the nurse or other people tell you. Keep looking for someone who can help you correct the baby's position. If, once your milk becomes abundant, the baby is only making small sucking motions and not doing the "open mouth wide–pause–close mouth" type of suckling that shows you he is swallowing mouthfuls of milk, he is probably not latched on well, and you may need to look for someone to help you. And if your baby is spending long hours at the breast and still seems dissatisfied, you probably need help.

It's easy to say "The latch is fine," but if you are still experiencing one or more of these challenges, it's probably not true.

To get milk from the breast well, the baby must latch on to the breast well. The greater the mother's milk supply, the less the baby needs to latch on well, but the mother may pay a price. For example, sore nipples are almost always due to a poor latch. Even when there is an abundant supply of milk, a baby who latches on poorly may be on the breast for long periods of time or want to nurse very frequently, or both—often leading his mother to believe her milk supply is inadequate.

It may be helpful to use a bottle-feeding comparison, since, in our bottle-feeding culture, we understand bottle-feeding much better than breastfeeding. When a baby latches on poorly, it is similar to his being fed a bottle with a nipple hole that is too small. The bottle is full of milk, but the baby will have difficulties getting that milk. The baby may suck for a long time and he may fall asleep while sucking, only to wake up soon after the bottle has been withdrawn from his mouth. Why does he wake up? Because he hasn't taken much. The smaller the nipple hole, the less milk he will get, and the longer it will take for him to get that milk. At the extreme (no nipple hole at all), the baby will get no milk, and eventually become sleepier and sleepier as he becomes more dehydrated, despite the fact that there was plenty of milk available, at least in theory.

It could be argued that women all over the world, since the beginning of human time on earth, have breastfed their babies, usually quite successfully, without paying much attention to exactly how the baby was latched on. This is undoubtedly true, but it does not mean the latch is not important. Because most women have more than enough milk, their babies almost always grew reasonably well, despite less than ideal latches. In traditional cultures, however, the fact that the baby was on the breast many hours of the day, sometimes constantly, did not cause a great commotion. Babies were expected to be on the breast much of the time, and nobody gave mothers a hard time about their milk being too weak, or inadequate in quantity. Nobody accused mothers of spoiling the baby by having him on the breast too much or carrying him too much or sleeping with him at the breast. With a generous milk supply available to them, with free access to the breast, most babies gained weight just fine.

In addition, in more traditional cultures, mothers have from the time they were toddlers watched babies being breastfed. It is as normal in their minds as breathing. They have a subconscious image of the way breastfeeding works, how babies are to be held and how they take the breast.

It is just the opposite in our society, where the mental picture most women have of infant feeding is not breastfeeding but bottle-feeding. In our society, the bottle is the cliché image of babyhood. Our using the bottle-fed baby as our model has led to difficulty in understanding how breastfeeding works. And thanks to an obsession with numbers and the clock, and with scientific medicine's increasing involvement in infant feeding, this more relaxed and usually successful approach—breastfeeding—was largely discarded.

By the early years of the twentieth century, pediatricians were advising mothers to feed by the clock—so many minutes on each side every so many hours. Each pediatrician recommended a different number of minutes as the ideal feeding time, and usually three to four hours as the ideal feeding interval. "Scientific" infant feeding (from which the specialty of modern pediatrics grew, incidentally) often enough did not work, so that, more and more, supplemental milk was "required." Surprisingly, though, given the obstacles the scheduled feedings put in the way of successful breastfeeding, breastfeeding sometimes still worked. When the mother's supply is abundant, sometimes even the most bizarre of rules will not derail the process. Also, of course, there have always been some mothers who simply ignored their doctor's advice (because going by the schedule was not working, or because they couldn't be bothered to follow the schedule, which in a way takes more effort) and breastfed the way their own mothers had. This is lucky; otherwise, the art of breastfeeding might have been lost completely in the industrialized world.

We now know that there are more efficient and less efficient ways of having a baby take the breast. Observations by experienced mothers and interested health professionals have shown us that babies can do well or less well at the breast depending on how they are latched on.

When the amount of time the baby spends at the breast, or the frequency with which the baby takes the breast, are not considerations, how well the baby takes the breast may not be that important. But when society, and the mother herself, and the "experts" expect the baby to feed 20 minutes on each side every three hours, a poor latch can result in the baby's finding it difficult to get enough milk within the time limits. Furthermore, the less milk a mother has, even if the amount is sufficient to nourish her baby adequately, the better the latch must be in order for her baby to get enough milk.

- good latch + abundant milk supply = good weight gain, pain-free nursing, "short" feedings, feedings that are not frequent
- adequate latch + abundant milk supply = good weight gain, pain-free nursing, more frequent and longer feedings
- poor latch + abundant milk supply = slower weight gain and/or sore nipples. As the latch becomes poorer, there may be no weight gain, some weight loss, or, on occasion, even severe weight loss and dehydration despite the presence of an abundant milk supply.
- good latch + average milk supply = good weight gain, pain-free nursing, "short" feedings, feedings that are not usually frequent.
- poor latch + average milk supply = slow weight gain, sore nipples. Weight gain will probably not be adequate, feedings may be very frequent and long, baby may become dehydrated.

One reason women worry so much about not having enough milk is recent media coverage of cases in which "breastfed" babies became dehydrated. Note that dehydration may occur even in babies whose mothers have an abundant milk supply. In my experience, most of the mothers whose babies have become dehydrated have more than adequate milk supplies, and if they persist with breastfeeding and are helped to improve their techniques, they are usually able to go on to breastfeed exclusively.

The principle always holds: the better the latch, the more easily the baby gets the mother's milk. Even in the unusual instances when a mother is truly incapable of producing enough milk, the baby will still get more of her milk when he is well latched on than when he is poorly latched on.

If you are a nursing mother, you can try this test yourself. Pretend your thumb and index finger are your baby's gums. Put your thumb over the top of one of your nipples, and your index finger under the nipple. Now squeeze. You may feel pain, and notice how little comes out. Now move your fingers back two or three centimeters (an inch or so) and squeeze. You probably feel no pain, and quite possibly your milk will spray. Notice what a big difference such a short distance can make.

It is exaggerating only a little to put it this way, but that's all there is to breastfeeding—getting the baby to latch on properly.

What Is a Good Latch?

The answer to this question has changed over the years as more and more observations of babies breastfeeding have been made by knowledgeable observers. It was often written, for example, that the baby was well latched on if he had most or all of the areola in his mouth. (The areola is the

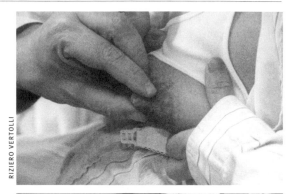

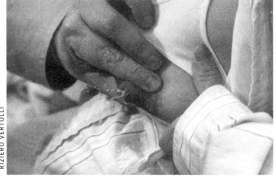

When a baby latches on over the nipple (upper photo), the baby cannot get milk easily. When the baby latches on over the areola, he gets milk better (lower photo). Both photos taken within seconds of each other *after the baby had finished nursing.*

pigmented area surrounding the nipple.) As a general rule, it is probably good if the baby has most of the areola covered by his mouth, but this does not guarantee that he has a good latch. A baby may cover most of a small areola and still not be well latched on. Similarly, a baby may cover nowhere near most of a large areola and be beautifully latched on. (Some women have areolas that cover well over a third of their entire breasts.) Other writers have said that the baby should have both his nose and his chin just touching the breast, and if his lips were also flanged back, the baby was well latched on. This refinement has led to more mothers and babies having an easier time with breastfeeding.

In my experience, even more mothers and

In the process of latching on. The baby hits the breast with his chin first, and the nose is usually not touching the breast. His mouth should open wide before the mother brings him onto the breast. In the upper picture, mother has moved her hand too close to the nipple. Note that the position of the baby's head relative to the breast does not change. The mother does not bring the baby's head up and over, and does not bend his neck to bring him onto the breast. Note also that these could be photos of the "football" hold, or even the baby coming onto the breast with the mother lying down.

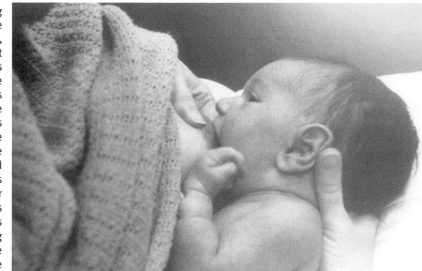

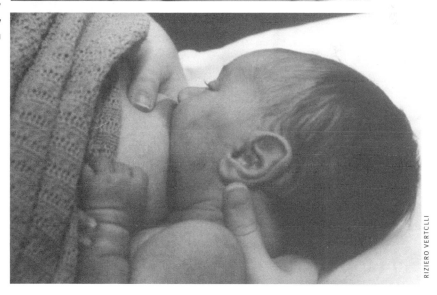

babies will have an easier time breastfeeding if the baby comes to the breast and latches on asymmetrically, covering more of the areola with his lower lip than with his upper lip. In this position, he can get his lower jaw under the milk sinuses and extract milk from the breast in a more efficient manner. He will get the milk he needs, and breastfeeding will be painless. (However, a pain-free latch doesn't necessarily mean the latch is good.)

How do you achieve this asymmetrical latch? I usually suggest mothers start by using the cross-cradle hold. Most mothers find this the easiest way to achieve the best latch, especially with a newborn. But it is not the only way. The best latch can also be achieved using the cradle hold, the football hold, or while lying down. (I'll explain how to latch the baby on in those positions in a minute.)

Let's imagine you are putting the baby to your left breast using the cross-cradle hold.

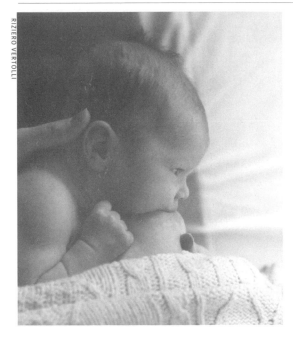

RIZIERO VERTOLLI

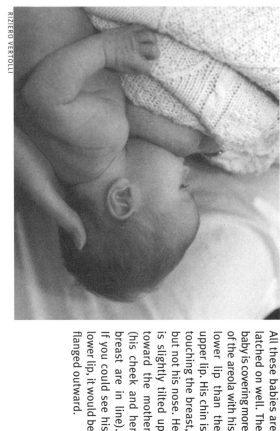

RIZIERO VERTOLLI

All these babies are latched on well. The baby is covering more of the areola with his lower lip than the upper lip. His chin is touching the breast, but not his nose. He is slightly tilted up toward the mother (his cheek and her breast are in line). If you could see his lower lip, it would be flanged outward.

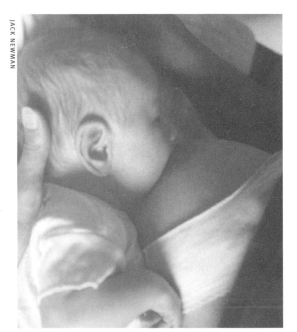

JACK NEWMAN

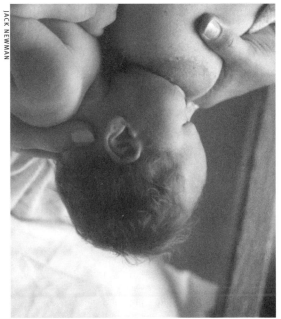

JACK NEWMAN

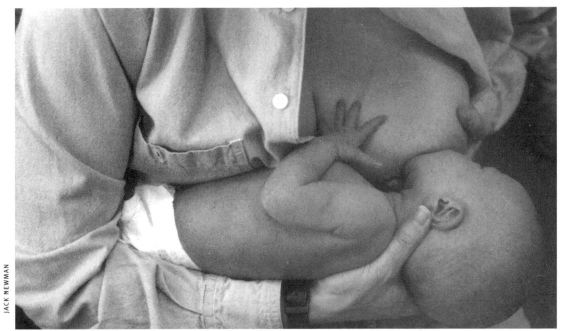

JACK NEWMAN

The cross-cradle hold.

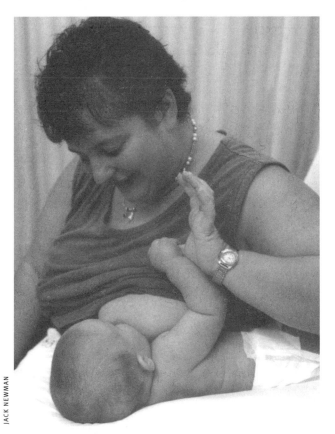

JACK NEWMAN

The football hold. As with the cradle hold and cross-cradle hold, the baby comes onto the breast with the nipple pointing to the roof of his mouth. He covers more of the areola with his lower lip than his upper lip.

• Hold your baby, lying on his side so his tummy is toward your tummy, with your right arm. Your baby's weight is supported by your forearm (and not by your hand or fingers).

• Push the baby's bottom into your body, with his legs underneath your arm, with the side of your forearm (the palm of your hand will face toward the ceiling). Don't worry, you won't hurt him.

• Your right hand is "under" the baby's face, palm up, with the web between your thumb and fingers at the nape of the baby's neck and your fingers "under" the baby's ears.

• Support your breast with your left hand, and place your thumb on top of the breast and all your fingers below the breast. Lightly brush the baby's upper lip with your nipple, running your nipple from one corner of the baby's mouth to the other. Be sure your fingers and thumb are well back from the nipple.

• Wait for the baby to open his mouth very wide, like a yawn, then quickly bring the baby onto the breast using your forearm, not just your hand or wrist, to move him. By moving your arm you will keep his bottom and feet tucked in close to your body.

• The baby should come onto the breast at an angle so that your nipple points toward the roof of his mouth.

If the baby has latched on well:

• he will cover more of the areola with his lower lip than his upper lip.
• his lips will be turned outward.
• his chin, but not his nose, will be touching your breast.
• his body will be slightly rotated upward so that he is looking at you.

If the baby hasn't latched on well, check to see if you are making one of these common mistakes:

• You used your hand or wrist to push only the baby's head toward your breast. If you do that, his head will tip forward and he may end up with more of his top lip covering the areola than his bottom lip—just the opposite of what you want. Use your whole forearm to move the baby, tucking his legs into your body with your elbow.

• You have your baby positioned with his head too far over on your left side. The baby should be positioned so that his mouth is right at the nipple, or a bit to the right of it, so that it is aimed toward the top of his mouth.

• Your baby is lying on his back rather than his side. In this position, he has to turn his head sideways to latch on to the breast—not a very comfortable position for drinking!

• You didn't wait until the baby's mouth was open wide enough before moving him onto the breast. His mouth needs to be very wide open, like a yawn. Be patient.

• Instead of moving the baby onto the breast, you tried to put the breast in the baby's mouth, as though you were feeding him a bottle.

Now your baby is latched on! How do you know if he is getting milk?

This is easy to recognize once you have seen it, but difficult to describe. The baby who is getting milk in substantial quantities will demonstrate a very definite pause in the movement of his chin as he opens his mouth to the maximum while sucking. As he pauses, his mouth is filling up with milk. You will see the baby open his mouth wide, keeping it wide open for a second or two, then close it again before opening it wide once more,

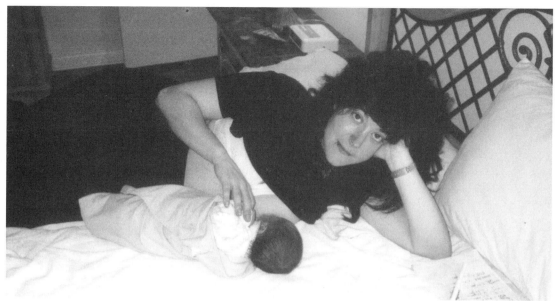

RONI CHASTAIN

Lying down to breastfeed.

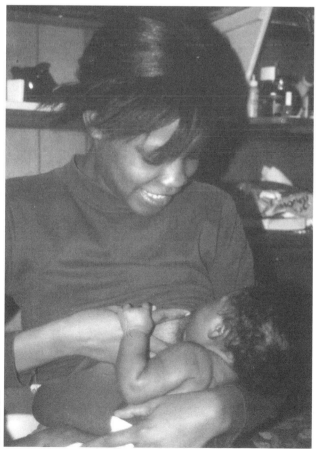

RONI CHASTAIN

The cradle hold. This baby's body could be wrapped more closely around the mother's body. Notice that the baby's head is on her forearm, not in the crook of her arm. If he were in the crook of her arm, his head would be too far to the side of the breast.

pausing while his mouth is open, then closing it again. The baby who is not getting much milk will have a fast sucking pattern without any of these wide-open-mouth pauses—just open-close, open-close, open-close (no pauses).

In the first two or three days, when your breasts are making colostrum, you may not see these pauses in your baby's sucking. Colostrum is generally produced in fairly small but adequate quantities and so the length of the pause is shorter than when the milk production is more abundant and may be difficult to notice. However, if your baby's latch is very good and you have lots of colostrum, you may see these pauses that indicate the baby is getting plenty of milk. You should certainly expect to see this once your milk "comes in."

Other Positions

To latch your baby on using the "football" hold, have your baby lying at your side, with his feet pointing toward the back of the chair you are sitting on. Support his weight on your forearm with your hand under the back of his head, palm up. Use your other hand to support your breast and to tickle the baby's upper lip with your nipple just as with the cross-cradle hold. As he opens his mouth wide, use your arm to bring him straight onto the breast. Do not bend his neck to bring him around.

In this position it is easy to make the mistake of pushing the baby "nose first" into the breast. Help him to latch on asymmetrically by using your arm, not just your hand and wrist. You might find it helps to have a pillow beside you and under the baby's body.

The cradle hold is the position you have probably seen in hundreds of classical paintings and used by mothers in the mall and at the park. To feed your baby on the left breast in this position, hold him in your left arm with his head just below the crook of your elbow and your left hand supporting his bottom. Be sure he is level with your nipple. Use your right hand to support your breast and run the nipple lightly along his upper lip from one corner to the other. When he opens wide, bring him in—moving your arm—so he can latch on.

You can also latch the baby on in the cross-cradle position and then switch the position of your arms so you are holding him in the cradle position. You may find this position more comfortable for longer feedings, especially as your baby grows.

To breastfeed lying down, lie your baby on his side, facing you, with his mouth level with your nipple. Use pillows behind your back and under your head to help you lie comfortably on your left side. If your breasts are small, you may want to put your baby on a firm pillow or folded towels so that he will be able to reach the nipple easily. Support your breast with your right hand and the baby with your left hand, moving him in to latch on when he opens his mouth wide. Be sure that as you move the baby on, you tuck his feet and legs toward your tummy, so that he latches asymmetrically.

Understanding latch seems pretty straightforward. So why do so many women have trouble with breastfeeding and getting their babies to nurse well? Common problems and solutions are discussed in the next chapter.

III

Common Problems and Solutions

5

Not Enough Milk

Myth: Many women are not capable of producing enough milk to feed their babies.

Fact: The majority of women are perfectly capable of producing all the milk their babies need for at least four to six months, and can continue producing plenty of milk for months and years as their babies add other foods to their diets. Most women are capable of feeding twins or even triplets, and some women have an over abundance of milk (which can cause problems, too (see Chapter 9, Colic). Only a small number of women truly do not produce enough milk for their babies. Even these women can still breastfeed, though not exclusively with their own milk.

Many women living in affluent societies believe they are not able to produce enough milk for their babies. How is it that women all over the world—women living in poor countries or in difficult conditions, women suffering from chronic illnesses (including nutritional deficiencies)—usually manage to breastfeed quite adequately and produce enough milk, while well-nourished, generally healthy women in affluent societies have so much trouble?

Is There Really a Problem?

Sometimes women become concerned about their milk supply when everything is, in fact, going well. Their concerns are based on the following:

The Baby's Behavior

Sometimes mothers think they don't have enough milk because of the way their babies behave. If the baby feeds frequently, or stays on the breast for long periods of time and does not seem content, many mothers (and their families) will conclude that the mother doesn't have enough milk, or that her milk is "weak" or "inadequate."

Interestingly, women who have "too much milk" also report that their babies feed frequently, stay on the breast for long periods of time, and are often unhappy or fussy. These babies not only gain weight well, but gain at a faster-than-average rate.

On the other hand, the baby who sleeps a lot, especially in the first week, may not be doing well at all. His mother may be fooled into thinking he is content and getting lots of milk when, in fact, he isn't. We will discuss this in more detail later.

The baby who won't follow a schedule can also worry a new mother. After many years of moving away from the idea of scheduling feedings, this approach is unfortunately making a comeback. Trying to stick to a schedule can make many mothers concerned that they don't have enough milk. If the baby wants to eat sooner than the schedule says, and cries (as he will), then the mother often assumes her baby didn't get enough to eat at the previous feeding. The problem is not her milk supply, though—it is the schedule. Breastfeeding works best when babies are fed when they want to be fed, so that the mother's supply adjusts to the baby's needs.

Weight Gain

Mothers also become concerned about their milk supplies after they have had the baby's weight checked and charted, and have discovered the baby isn't exactly where they feel he should be on the chart. There is an awful lot of concern about weight gain amongst physicians, especially pediatricians, as well as public health nurses and, of course, new mothers and their families.

The first question we should be asking is, Why are we concerned about weight gain? More particularly, why is it necessary for babies to gain a certain amount of weight each day or each week or each month?

Most physicians would say that it is normal for a baby to lose weight during the first few days, and then regain that weight by 10 days of age. Actually, my experience in Africa, where babies were with their mothers and in their beds during the entire hospital stay of a couple of days, was that many babies did not seem to lose weight at all. Midwives also report that babies born at home and breastfed without restrictions will often be over their birthweights by four or five days of age. After that, a baby typically gains about 30 g (about one oz) each day for the first two months or so, and then 15 g (or about half an ounce) per day until about six months of age. Thus, a baby who is born at 3.3 kg (about 7 lb 4 oz) will lose some weight during the first days, and then, by 10 days of age, will be back at 3.3 kg. By one month, he should weigh 3.9 kg (8 lb 9 oz). By two months, he should weigh another

900 g, or 4.8 kg (10 lb 9 oz). But now his rate of weight gain will usually slow down. By about three months, he will weigh about 5.25 kg (11 lb 9 oz). And by about six months the baby will weigh 6.57 kg (14 lb 7 oz). Some physicians mistakenly expect the baby to continue gaining at the same rate in the third to sixth month as he would normally gain in the first two months, in which case the baby would weigh a lot more than he needs to—8.85 kg (19 lb 8 oz) at six months of age.

But all growth rates are *guidelines*. What does it mean if a baby gains a little less or a little more quickly? What does it mean if the baby gains a lot less or a lot more quickly?

The fact is that many health professionals have forgotten what growth standards and growth charts are really for. When a baby or a child gains weight and grows in length (or height) at a rate that can be considered "normal" or "average," this is one sign of good health. A baby smiling by a certain age is also a sign of good health, just as is social interaction with other people, and just as is the absence of a heart murmur. None of these, or the myriad other signs we use, *alone* is a guarantee that a child actually is in good health. Thus, a child who smiles socially at four weeks of age is on track for development, but could easily have a heart problem. A baby could gain weight just fine, yet have a kidney problem.

Growth charts developed because they were an easy way of keeping track of large numbers of babies, particularly in poor areas, where medical care was not as available as in more affluent areas of the world. Weighing babies, measuring their lengths and head circumferences, is an easy way of screening large numbers of infants to see which of them needs extra care. The weight, which is the first of the three measures to go off when something is wrong, allowed health workers to separate those babies who needed interventions from those who probably did not. The intervention may just have required information about feeding the baby more frequently on the breast if that seemed to be the problem, or may have required more serious intervention, if the baby had heart disease, for example.

Growth charts are designed so the baby's weight is charted against his age in months, and the lines on the chart are called *percentile lines*. Many parents, and some physicians, seem to believe that only babies at the fiftieth percentile and above are normal. This is not true. Growth charts are made from data on *normal* babies (though the majority of them were formula-fed or not breastfed more than a few weeks, and they often had solids introduced fairly early). Thus if a baby is on the fiftieth percentile for his age, it means that 50 percent of all normal babies his age weigh more than he, and 50 percent weigh less. It does *not* mean this baby is normal just because he is on the fiftieth percentile. If a baby is on the third percentile, it means that 97 percent of normal babies his age weigh more than he does. But it does *not* mean he is unhealthy, and it does not mean he should weigh more. Somebody has got to be there on the third percentile.

Furthermore, a single weight does not tell anyone anything. A baby who was on the fiftieth percentile at six months of age, and is on the tenth percentile at 12 months, is a baby to be concerned about. A baby who was on the tenth percentile at two, four, six, eight, and 12 months of age is probably fine. And he is doing just what we expect him to do.

Growth charts always have to be interpreted. The person who is reading the information has to take into account that the data might not be appropriate to the child being weighed and put on that chart. Growth charts available in North America were developed using data from mostly Caucasian babies and children who were fed formula from early on in their lives and given solids relatively early on. Thus, these growth charts may not represent normal growth curves for Chinese babies, or Inuit babies, regardless of how they were fed. (In fact, growth charts were recently developed in Hong Kong for babies of Chinese origin. Their growth curves, in a population where malnutrition in babies is almost unknown, are quite different from the charts developed in North America.) The charts also may not represent normal growth curves for babies exclusively breastfed.

As with all tools, growth charts have to be used properly; otherwise they can be worse than useless. We must not only interpret them carefully, but be aware that mistakes can be made that give us inaccurate information. A child who is four months old, whose weight is at the fiftieth percentile, will look as if he is not doing well, if his weight is accidentally plotted on the line for a six-month-old. This is an easy mistake to make, by the way.

Incidentally, the birthweight is not the standard that determines where the baby should be. Some are born big and then settle into their percentile a bit later, which might make them seem to be growing too slowly. Trying to keep them on their birthweight percentile is not only futile, but may lead to supplementing, and undermine breastfeeding.

Once a baby has been charted on a certain percentile line, is it essential that he stays on that line? Remember our earlier discussion of weight gain as only one sign amongst many that give us information about how the baby is doing.

It is not okay for a baby to gain no weight at all

for an extended period of time—but slow or no weight gain can often be improved if breastfeeding techniques are improved. If the baby is content, developing normally and growing slowly but steadily, I would keep an eye on him but otherwise not be too concerned. On the other hand, if the baby is very fussy and unhappy, maybe another approach is necessary.

It may surprise people to know that many breastfed babies who are doing well actually gain weight faster than formula-fed babies, at least for the first few months. Not all do, and some gain at about the same rate, and some even more slowly. Then, between four and six months of age, some breastfed babies actually gain more slowly than formula-fed babies. So if the breastfed baby's weight is charted on the standard charts (based on babies fed formula), he may drop from the fiftieth percentile to the thirtieth, for example. If the growth chart was based on the weights of breastfed babies, the baby would stay at the fiftieth percentile.

The Baby's Fontanelle

This way of "knowing" about the baby's state of hydration is mentioned only to be condemned. The fontanelle is the "soft spot" on the top of the baby's head. Many physicians have difficulty judging whether a baby's fontanelle is sunken or not. Almost all babies have a "sunken" fontanelle if they are held in a sitting position, and this may confuse both the parents and the health care professional.

By the time a baby is dehydrated enough to have a truly sunken fontanelle, the situation is late indeed, and the baby must have been showing signs for some time that he was not getting enough milk.

Frequency of Feedings

Knowing the frequency of the baby's feedings is not very useful in determining how much milk the baby is getting. A baby may sleep longer than the now engraved-in-stone three hours, either because he has had a really good feeding, or because he got almost no milk at all and is becoming weak and lethargic! A baby who breastfeeds well will wake up when he is hungry. A baby who does not breastfeed at all may sleep for long periods of time, though this is usually a problem only in the first week or so.

Often people feel that more frequent feedings will help in this situation. But waking the baby up so that he will nibble at the breast—not truly feeding—eight times a day instead of six makes no sense. Eight times nothing is nothing, just as six times nothing is nothing. For that matter, so is 12 times nothing. It is true that babies who get very little to drink may sleep for long periods of time, and this is not a good thing. But if a baby is sleeping long periods because he is not drinking much at all, the idea is to fix the breastfeeding technique and get food into the baby, not just to wake the baby up more so that he drinks nothing more often. It should be emphasized again that just because a baby is on the breast frequently, that does not mean he is getting more milk than if he is on the breast less frequently. The same is true if the baby is on the breast for long periods of time.

This is a different situation from that of a baby who is feeding infrequently because he is being kept to a schedule. In this situation, the baby may well be waking up and crying to be fed, but the parents may insist that the baby wait until the clock says it's feeding time. Sometimes these babies eventually give up and stop crying, even though they are hungry. Some will give up and go back to sleep. In this case, assuming the baby is latched on properly, more frequent feeding may well be the solution.

Incidentally, a baby who has been doing well does not—unless he is sick—suddenly stop waking up for feedings when he is hungry. A baby who has been doing well for a couple of weeks or a couple of months, and then suddenly is getting less milk for some reason, will let his parents know he is hungry. He will cry until picked up and fed, or until he cries himself to sleep from exhaustion. It does sometimes happen, though, that the three- or four-month-old will merely suck his thumb or finger, quite content not to nurse.

So if these signs are not very reliable, what are the signs we *should* be looking for to indicate that the baby is not getting enough milk?

Signs to Look For

Insufficient Weight Gain

Yes, I've just pointed out many of the hazards of relying on weight charts and scales. And there are further limitations I want to point out here.

Scales need to be calibrated fairly often. If they are not calibrated, even the digital electronic scales do not give accurate weights. If the weight is not accurate, it can't tell us much about how the baby is doing.

Balance scales will vary with the person doing the weighing, depending on where they consider the weight to be "balanced." If a baby's weight is being followed on a daily basis, a weight increase of about 30 grams (about 1.0 oz) each day is the goal. But that is a very small amount, and weights done by different people could easily vary by that amount. This is less of a problem with digital readout scales.

The weights can vary with the baby, as well. When a baby cries vigorously on the scale, the weight jumps all over the place. With balance scales, the reader takes the most likely weight, but it is a ballpark figure. With digital readout scales, the "reader" is the scale itself, and it also takes a ballpark figure—a guess, really.

It should not be forgotten that babies' weights will vary according to whether or not they have just pooped or peed. If the weight is being followed every few weeks or longer, this is not a concern. But if the baby's weight is being followed closely for some reason, say every day, whether he emptied his bladder and bowels before or after the weighing could make a significant difference on the scale. A bowel movement could easily weigh the 30 grams (1.0 oz) we would like the baby to gain in a day.

In some offices, babies are weighed with their clothes on; in others not. If we want to know the baby's weight, we should not be weighing his clothes as well, particularly his diaper. I have personally weighed a heavy diaper at 260 grams (over half a pound). A baby should be weighed naked each time, or with a brand-new dry diaper put on just before the weighing.

Scales vary. One may be calibrated, the other may not be; but even if the other is, it may be true to itself, but not to other scales. Thus, when a baby is weighed on one scale and then on another, possible variation must be taken into account. Some of the easiest referrals I have ever had were from a physician who would send one- or two-week-old babies with a concern about "no weight gain" or "weight loss." It turned out her scale weighed about 500 grams (over a pound) less than anyone else's scale (including the hospital's). In our clinic, we weighed the baby on two different scales to make sure our scale was not out. Furthermore—and this is vital—babies are not assessed on weight alone, but on how well they are breastfeeding and whether they are getting milk. That physician's babies were obviously getting lots of breastmilk while they were breastfeeding.

Scales, even when accurate, can be read wrongly, or the weight may be noted down incorrectly. I have seen, with my own eyes, the weight on the digital scale of 3.62 kg (7 lb 15.5 oz) written down as 3.26 kg (not quite 7 lb 3 oz). Errors such as this occur frequently, but are not always caught.

I am not saying that the scale is useless. Indeed, in the breastfeeding clinics where I work, we do weigh babies and record the information. But weight is only one of the many factors that we take into consideration when we try to decide whether a baby is doing well on the breast. The scale is most helpful over an extended period of time when the limitations of the scale are less likely to have an effect on the interpretation of the information. In other words, if the baby gains 500 grams from age four months to age five months, this is not really significantly different from gaining 400 grams during the same period of time—both being good weight gains. But a difference of 100 grams in one week could very well be the difference between good weight gain and poor weight gain. A baby who gains 200 grams from week two to week three of his life is gaining well. A baby who gains 100 grams during that time is not, though this does not mean he needs to be supplemented. First we'll work at improving breastfeeding.

When the baby's weight is reliably measured, however, and the weight gain is very low or nonexistent, this is certainly a sign that there may be some problems.

Bowel Movements

Babies pass bowel movements called meconium during the first few days. Meconium is the substance that accumulates during the baby's time in the mother's uterus, and it is expelled during the first few days. It is very dark green, almost black, in color and usually quite sticky.

Colostrum, the milk a mother produces in the first few days after giving birth, is a laxative and helps the baby expel the meconium more quickly. This is why early and effective feeding will prevent unusually high levels of bilirubin (jaundice) in the breastfed baby in the first few days of life that so many physicians and nurses worry about. As the baby drinks more milk, the bowel movements become lighter and eventually turn to yellow-brown (mustard color). The more milk a baby gets in the first few days, the earlier the bowel movements will change color. Thus, some *exclusively* breastfeeding babies will start having lighter bowel movements by the second day of life, though this is unusual—many babies are not latched on well at the beginning. Many parents will notice lighter bowel movements by day three or four, with the bowel movements turning to yellow or mustardy on day four or five. This is the pattern of the baby who is doing well. The early change to mustard color (by the fourth day of life) is a good sign.

If a baby is still having meconium-like bowel movements on the fourth day of life, this is a real reason for concern, and I would not be reassured if my scale showed that the baby's weight was down only 5 percent or even less—or even, for that matter, that the weight was up—from birthweight. The change in color of the bowel movements is a better sign than the weight as to how well a baby is doing during these early days.

A baby still having meconium-like bowel movements on the fifth day of life urgently needs evaluation, preferably by someone who knows something about breastfeeding. It would never come to that, however, if we had good help for mothers in the hospital as well as good follow-up once they were out of hospital.

Breastfed babies also have frequent bowel movements. Once the meconium has been completely expelled, a baby who is doing well will have at least two or three substantial mustardy bowel movements a day, plus some stains at the bottom of the diaper, usually with every feeding. What is substantial? Well, many babies will actually leak poop out the side of their diapers. Leaking isn't a requirement, but most babies who are doing well will have an amount that requires at least some work to clean off their bottoms. During the first few weeks of life, the baby should continue to have substantial frequent bowel movements.

If a baby passes even 24 hours during this time without a substantial bowel movement, I would be concerned and would ask the mother to come in so that I could observe a feeding. Though there are definitely exceptions, when it is obvious that the baby is doing well even though he is not passing bowel movements every day, in the majority of cases, infrequent bowel movements at this age mean the baby is not getting enough milk.

After about three weeks of age, some babies do change their patterns from many bowel movements every day to only one bowel movement every few days. Indeed, sometimes the time between bowel movements is more than a few days! The longest time I am aware of is 31 days without a bowel movement in a healthy, normal, happy, exclusively breastfed baby who was gaining well. If the baby is happy and gaining weight, there is no need for concern and no need for treatment, because this is a normal pattern for some babies; there is no need to treat or be concerned about something that is normal. Physicians unused to breastfed babies, especially exclusively breastfed babies, may worry about

this pattern, but then, this is another example of taking the artificially fed baby as the model of normal.

Some mothers do complain that as the days go on without the baby having a bowel movement, the baby does start to become fussy and seems uncomfortable. Not the majority, but some. In such a case, the parents should perhaps help the baby have a bowel movement.

The most natural way to do this is to take advantage of what is called the "gastro-colic reflex." This reflex results in our wanting to have a bowel movement when the stomach fills up, and becomes most obvious in the morning after we eat breakfast. Babies tend to have a more active gastro-colic reflex, and often have a bowel movement with a feeding. Thus, what the mother can try, if the baby is trying to have a bowel movement and not succeeding and being very fussy, is to put him to the breast. If the baby feeds, he may have his bowel movement, and everyone will be happy, including the baby.

Unfortunately, this does not always work, because the baby may not be interested in taking the breast. Or because despite the gastro-colic reflex, the baby does *not* have a bowel movement. What now?

Well, not prune juice, nor any other oral laxatives, or even sugar water. They may work, but they may not, and can cause the baby quite severe cramps, particularly the prune juice and laxatives. If necessary, the baby can be induced to have a bowel movement with the tip of a children's glycerin suppository. These are available without a prescription at pharmacies. Take just the first 2 or 3 cm of the suppository (it cuts nicely with an ordinary kitchen knife) and pop it into the baby's anus. Keep his buttocks squeezed together for a few minutes, and usually the baby will have a bowel movement. I would not suggest this be done as a routine even if the baby has seven days between bowel movements or even longer. As long as the baby is content, don't do anything.

A normal exclusively breastfed baby almost never (never say never) has hard, constipated bowel movements. Hard, constipated bowel movements in an exclusively breastfed baby, even if he is gaining weight well, should be investigated.

The color of breastfed babies' bowel movements can vary considerably. They may be mustard color, they may be green, they may be orange. They may be one color one day, and another the next. Sometimes one part of the bowel movement is one color, and another part is a different color. Green bowel movements, even if every bowel movement is green, are normal, and no cause for concern if the baby is content and gaining weight well.

However, just like the numbers on the scale, knowing the history of the baby's bowel movements is only one piece of information, and basing decisions about the adequacy of breastmilk intake only on the bowel movements can be misleading. For example, some babies who are not getting enough milk may have frequent watery green or even yellow bowel movements. This may occur because they are getting mostly low-fat milk, which can result in their having many bowel movements without getting enough calories.

Urine Output

The number of wet diapers a baby has is probably the least useful of all the pieces of information we might use to decide if the baby is getting enough. A baby who is getting enough to maintain his weight but not enough to make him gain well, could still be getting enough fluid to make him urinate fairly frequently. Furthermore, with the ultra-absorbent disposable diapers that do not feel wet, a new mother may not know if the diaper is really wet. An experienced mother will know how a really wet, heavy diaper feels, but how can a new mother know what she is looking for?

In the early days, the urine output is an even less useful indicator than later on. Nobody knows what normal urine output should be in the exclusively breastfed baby during the first few days, when most are getting small amounts of colostrum and many are getting virtually nothing (because they are not latched on well). We have for so long taken the formula-fed baby as the model of normal that the tremendous urine output of those babies is taken as the rule. Even breastfed babies were so often supplemented (and still are, almost always unnecessarily) in the first few days, that we still do not have a notion of what the normal urine output of babies on days one, two, or three after birth should be.

What about brick-colored urine in the first few days? The appearance of red urine in the first few days is enough to convince some nurses and doctors that "The baby is dehydrated!" In truth, nobody really knows what it means. Textbooks written at the beginning of the century, when supplements were only rarely given to breastfed babies, say that it is normal for newborns to have red urine. I don't think it is, though, because most of those babies were not fed as they should have been. There was a six-hour and sometimes even a 24-hour separation between mother and baby after the birth at that time, and babies were fed by the clock only every four hours and only five minutes on each side on the first day, 10 minutes the second day and so on. Later, supplementation of newborns during the first few days became routine, and red urine was seen as abnormal, so if a mother dared to insist that her baby not be supplemented, she would be shown the evidence of her baby's need for the supplement in the red-stained diaper.

In general, an exclusively breastfed baby should have one wet diaper on the first day of life, two wet diapers on the second, and three on the third. (Numbers again!) Thereafter, the number should increase rapidly so that by the end of the first week, the baby will have six soaking wet diapers in a 24-hour day. Six *wet* diapers is not enough, they should be *soaking wet*. A baby having only six wet, but not soaking or heavy, diapers in a 24-hour day at a week of age or older is probably not getting enough milk.

Changes in the Mother's Breasts

The mother's feeling full before a feeding, and less full after a feeding, is not bad as a sign of the baby's milk intake, but the mother has to be feeling full in order for this to be useful. In the first three or four days, some mothers just do not feel full at all, so this is not too helpful at this point. Also, while some women feel the milk "letting down" very strongly, others don't, so this may not be a good indication, either.

Investigating the Situation

My five-day-old baby has lost more than 10 percent of his birthweight. What do I do?

The weight loss is only one piece of the puzzle. If a mother came to me with this question, this is what I would do:

1. I would do a general history and a history of the baby's feeding, asking specifically about the baby's drinking, bowel movements, and urine output.
2. I would weigh the baby and do a general physical examination.

3. I would observe a feeding. I would watch for the open mouth wide–pause–close mouth type of sucking (as described in on page 60) and would point that out to the mother, so *she* knows how to be sure the baby is getting milk. Without observing a feeding, any physician, pediatrician, nurse, or midwife who tells the mother she needs to supplement, or reassures the mother that all is fine, is doing so based on insufficient information, and that is both inappropriate and potentially dangerous.

4. If the baby is drinking lots, I would reassure the mother, and make an appointment to check the baby again in the next day or two. If the mother has sore nipples, I would help her latch the baby on better.

5. If the baby is not drinking lots, I would help the mother latch the baby on so he could get more milk. I would also show the mother how to use "breast compression" (described on page 72) to increase the amount of milk the baby gets at the breast. I would encourage the mother to keep the baby on the first breast until the baby is no longer drinking even with compression, and then change sides and repeat the process. Finally, I would discuss the use of herbs to increase the mother's milk supply or flow. If the open mouth wide–pause–close mouth type of sucking increased with this help (as it usually does), I would ask her to bring the baby back in the next day or two, or, if things improved a lot, in a week.

6. If we have tried these steps, and the baby is still either not drinking at all or drinking only a little (and this is a judgment call), I will suggest to the mother that she needs to supplement breastfeeding. The mother's expressed milk would be the ideal first choice, and banked human milk is a very good second choice, but these may be hard to

get. The only choice may be artificial baby milk. The methods of supplementation are described later.

Let's look at the steps I would go through in more detail.

Improving the Baby's Latch

This is extremely important, and is discussed in Chapter 4, Getting Off to the Best Start. It is often all that is needed to get the baby feeding well enough to get as much as he needs.

Breast Compression

Breast compression is a technique that can help the baby get more milk. It is used, in one way or another, all over the world, and I personally noticed women doing something similar in southern Africa when I worked there. Often I would see them walking along the street, with the baby at the breast, and pressing that breast with their hands. I never really thought too much about it, until a woman from South America came to the clinic with her baby, and she was gently squeezing or compressing her breast while the baby was breastfeeding. I asked why, and her first response was that her mother had suggested she do it. Now that is a good reason, since the passing on of breastfeeding knowledge to the new generation used to be the domain of the more experienced mothers around the new mother. When I asked why her mother had suggested it, she looked at me as if I were from a different planet, and said, "Because the baby gets more milk." And the penny dropped for me. Of course, the baby gets more milk. It's so obvious. This technique does not, by the way, increase the risk of the mother getting blocked ducts, as many mothers are told in the hospital.

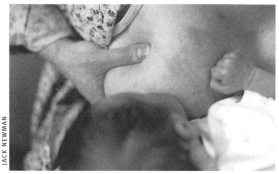

Breast compression: The mother compresses to keep the baby drinking milk. The idea is to "finish" the first side before offering the second.

Here is how I suggest to mothers that they use breast compression:

1. The mother needs to know when the baby is getting milk (open mouth wide–pause–close mouth type of sucking).

2. When the baby is drinking milk, the mother does not need to use any breast compression.

3. Once the baby is sucking but not drinking, just nibbling, the mother should start with the breast compression.

4. The baby should be sucking, but not actually drinking (open mouth wide–pause–close type of sucking). As the baby sucks, the mother, who is holding her breast with one hand, the thumb on one side and her other fingers on the other side of the breast, with a good amount of breast in her hand, should just bring her thumb and fingers together, compressing the breast. This should be done firmly, but not so hard that it hurts.

5. The baby may start to drink again (open mouth wide–pause–close mouth type of sucking). If so, the mother should keep up the pressure until the baby is back to nibbling. Once the baby is nibbling only, the mother should release the pressure on the breast so her hand does not get tired, and allow milk to start flowing again.

6. When the mother releases the pressure, a young baby, say under two or three weeks of age, will stop sucking. He will restart sucking when he tastes milk again. An older baby may continue to suck. If the baby drinks, fine. If he sucks but does not drink, the mother should restart the compression.

7. If compression has no effect at a particular moment, this does not mean the mother must immediately switch sides. Sometimes compression will work, other times not. But as the baby has nursed longer and longer, it will work less and less, as the flow of milk slows. This means not that the breast is "empty," but that the baby is getting less and less. Babies respond to flow of milk.

8. If compression is no longer having an effect, and the baby is getting sleepy, or starting to fuss because flow is slow, the mother should take the baby off the breast and offer the other side. She should then repeat the process.

9. The mother should experiment. I have found the above technique to be best, at least among the mothers being shown how at the clinic, but mothers should do whatever works best for them. As long as it does not hurt the mother to compress the breast, and the baby gets milk, the technique is working.

The idea of keeping the baby on just one breast at each feeding makes no sense. The mother should "finish" the first breast, and, if the baby wants more, offer the other. A baby has finished one side when he is falling asleep at the breast and doing no more, or very little, of the open mouth wide–pause–close mouth type of sucking. A baby may let go of the breast when he is getting little milk from it, but not necessarily. Sometimes he will just let go because he wants a break, or is distracted by something, or for reasons we don't

know. If the baby comes off the breast on his own, and then seems to want more, it may be worthwhile to try him again on the side he just let go of, to see if he will drink some more. If not, change him over to the other breast.

Herbs

From the beginning of time, mothers have used various herbs to increase their milk supply. This is just a confirmation of the fact that some mothers, indeed, do not produce enough. Do these herbs work? Maybe. There are modern drugs that definitely increase the milk supply, so there is no reason not to believe that in nature there are plants producing compounds that act in a similar way to those modern drugs (which all act in a similar way), or perhaps in different ways altogether. Every culture had its own favorite herbal remedy. Some cultures had their special gods to whom new mothers prayed for a bountiful supply of milk. It is possible that some of these methods really worked, while some worked only by giving the mother confidence—which is helpful, but not absolutely necessary, in breastfeeding. (A lack of confidence may be one reason, incidentally, that so many women in modern societies have breastfeeding problems, and one that the formula companies exploit in their "helpful" information booklets.)

In northern Europe, brewer's yeast and beer were thought to increase milk supply. In southern China, fish and papaya soup. In various places, different herbs, probably depending on what was available locally. Borage, alfalfa, fenugreek, raspberry leaf, fennel, blessed thistle, goat's rue—these are just some of the various herbs that have been thought to increase milk supply.

It should be said that if an herb works to increase milk supply—*really* works—by stimulating some receptor in the mother's breast or some hormone which she secretes, then that herb is a drug, despite the fact that it is a natural-source drug. Digitalis, which can be rapidly fatal if taken in too large amounts, has been used for the treatment of heart problems for many years, and came originally from a plant, foxglove. All knowledgeable gardeners know that foxglove is poison. Furthermore, a problem with herbal remedies is that there is no quality control over how much of what active ingredient (or, more likely, active *ingredients*) is in any preparation. The amounts may vary not only from the preparation of one company to that of another, but also from lot to lot of the same company. Indeed, because in many cases we don't know what the active ingredient in the herb even is, it is difficult to know how much of any herb should be taken.

It is our experience, however, that fenugreek and blessed thistle do seem to work for a lot of mothers, both in increasing the milk supply and in increasing the rate of milk flow. These two herbal remedies seem to work better in the early weeks than later on, but in some cases have seemed to work later, as well.

Fenugreek (*Trigonella foenum-graecum*) is used to increase the milk supply in both India and Egypt. Several Egyptian and Indian women have told me that all nursing mothers in their countries take fenugreek tea when they are nursing. Fenugreek is an ingredient of curry, and sometimes it is quite evident that a mother is taking it because of the smell it gives her skin. I now tell the mothers that the amounts of fenugreek vary considerably from preparation to preparation regardless of what it says on the bottle. That if they don't smell fenugreek on their skin, they should take more. Not all mothers like that smell, but as someone who quite appreciates Indian food, I like it a lot. Indeed, fenugreek is a natural deodorant. Side effects have been very few in the mothers we have

suggested use it. It is said that in large doses it can cause cramps and diarrhea, but we have not heard many women mention this.

Blessed thistle (*Cnicus benedictus*) has also been used for a long time to increase milk supply, but it is a difficult herb on which to get reliable information. Most of the mothers who have taken it at the suggestion of our clinic have had no obvious side effects. The main complaint is that the tea and the tincture taste awful.

We have generally suggested that mothers take the herbs in capsule form, using both fenugreek and blessed thistle, three capsules of each three times a day. The response, if it occurs, is quite rapid—mothers often notice a difference in less than 24 hours. The response almost always takes less than a week. As with all medications, some people respond better than others, and some women do not respond at all. Some mothers who initially had a problem with milk supply, now seem not to know what to do with all the milk they produce!

There is unlikely to be any effect on the baby, as is the case with most medication (see Chapter 11, Breastfeeding While on Medication).

Other Drugs
for Increasing the Milk Supply

Many drugs will increase a mother's milk supply. None was specifically manufactured with this effect in mind, but most have been available for many years. Some drugs produce milk as a secondary effect only in the occasional user. Digitalis is one of these. Other drugs will have this effect on a fairly consistent basis. These drugs work by increasing the amount of prolactin (the hormone that stimulates milk production by the milk cells of the breast) produced by the mother's pituitary gland. They do this by inhibiting the secretion of dopamine by the mother's hypothalamus. Dopamine inhibits the release of prolactin. These will be discussed below.

Major tranquilizers

This group of drugs was first introduced in the early 1950s as a treatment for schizophrenia, and is still being used for this reason. The group includes chlorpromazine (Largactil, Thorazine), haloperidol (Haldol), and prochlorperazine (Compazine, Stemetil). The latter is used mainly as a treatment for nausea and vomiting, another effect of this group.

This group of drugs does increase the milk supply fairly consistently, but because of the possible side effects on the mother, is rarely used for this reason anymore. Side effects that occur fairly regularly are sedation and fatigue. Others, including neurological symptoms such as tremor and uncontrollable movements of the eyes and limbs, occur less frequently, but are quite distressing, though rarely permanent. Usually the symptoms disappear with discontinuation of the drug, but the risks are too great for the mother to use these drugs to increase milk supply.

Methyldopa

Methyldopa (Aldomet) is a drug frequently used to treat high blood pressure. It also interferes with secretion of dopamine and therefore results in increased prolactin secretion. Its effect on milk supply, however, is not great enough to justify its use for this reason in women who are not also hypertensive.

Sulpiride

This drug is not available in Canada or the United States. Used as an antipsychotic, it inhibits the secretion of dopamine and has been shown to increase milk production. It has side effects similar to those of the major tranquilizers, however, and is probably best not used to increase milk supply.

Metoclopramide

This drug (Reglan, Maxeran) has been used to increase milk supply—and quite successfully. I don't use it anymore because of the side effects on the mother, and because I find domperidone (see next) far more helpful.

Domperidone

Domperidone (Motilium) has been very helpful in increasing milk supply for many breastfeeding mothers. It is readily available in most countries; in the United States it must usually be made up by a "compounding pharmacy." Almost every U.S. city has at least one compounding pharmacy.

Domperidone is generally used for disorders of the gastrointestinal tract (gut) and has not been released in Canada, or any other country, as far as I know, for use as a stimulant for milk production. This does not mean that it cannot be prescribed for this reason, but, rather, that the manufacturer does not back its use for increasing milk production. It has been used, for several years, in small infants who spit up and lose weight.

Domperidone's ability to increase milk production has been recognized since it first became available. Another related, but older, medication, metoclopramide (Maxeran), is also known to increase milk production, but it has frequent side effects that make its use for many nursing mothers unacceptable (fatigue, irritability, depression). Domperidone has fewer side effects because it does not enter the brain tissue (pass the blood-brain barrier) in significant amounts.

When is it appropriate to use domperidone?

Domperidone must never be used as the first approach to correcting breastfeeding difficulties. It must not be used unless all other factors that may result in insufficient milk supply have been dealt with first. These include the following:

- correcting the baby's latch so that the baby can obtain as efficiently as possible the milk that the mother has available. Correcting the latch may be all that is necessary to change a situation of "not enough milk" to one of "plenty of milk."
- using breast compression to increase the intake of milk
- using milk expression after feedings to increase the supply
- correcting sucking problems, stopping the use of artificial nipples and other stratagems.

Domperidone works particularly well to increase milk production under the following circumstances:

- when a mother who is pumping milk for a sick or premature baby in the hospital has a decrease in the amount she pumps around four or five weeks after the baby is born. The reasons for this are probably many, but domperidone generally brings the amount of milk pumped back to where it was, or even to higher levels.
- when a mother has a decrease in milk supply, often associated with the use of birth control pills (mothers should avoid estrogen-containing birth control pills while breastfeeding), or on occasion for no obvious reason when the baby is three or four months old, domperidone will often bring the supply back to normal.

- when the mother has had her milk decrease because of "emotional stress." Some will dispute that this can occur, but it occasionally does.

Domperidone still works, but often less dramatically, under these circumstances:

- when the mother is pumping for a sick or premature baby but has not managed to develop a full milk supply
- when the mother is trying to develop a full milk supply while nursing an adopted baby
- when the mother is trying to wean the baby from supplements.

Domperidone seems to work better when the mother is more than six weeks past the birth of the baby, but is sometimes helpful as early as two or three weeks after the baby arrives.

Are there side effects to using domperidone?

As with all medications, side effects are possible, and many have been reported with domperidone (textbooks often list any side effect ever reported, but symptoms reported are not necessarily due to the drug a person is taking). There is no such thing as a 100 percent safe drug. However, our clinical experience has been that side effects in the mother are extremely uncommon, except for increasing milk supply. Some side effects reported (very uncommonly) by mothers we have treated are the following:

- dry mouth
- headache, which disappeared when the dose was reduced
- abdominal cramps.

The amount that gets into the milk is so tiny that side effects in the baby should not be expected. Mothers have not reported any to us, in many years of use. Certainly the amount the baby gets through the milk is a tiny percentage of what babies would get if being treated for spitting up.

Are there concerns about the long-term use of domperidone?

The manufacturer states in its literature that chronic treatment with domperidone in rodents has resulted in increased numbers of breast tumors. The literature goes on to state that this has never been documented in humans. Note that toxicity studies of medication usually require treatment with huge doses over periods of time involving most or all of the animal's lifetime. Note also that *not* breastfeeding increases the risk of breast cancer, and breast cancer risk decreases the longer you breastfeed.

How much do I take?

Generally, we start domperidone at 20 mg (two 10-mg tablets) four times a day. Printouts from the pharmacy often suggest taking domperidone 30 minutes before eating, but that is because of its use for digestive intolerance. The mother can take the domperidone about every six hours, when it is convenient (there is no need to wake up to keep to a six-hour schedule—it does not make any difference). Most mothers take the domperidone for three to eight weeks. Mothers who are nursing adopted babies may have to take the drug much longer.

After starting domperidone, you may not notice an effect for three or four days, though some mothers do so within 24 hours. It appears to take two to three weeks to get a maximum effect.

After two or three weeks on the domperi-done, the mother may or may not have noticed the desired effect. If not, she should continue the domperidone for another two or three weeks. If there has been no effect after that time, she should stop the domperidone. If the milk supply has increased as desired, the mother should slowly decrease the amount of domperidone she takes. Thus, if the result has been very good while taking 20 mg four times a day, the mother should decrease the dose to 20 mg three times a day for a week or so. If there has been no decrease in the milk supply (the usual situation), the mother can continue decreasing the amount of domperidone by a pill at a time, staying on the reduced dose for four or five days before dropping another pill. If the mother gets down to no medication, great. However, if the milk supply decreases at a certain point, the mother should up the dose of domperidone to the previous effective dose and stay there for a couple of weeks. Then she should try again to decrease the dose. Often the attempt will work the second time, or the third time, when it didn't work the first. Some mothers find they need to be on the domperidone for several months, particularly if they are using it to maintain the milk supply for an adopted baby.

Other Reasons for Low Milk Supply

Herbs

It is said that sage and parsley decrease the milk supply. I don't know anything about this. I have also heard that borage decreases the supply, but if you go back to the section on herbs to increase supply, you will see that borage is mentioned there as well. Borage does seem to decrease engorgement.

Drugs

Estrogens definitely can decrease the milk supply. They are most likely to be taken by nursing mothers as one of the ingredients in the birth control pill. Oral estrogens should be avoided by nursing mothers whenever possible. Locally applied estrogens should not be a problem, under normal circumstances. There is rarely a need, in any case, for a nursing mother to take estrogens. If the mother really does require the birth control pill for contraception, progesterone-only pills are available.

However, the pill is not the only method of "child spacing" available to nursing mothers. In fact, breastfeeding is a good method of child spacing. Under the following circumstances, the chances of a breastfeeding mother becoming pregnant are about 2 percent (compared to a pregnancy rate of 1 percent with the birth control pill):

- the baby is breastfeeding exclusively, or virtually exclusively
- the baby is younger than six months of age
- the mother has not had a normal menstrual period (bleeding during the first eight to twelve weeks does not really count)

After the baby is six months of age, or if he is taking other foods in addition to breastfeeding, then the protection against pregnancy afforded by breastfeeding becomes less, but still not negligible. On average, a mother who breastfeeds into at least the second year of her baby's life, and does not use any form of artificial birth control, will have a baby about every 24 to 30 months. If the mother wants to be surer, there are barrier methods of birth control, the IUD, and others. The pill is not for everyone, and sometimes other methods are definitely preferred by couples.

Some physicians will say that after six or eight weeks, or even four months, there is no concern that the milk supply will decrease with the estrogens, but this is not true. It is always a risk, and not a negligible one. It is true that not *all* mothers seem to have a decrease, but a significant number do. The effect of the birth control pill is unpredictable. We have had mothers take the same pill starting at the same time, without problems in milk supply for one or two babies, but with a significant decrease for subsequent babies.

Progesterones are not supposed to decrease the milk supply. Indeed, it has been said, without too much proof, that they may increase the supply. However, there are some anecdotal reports of progesterones decreasing the supply. One relatively new method of birth control, long-acting injected medroxyprogesterone (Depo-Provera) is being used more and more. Even though the company that makes it states that it should only be given to breastfeeding mothers six weeks or more after the birth, many mothers are getting the injection within a day or two of the birth. This may cause a significant decrease in milk supply.

Research in Australia has suggested that the drop in progesterone that occurs with the birth of the placenta is what sensitizes the milk-producing cells of the breast to the action of prolactin. If the progesterone does not drop, the breasts do not produce milk. This may be the reason why a mother who has a piece of placenta remaining in her uterus does not get the increase in milk supply that is generally seen three or four days after birth. This may also explain why some women who got the injection of progesterone immediately after the birth of the baby did not produce enough milk. This is anecdotal, and may not be true, but it is best to avoid the injection in the mother just after she gives birth. Indeed, I would suggest that if a mother is considering using progesterones for birth control, she should first try a month of the progesterone-only pill, so that if there is a decrease in the milk supply, she can stop the pill. If there appears to be no negative effect from the pill, the mother can then get the injection. The injection, once given, cannot be turned off, and the effect lasts at least three months.

Some drugs used to induce fertility in women may decrease the milk supply. Clomiphene (Clomid) is one such medication. It probably decreases the milk supply by stimulating the production of estrogens in the mother. The drug is not contraindicated for a breastfeeding mother, as many gynecologists claim, but the fact that the milk supply may be significantly depressed needs to be taken into account.

Another such drug is bromocriptine (Parlodel). Some women produce too much prolactin, due to a small tumor in the pituitary, and the increased amount of prolactin interferes with their ability to become pregnant. Some of these women also produce milk because of the high prolactin levels. However, some mothers who have been treated for this condition, once they become pregnant and give birth, seem *not* to produce enough milk. Perhaps the long-term use of bromocriptine has interfered with their ability to produce milk. This does not occur with all mothers who are on long-term bromocriptine. Bromocriptine will also interfere with breastfeeding if used while the mother is breastfeeding. But there does not appear to be any need to use bromocriptine during lactation, since the main reason for using it is to decrease prolactin secretion, unnecessary if the mother is breastfeeding. There is no evidence that bromocriptine slows the growth of the pituitary tumor, which, in any case, is generally tiny and does not grow enough to cause problems other than infertility. On rare occasions, the tumor does grow and may need surgical treatment.

There is no evidence, however, that breastfeeding increases the size of the tumor.

Breast Surgery

Some women experience decreased milk supply as a result of surgical procedures on the breast. The most common of these is breast reduction surgery, but any surgery performed with an incision around the areola risks decreasing the milk supply significantly. Nevertheless, some women who have had breast reduction surgery have managed to breastfeed exclusively without problems.

Breast augmentation surgery is usually done with the incision near the woman's chest wall, and when done this way, does not interfere with milk production. However, some surgeons, for reasons I cannot understand, will do the breast augmentation by making the incisions around the areolas. And some surgeons, for something as minor as a breast biopsy, will do an incision around the areola. The argument, I suppose, is that the "aesthetic result" is better. That's debatable, but the bigger concern is that this type of incision might considerably decrease the amount of milk the mother produces on the side where the surgery is done. It is a mark of how breasts are perceived in our society that a surgeon would sacrifice the function of a part of the body for the "aesthetic result." Imagine a plastic surgeon doing surgery on a nose to make it "look better," but leaving the patient unable to breathe. No surgeon would ever deliberately aim for such a result—except when the breast is the part being operated on.

The same can be said in many situations where a mother wants to have breasts of the same size, where one breast is much smaller than the other. In many cases, instead of augmenting the smaller breast—the breast that is not likely to produce enough because it hasn't developed properly—the surgeon does a reduction on the larger breast, and thus destroys the function of the breast which probably *would* have produced plenty of milk.

Radiation to the breast for the treatment of cancer is likely to decrease the milk supply—even to turn it off completely because the milk-producing cells are killed by the radiation. But this happens only if the breast is irradiated directly. Irradiation to the abdomen, for example, should not interfere with lactation.

Retained Placenta

An uncommon cause of a decreased milk supply is the retention in the womb of fragments of placenta. Because these fragments produce hormones, including estrogens and progesterone, breastmilk production may be very low. The mother who has a retained placental fragment will have longer than expected bleeding and cramping, or may have a return of cramping and bleeding later. There are blood tests (measuring human chorionic gonadotropin) and ultrasound examinations that can make the diagnosis. The treatment is to remove the fragments, and if removal has not been delayed too long, the milk supply will usually rise fairly dramatically.

Are some women truly incapable of producing enough milk?

There is no doubt that some women are unable to produce enough milk, just as some people do not produce enough insulin or thyroid hormone. But this does not mean these mothers cannot, or should not, breastfeed. Many mothers have breastfed their babies for two or more years, using a nursing supplementer (lactation aid). Though breastmilk is important, there is more to breastfeeding than breastmilk. Besides, "not enough milk" does not mean "no milk," and the baby will continue to get breastmilk as long as

the mother is putting him to the breast. I cannot fathom, really, the idea that "if I can't breastfeed exclusively, I might as well not breastfeed at all." Some breastmilk is better than none.

Supplementing the Baby Who Needs More Milk

Sometimes the baby does need supplements. I would like to emphasize, however, that supplements are being given far too often, and quite unnecessarily, as infant formula, rather than expressed milk or sugar water. Most babies do not need formula in the first 24 or 48 hours of life. They can manage with small amounts of colostrum, perhaps with a little sugar water added in some cases. Nevertheless, if supplements are truly necessary, we now have methods of supplementing the baby without using an artificial nipple.

Is there such a thing as nipple confusion? In fact, we don't need to use artificial nipples to supplement breastfed babies, but let us consider the question anyway.

The term *nipple confusion* (or *nipple preference*) is used to describe a situation in which a breastfed baby has been fed with a bottle (or given a pacifier) and then tries to nurse at the breast using the same sucking technique he used when sucking on the bottle.

Nipple confusion is not an all-or-nothing situation. As mentioned earlier, the basis of successful breastfeeding is a good latch. If the mother has a bountiful supply, the latch does not have to be great for the baby to do well. If the mother's supply is just abundant enough, the baby really must have a good latch in order to do well.

Babies are not complicated. They want milk. If they go to the breast and get lots to drink, and then get lots to drink from a bottle, they will usually do both breast and bottle. But if the baby goes to the breast and gets only a little, and then goes to a bottle and gets lots, it is obvious that sooner or later the baby will catch on. If he is not too hungry he may still take the breast, but if he is ravenous he may refuse the breast. Indeed, some babies refuse the breast without ever having had an artificial nipple—if they do not get good flow from the breast.

For a baby to get milk from a bottle, he does not have to open his mouth particularly wide. So if the baby has had some experience with bottles, he may open his mouth only a little when he goes to the breast. He may continue taking the breast, but he won't get milk quite as well. If the baby latches less well than he could, he depends more on the rapid flow of milk (caused by the "letdown" or milk ejection reflex) than on actually extracting milk from the breast. When the flow slows, he no longer drinks. Because the baby suckles less well, sooner or later the milk supply will decrease, and the baby will stop nursing earlier and earlier. Furthermore, the early use of bottles can lead to sore nipples, because the baby tends not to open his mouth as well when he comes to the breast and as a result sucks on the nipple.

It is interesting that some of the loudest mockers of "nipple confusion" are often the same people who encourage the mother to start bottles early, saying that otherwise "the baby will never take one." And it is sometimes true that a baby who is breastfeeding only will refuse to take a bottle or pacifier. This may occur as early as a few weeks of age, or only after three or four months of age. It may also occur even if the baby is getting regular bottles from early on. Suddenly a baby who has been taking both will stop taking the bottle when he is three or four months old. Or, unfortunately, a baby who was taking both breast and bottle stops taking the breast. It is also obvious that some babies who seem to be doing both breast and bottle are *not*. In fact, they "pacify" on the breast—getting virtually no milk—but actually feed from the bottle.

One example: Lise is breastfeeding her five-week-old baby and is doing fine, as is the baby who is gaining weight very well. The mother has no problems with nipple soreness or milk supply. She is prescribed metronidazole (Flagyl) for a problem unrelated to breastfeeding and is *incorrectly* told she must stop breastfeeding during the 10 days she is on it. The mother takes the baby off the breast; she maintains her milk supply very well with pumping. After a week, she finds out that she did not have to take the baby off the breast. But all efforts to put the baby back to the breast fail. How do we explain this phenomenon? Is it low milk supply? No, because the baby was able to grow subsequently on expressed milk (with no formula) at a tremendous rate. I believe the conclusion is obvious.

Nipple confusion is not a black-and-white issue. The use of artificial nipples may cause no problems for some babies, tremendous problems for others, and everything in between. Since it is rarely necessary to use bottles to feed babies (more on this later) even if they need supplementation, and since it is not always possible to know which baby will be affected, we should do everything to avoid the use of bottles until breastfeeding is well established. And that certainly means no bottles in the first few days. Each baby is different. Each baby is an individual, and a mother who "fed her others both breast and bottle, and the babies did well" may not do as well with a new baby.

Supplementing Without Bottles

There are several methods of supplementing that do not require the baby to receive an artificial nipple. The best is what I call a "lactation aid," or others call a "nursing supplementer." This device is best because

- babies learn to breastfeed by breastfeeding.
- mothers learn to breastfeed by breastfeeding.
- the baby continues to get milk from the mother's breast even while being supplemented, thereby increasing her milk supply.
- the baby will not reject the breast.
- there is more to breastfeeding than milk alone.

The Lactation Aid

This device can be made up from hospital materials—an ordinary feeding bottle with the nipple hole enlarged with scissors so that a 5 French, 91-cm (36-inch) feeding tube can pass through the hole—or it can be bought ready made. In most cases, especially in the first day or so, there is no need to buy the manufactured device; the supplement may be required for only a few feedings.

To prepare to use your homemade lactation aid, you put the supplement in the feeding bottle, screw the rubber nipple onto the bottle, and stick one end of the tube through the enlarged hole that you have made in the nipple. Push the tube in so that it is at the bottom of the bottle, but not bent. Set the bottle on a table close to where you are feeding the baby, or have someone else hold it or put it in a shirt pocket. The other end of the tube should lie alongside the mother's nipple and go into the baby's mouth when he begins to suck. You can first latch the baby onto the breast, then slide the tube into the corner of the baby's mouth. The baby's suction will make the milk flow.

Generally, a lactation aid is used as follows:

- *The baby must be latched on as well as possible.* Of course, not all babies latch on perfectly in the first few days, but using a lactation aid to supplement before fixing the latch is unwise. This is key. In the first place, the better the baby latches on, the less likely it is that the supplement will actually be necessary.

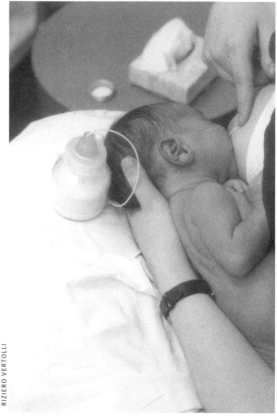

RIZIERO VERTOLLI

Using a lactation aid. The mother's hand position is not as we usually teach it, but since the baby is being supported on the pillow, this is fine.

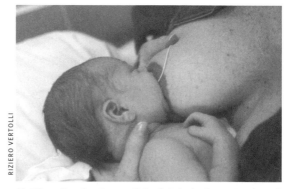

RIZIERO VERTOLLI

Getting the best possible latch is important and should be done *before* introducing supplements. The better the latch, the less likely the need for a lactation aid. The better the latch, the easier it is to use. The better the latch, the faster the mother and baby will be able to do without it.

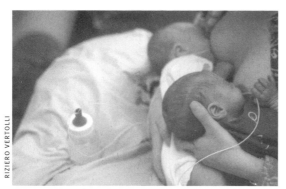

RIZIERO VERTOLLI

Twins using a lactation aid. One is in the football hold and the other in the cradle hold.

Second, the better the baby latches on, the easier the lactation aid is to use. Third, the better the baby latches on, the shorter the time the device will be necessary.

• *The mother must be able to tell whether the baby is getting milk.* This is easy to recognize once you've seen it, but difficult to describe. A baby who is getting milk in substantial quantities demonstrates a very definite *pause* in the movement of his chin as he opens his mouth to the maximum while he is sucking. The baby opens his mouth and, as the "opening" phase of the suck comes to an end and he has opened wide (to the maximum opening), there is a delay, or a pause, just before he closes his mouth again. That pause tells you that the baby just got a mouthful of milk. The longer the pause, the more milk he got; the shorter the pause, the less—but if there is definitely a pause there, the baby got a significant amount of milk. This pause can be seen on the first day of life if the baby is latched on well. You will see the pause when your milk supply is more abundant than on the first day or so, even without a good latch. But if you see it on day one, the baby must be latched on well, or else you have quite a lot of colostrum. This pause, when you see it, is your guarantee that the baby just got milk. You don't have to hear the baby swallow, unlikely in any case during the first days. Also, I mistrust going on "hearing the baby swallow," though, like the pause, once you hear it you know what it is. The trouble is that babies can make all sorts of noises while on the breast that can be mistaken for swallowing. The pause is more reliable.

If you are having trouble recognizing when the baby is swallowing milk, try this: Get yourself a straw and a glass of water. Put one hand under your chin and begin to drink the water through the straw. As you draw the water through the straw and into your mouth, you will notice that your chin drops and stays down as long as you are filling your mouth with water. When you stop, your chin comes back up. This is what you are looking for when the baby is at the breast—an open-mouthed pause that means the baby is getting a mouthful of milk. The longer the pause, the more the baby got. The length of time the baby is at the breast is not important—a baby who sucks this way, with pauses, for twenty minutes will probably not take the second breast. The baby who just nibbles at the breast—making quick, fluttery sucks with no pauses—will still be hungry after an hour. So rules like "feed the baby for twenty minutes on each breast" make no sense.

• *The lactation aid should be introduced only after the baby has nursed on both sides.* A baby who is reasonably latched on should not have the tube introduced immediately. The mother should feed the baby on the first side until the baby does not appear to be drinking anymore (no more pauses, even when she uses breast compression). Then she should change sides and feed the baby some more, until the baby no longer drinks. If she wishes, she can offer the first side again—or even go back and forth a few times—but she should feed at least both sides before offering the supplement with the tube. The supplement is then given, and the baby takes what he wants. As things improve, the mother will be introducing the tube later and later in the feeding, until, eventually the baby actually refuses the supplement.

Cup-Feeding

Cup-feeding has been around for thousands of years. In fact, cups for feeding infants have even been found in ancient Egyptian tombs. Around the world, women feed their babies water (unnecessarily) using the oldest cup around: the human hand. It works just fine. I have seen a mother give her one-day-old baby water with the cup of her hand, and the baby drank it quite nicely. Giving water to young babies is, in fact, not a good idea, especially in those parts of the world where it is most common, because the water supply is often unsafe, and breastmilk is far superior to slake a baby's thirst. Well-designed studies have shown that even in the hottest of climates, enough breastmilk also means enough water—breastmilk is approximately 90 percent water.

Cup-feeding should not, in general, be used when the baby is latching on to the breast and needs a supplement. It should be used only if the baby is *not* latching on, or when the mother must be separated from the baby. If the mother is present, the baby is latching on, and a supplement is truly necessary, it should be given with the lactation aid. As mentioned earlier, babies learn to breastfeed by breastfeeding; babies do not learn to breastfeed by cup-feeding, finger-feeding, or any other feeding. Babies can learn to bring their tongues forward by cup feeding; they can be stimulated to suck in a manner similar to what they

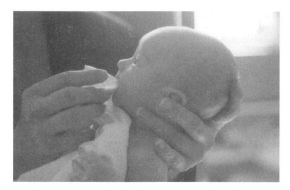

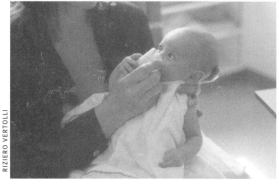

RIZIERO VERTOLLI

Cup-feeding a baby under one month of age. Note that the mother is not pouring the milk down his throat, but rather tipping the cup until the baby tastes the milk. The baby then laps the milk up with his tongue.

would normally do on the breast with finger-feeding; but babies learn to breastfeed by breastfeeding. Strange as it may seem, there are many who don't understand this. There is only one way to learn how to ride a bicycle, and that is to get on it and keep trying until it works. You can't learn by reading about it, or even practicing on an exercise bicycle, though both might be helpful.

The cup is a good way of feeding the baby when the mother is separated from her baby, for whatever reason. It does not seem to interfere with breastfeeding as much as a bottle does, and it is faster than finger-feeding. The technique can be used if the lactation aid does not work, as is sometimes the case. It is also simple to learn and safe to do.

An open cup, such as a 30-ml (1-oz) medicine

cup, should be used, though manufactured cups specifically designed for cup-feeding premature babies and very young babies have started to show up on the market. Parents at home can use a shot glass or any other small cup. The "sippy cups" and similar cups with lids often used with toddlers don't work well, because the baby will pucker up his lips to drink, just as he does with a bottle.

To feed the baby, sit him up on your lap with his head and back supported. Bring the cup, filled with whatever liquid is to be given (expressed breastmilk is, of course, the best supplement in all but extraordinary cases) to the baby's lips. Press the rim of the cup lightly on the baby's lower gum margin, then tilt the cup until the baby receives a little milk on his tongue or in his mouth. When the baby tastes that little bit of milk, he will start, usually, to stick out his tongue and try to lap up the milk. It is an amazing thing to watch, especially for those of us who were taught that babies cannot really start drinking from a cup until they are six months of age or older. Usually the baby drinks very quickly. Indeed, a baby, even a premature baby, can often cup-feed much faster than he can drink from a bottle.

Is cup-feeding safe? Is it stressful for babies?
A 1999 study by Cynthia Howard and other researchers, as reported in *Pediatrics* (Vol. 104 #5) looked at breastfeeding, bottle-feeding and cup-feeding and how infants responded. They monitored the heart rates, levels of oxygen, and breathing rates in the babies when they were fed in these three different ways. They also measured how long it took for the baby to complete a feeding.

They found that breastfeeding took longer than the other two methods, but the babies had higher oxygen levels, and better heart rates and breathing rates when breastfeeding than when fed by either of the other two methods. It took the same amount of time to feed the baby by cup as by bottle, and the heart rates, breathing rates, and oxygen levels were the same in the cup-fed and bottle-fed babies.

Finger-Feeding

Finger-feeding is a technique that can be quite useful and helpful for the mother having difficulties latching a baby onto her breast. As with all techniques, however, it can be used in situations that are inappropriate, and the technique itself can be done incorrectly. It will not work as well, and can even be harmful, if done for the wrong reasons or in the wrong way. Some have condemned the use of finger-feeding, usually for no specific reason, and often without having tried the technique or tried it properly. I think finger-feeding definitely has its uses.

To finger-feed, you need the same equipment you would need for a lactation aid. However, you would use finger-feeding rather than the tube at the breast in cases where the baby is refusing the breast or not latching on.

The reasons for finger-feeding in these situations are as follows:

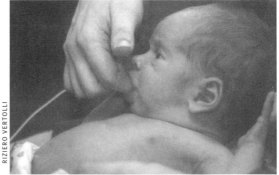

RIZIERO VERTOLLI

Finger-feeding. The finger should not be pointed up to the roof of the baby's mouth but should be flat, keeping the tongue flat and forward. The further the mother's (father's) finger is in the baby's mouth, the better.

- To calm the angry baby who is refusing the breast
- To encourage him to suck in a fashion similar to that he should use at the breast, and thus help him to latch on to the breast
- To wake up a sleepy baby, particularly in the first few days of life when some babies sleep for long periods—especially if the sleepiness is due to poor feeding

The larger the finger used the better, to encourage the baby to open his mouth wide. From the point of view of size and convenience, the index finger is the one I find the best. Some lactation consultants use their thumb, which I find difficult. I believe the baby finger, which is often taught, is probably the worst of choices. Not only is it awkward, but it doesn't encourage the baby to open his mouth wide.

The tube of the lactation aid can be held between the thumb and the middle finger at about the position of the first joint in the finger closest to the knuckle. If the person doing the finger-feeding holds the tube like this, the tube will lie along her index finger so that no tape is necessary to keep the tube in position. The baby can be held in any comfortable position, but I prefer holding the baby facing me, my left hand (since I use my right-hand index finger to finger-feed) supporting the back of the baby's shoulders and neck. This allows me to keep my finger flat (not pointed upward to the roof of the baby's mouth), so as to keep the baby's tongue forward and flat—which is what we want. The finger-feeding finger should also be as far into the baby's mouth as possible. (Most babies do not mind the finger quite far into their mouths.) The baby will start sucking when he feels the finger in his mouth, and if he sucks effectively, the supplement to be fed will be drawn up into the tube and into the baby's mouth. At

first some babies suck in a very ineffective manner, but once they start to get fluid, they start to suck in a manner much more similar to breast-feeding. That is, they will wrap their tongues around your finger, and you will feel a tugging toward the baby's throat. Once the baby "gets" this, the feeding goes much more quickly. The idea is not to feed the baby, however, but to prepare the baby to take the breast. Thus, once the baby is calm and sucking well, the finger-feeding should be stopped, and the baby should be tried on the breast. It rarely takes more than a minute or two for the baby to suck well on the finger and be ready to try the breast.

Unfortunately, finger-feeding is often used incorrectly. Since the idea is to get the baby to the breast, finger-feeding should not be done *after* many minutes or longer of unsuccessful attempts on the breast, but rather before everyone is fed up and tired. It takes only a few minutes to know the baby is not going to take the breast, so efforts should be stopped and the baby finger-fed. Once finger-feeding has calmed the baby and improved his sucking technique, there is a better chance of getting him to take the breast. If not, efforts should be halted temporarily for another minute or two of finger-feeding, and then the baby brought back to the breast.

If the baby does not take the breast at that feeding, the whole feeding may be done as finger-feeding. This is fairly easy during the first few days because the baby does not need very much. The main disadvantage of finger-feeding is that it may be quite slow, so that as the baby gets older, finger-feeding may take longer and longer. However, some babies finger-feed as quickly as they would feed with any other method.

As with all methods that feed babies away from the breast, finger-feeding can teach the baby to prefer the finger to the breast—which is a good reason not to supplement this way. But the preference seems to develop slowly, at least partly because finger-feeding does not provide the rapid flow that comes from a bottle.

Other Methods

Spoon-feeding is a very old method (probably as old as spoons) and an easy method, used by mothers around the world. I find no advantage to spoon-feeding or syringe-feeding over the methods mentioned above. Mothers often like it because it requires no special equipment—everyone has spoons—and it can be used in an emergency situation. For example, when one mother had to rush to the hospital because her older child had been injured, her friend was able to spoon-feed the baby expressed breastmilk and keep the baby content until Mom returned five hours later. Of course, it would have been better if the mother had taken her baby with her to the emergency department. A breastfeeding baby can go with his mother anywhere, anytime.

Some mothers have also used sterile syringes (with no needle, of course) to supplement their babies. They simply squirt a small amount of milk into the baby's mouth, wait for him to swallow, then squirt a little more into his mouth. A syringe can also be used while the baby is at the breast, but has no advantage over a lactation aid and is more difficult to manage.

The point is that there are many different ways to supplement your baby, even if you are temporarily separated, that do not involve using artificial nipples.

On the other hand, I believe that feeding a baby with a tube in his stomach (as is sometimes done with premature babies), when other methods will do, is unnecessarily risky and no improvement over other methods. Of course, if there is no option, this is a good technique and

usually preferable to intravenous feeding. However, for a full-term, healthy baby, a tube in his stomach to avoid bottles makes no sense.

If no other methods work, is it okay to use a bottle? Well, of course, but the bottle is at the bottom of the list of choices, in my opinion. It is rare for a bottle to work in feeding a baby when no other method will work. If a baby won't cup-feed or finger-feed, it is unlikely he will take a bottle and feed from it, either. About once a year I advise a mother to use a bottle because the other options are not working. But I see about 1,200 mothers with their babies every year, just for breastfeeding problems. And these babies are relatively old. In the first few days, it is rare to have to use a bottle, even for a baby with a cleft palate, for example, who, if he won't latch on, can drink very well from a cup.

Most health professionals who don't consider the alternatives to a bottle do so simply because they do not have experience with the other methods. Or, in some cases, unfortunately, because it may just seem easier to recommend going to bottle-feeding.

Of course, none of these methods is always easy to use. And of course, there are some mothers who have difficulty using a lactation aid, or finger-feeding or cup-feeding. But the more experience the helper has, the easier it becomes to instruct the mother correctly—especially when the mother should be able get help at most feedings, while she and the baby are still in the hospital.

Expressed Milk Is the Best Supplement

Sometimes babies do need to receive supplements. As noted above, this does not mean they need to receive bottles. But if the baby does need a supplement, which is the best supplement to give?

There is no doubt that the first choice, under

all but the most extraordinary circumstances, is the mother's own freshly expressed milk. Sometimes it is not easy to get the baby to latch on well right away, or even in the first few days, no matter how experienced the helper. If it is becoming urgent to feed the baby, the mother should be starting to express her milk for feeding her baby as soon as alternative feedings are being considered. Most of the time, when a baby is not getting enough milk, it is not because the milk is not there, but because the baby is not able to remove it from the breast. He may be able to get that milk more easily using other methods, though I believe there is often unseemly haste in starting alternative feedings. Remember that not long ago hospital policies dictated that babies were not to be fed at all for the first 24 hours of their lives.

Expression of milk using a pump may not always be the best policy during the first few days. Many mothers, properly instructed, can express more milk by hand—when there is only a little to express—than they can from even an industrial-grade electric pump. Often mothers feel that if they cannot express more than a few drops, they will not produce enough milk. This is false. A pump is not a well-latched-on vigorous baby; a baby suckling properly with a good latch can get more milk than a pump, especially in the first few days. Also, mothers pumping their milk in these circumstances often feel stressed and worried about their babies, something that can make it more difficult to get much milk by pumping.

So, the first choice for a supplement is the mother's own milk (colostrum in the first few days—and colostrum, despite having a different name, is still milk—just the first type of milk). If only a small quantity can be expressed in the first few days, it can be diluted in sugar water. In other words, colostrum diluted in sugar water

will be the second choice at least for the first 24 to 48 hours. Diluted colostrum, even a few drops of it, still has antibodies, white cells, and protein to help the baby fight infection and get some of the appropriate protein and fat he needs.

What if colostrum is not available at all? There are some mothers (who, by the way, almost always go on to produce tons of milk) who have difficulty expressing any colostrum at all, even a few drops.

The third choice is plain sugar water, which can be used for about 24 to 48 hours. The baby will remain well hydrated, will get some calories, and, if the sugar water is used properly, will, we hope, be breastfeeding by 24 hours of age. Some worry about babies becoming jaundiced because of the sugar water, but I don't see this as an issue. The proper management of breastfeeding will prevent the development of excessive jaundice caused by inadequate intake of calories.

The fourth choice—and it is only fourth because it is not easy to get in most regions—is banked breastmilk. Unfortunately, there are only nine breastmilk banks in the United States, and, at this time, only one in Canada. This really is unfortunate, because banked milk could be useful for many situations in which we now use formula.

Which brings us to the fifth choice, formula, which unfortunately is all too often used as a first choice. And it is used as a first choice because of "convenience" (no expressing necessary, no waiting, it's always available thanks to the "generosity" of the formula companies) and because too many health professionals do not realize that they are using it as a drug. As with all drugs, we must be careful. There are side effects associated with using formula (see Chapter 1, Why Breastfeeding Is Important). Some babies do not tolerate formulas, especially in the first few days. And, since formula is not necessary most of the time, we should not be using it unless there is no alternative.

Some have accused me of being "against formula." This is not true. I am no more against formula than I am against ampicillin, or any other drug, for that matter. A drug can be life-saving; a drug can be useful. But like so many drugs, formula is overused, used too early, and too often employed before alternatives have been explored.

When a health professional pushes (and this is frequently the correct word for what is done in North American maternity or postpartum units) formula on a breastfeeding baby and his mother, the parents are given a very clear message: This stuff is not only harmless (it is not), it is good medicine. Furthermore, the mother is told that she doesn't have enough milk. Mothers tend to be more emotional and vulnerable during the first few days after giving birth, and they are naturally concerned to be doing the best thing for this very new, very precious baby. The mother who is well informed about breastfeeding and who is commit-ted to succeeding may not be affected by this message, though even the strongest of the strong can be shaken. But not all breastfeeding mothers are strongly committed to breastfeeding. They are "trying it out." This is one reason formula companies fight each other tooth and nail to become exclusive providers for a hospital. The formula companies even pay huge amounts to the hospital for this privilege. They do it because they know it will pay off for them—most women will use the formula used in the hospital.

I am not saying that formula is never necessary. I am saying that it is only fifth choice. This does not mean that every other choice has to be tried and shown not to work before we try formula, but health professionals who are helping the mother with breastfeeding and taking care of the baby should at least consider the other options before jumping to formula. This, I guarantee you, is not being done in the majority of hospitals in North America or Europe. And unfortunately, more and more it is not being done in the rest of the world, either. Too many health professionals are happy to adopt the "western" approach.

Late-Onset Slow Weight Gain

Some babies gain well during the first two to four months, and then problems with weight gain seem to begin. There are several possible reasons for this.

Probably one of the most common goes back to a poor latch (as do so many breastfeeding problems). The baby has not really been nursing well from the beginning, but because the mother has a good milk supply, the baby gains weight well for a while. As mentioned earlier, babies do not have to latch on well to get lots of milk. They wait for the milk ejection reflex (letdown reflex) and then they drink and drink. Once the flow slows down, the baby tends to sleep at the breast, and when the next milk ejection reflex comes, the baby drinks again for a while.

The problem arises as the baby gets older and smarter. After four or five weeks of age, while some babies continue to be content to sleep at the breast when the flow slows down, most start to get impatient with the milk coming so slowly. The baby who is content to sleep at the breast may get several more letdown reflexes of milk pouring into his mouth and may do well as far as weight gain is concerned. As for the others, as the milk flow slows, they will pull at the breast, coming on and off the breast, obviously not content. Usually, if the mother switches sides, the baby will be content again for a period of time, only to repeat the pulling at the breast once the flow slows down. As time passes, the milk supply actually might decrease, since the baby drinks less and less from the breast. As they get older, these babies may pull off the breast and suck their hands rather than continue on the breast.

What can be done? Once again, the best treatment is prevention: getting the latch right in the beginning. However, the baby in this situation can often be kept on the breast longer using the breast compression technique. The mother should use this to keep the baby on the first side until he is obviously no longer drinking, or is pulling off. The mother should then switch sides. Indeed, she can switch back and forth for as long as she can keep the baby drinking (open mouth wide–pause–close mouth type of suck).

Some mothers also seem to have a real decrease in their milk supplies about three or four months after the baby is born. This is not the "growth spurt" that may occur around that time, since the baby may actually lose weight, or not gain weight, something that does not occur with a growth spurt. It is obvious that the baby is getting less, as he pulls at the breast in frustration, coming on and off the breast and always wanting to drink more, but obviously not getting it. Sometimes this drop in milk supply is due to the birth control pill, but sometimes there is no obvious reason.

If the mother's supply is down because she is on the birth control pill, she should stop the pill immediately. Domperidone often brings the milk supply back quickly.

There may be other things to consider, too. Has the baby recently been trained to sleep through the night? The baby may need those night feedings to get enough milk to keep up the milk supply. Has the mother started to stretch out the time between feedings in recent weeks, hoping to get the baby on a more predictable schedule, or because she's busier?

Some babies at this age are so easily distracted by any activity going on around them that they do not nurse well. Some babies won't nurse if there is even a TV or radio on in the same room. For these babies, it helps to find a quiet place for some relaxed feedings every day.

And finally, has the baby been getting bottles? Some babies who managed to switch between breast and bottle earlier on will now decide they prefer the bottle. While the mother may have had lots of milk in the beginning, as the baby continues to get at least part of his daily intake from bottles, her milk supply gradually decreases. On days when the baby seemed hungrier than usual, she probably gave extra bottles, rather than nursing more frequently to build up her milk supply. This causes a further decrease in milk production.

If the milk supply has dropped, for whatever reason, breast compression and switching back and forth from one breast to the other may help. But if it does not improve fairly quickly, I will usually prescribe domperidone for the mother. This almost always brings a rapid increase in the mother's supply and sets things right. After a two-week treatment, the mother can usually decrease the dose slowly (see page 75) until she is off the medication. Usually, the milk supply will remain good and not decrease as the mother goes off the domperidone.

The one thing not to do at this point, if the mother wants to continue breastfeeding, is start bottles, even of expressed milk. The baby will very quickly catch on. Some will continue "pacifying" at the breast, but most will soon reject the breast completely.

If the baby is more than four months old (though sometimes I have suggested this at three months), solids can be introduced. This will almost always result in an increase in weight gain, but some babies may still not be patient at the breast. Again, babies like the milk to flow quickly, and not all babies just like to suck at the breast if little milk is coming. They may be more patient if they are less hungry, so feeding them solids before putting them to the breast may help (see Chapter 15, Breastfeeding and Other Foods).

MOTHERS' STORIES

Below are a number of stories of mothers and babies who were brought to the clinic for help with breastfeeding. The names are not the mothers' real names and the baby was not always a boy, but will always be referred to as "he" since the mother is, obviously, always "she" and this avoids confusion. Their stories will not be the same as yours, but the general principles remain the same.

1. Fix the latch. The better the baby latches on, the more he will get of his mother's milk, no matter how little she produces.
2. Teach the mother how to know the baby is getting milk.
3. "Finish" one side (the baby does not drink much even with compression), then switch sides and repeat. In fact, as long as the baby gets reasonable amounts of milk, and her nipples are not sore, the mother can go back to side one after the baby does not drink on the second side, and back to the second side again.
4. Using fenugreek and blessed thistle may be helpful.
5. If the baby does not drink well, or weight gain does not occur, supplementation likely becomes necessary, best done by far with a lactation aid at the breast.
6. Work to do away with the supplementation. Encourage the mother, because it is not always easy to keep going, especially with pressure from all around.

SUSAN

This baby was brought to our clinic on his fourth day of life. The problem, according to his mother Susan, was that the baby would not latch on to the right breast. In reality, the baby was not taking the left breast, either; he only seemed to take the left breast. The mother had sore nipples, but like so many mothers, did not consider this a problem because "breastfeeding is supposed to hurt" at first. [*No, it is not! This is a common misconception that arises from the fact that women have been given such poor information and help for so long that the abnormal has come to be seen as the normal (see Chapter 6, Sore Nipples).*]

According to the mother, the baby was feeding about eight times a day, every three hours. He would spend 15 to 20 minutes on the left side. [*The baby seemed to be breastfeeding every three hours, but he was not. He was on the breast for 15 or 20 minutes, but he was not feeding. This case demonstrates the folly of depending on these rules. It is not how long or how often the baby goes to the breast, but how well he nurses when he is there. This point cannot be overemphasized.*]

The baby was calm after the feedings. [*Calm may not be a good sign in the first week. Indeed, babies who are not getting enough may be quite lethargic. A baby who drinks well and then sleeps is fine. A baby who does not drink and then sleeps is in trouble. This is the reason that mothers are told to wake their babies to feed, but a baby who gets nothing every three hours is no better off than the baby who drinks nothing every four hours.*]

The baby had, in the last 24 hours, two black bowel movements, and six wet—but only just moist—diapers. [*The information about the bowel movements was worrisome. The bowel movements should not still be black on the fourth day. The number of wet diapers was difficult to interpret, but certainly didn't seem to indicate the baby was getting lots of milk.*]

This was the first pregnancy for this 31-year-old mother, who is a physician. [*The fact that the mother is a physician didn't help her to know how to identify the problem or how to get her baby feeding. She thought the baby was simply refusing the right breast, when in fact the baby wasn't breastfeeding at all.*]

The pregnancy had been unremarkable, the labor had started spontaneously at 38 weeks, and lasted only four hours. Susan received no pain medication, and the baby was fine when he was born. He weighed 3.07 kg (6 lb 12 oz) at birth. He was not tried on the breast until a few hours after birth. [*This is precisely a few hours too late.*]

The hospital stay was about 24 hours, during which time the baby got some sugar water once by cup. [*Why was this baby given water? The mother was not sure. Was the nurse concerned about something? If so, the appropriate thing to have done was to fix the breastfeeding, not give water. The nurse may have felt she was being supportive of breastfeeding because she didn't use a bottle, but getting the baby latched on well would have been much more helpful. If the baby did truly need supplementation, then it should have been given by a lactation aid rather than a cup. Babies learn to breastfeed by breastfeeding.*

If the nurse used a cup because the baby wasn't latching on well, she should at least have attempted to get the baby nursing properly. According to the mother, the nurse didn't. And if the baby wasn't nursing well, but mother and baby had to be discharged from the hospital, the nurse should have referred the mother urgently to a breastfeeding clinic. The mother was not even told about the breastfeeding clinic by the hospital, but heard about it from a friend—even though the clinic is in the hospital where the baby was born!]

During the first visit to the clinic, the baby was moderately jaundiced. [*This jaundice is what I call not-enough-breastmilk jaundice. The baby was more jaundiced than average because he was not feeding well. See Chaper 8, Jaundice.*]

His weight was 2.64 kg (5 lb 13 oz). [*This represents a loss of 14 percent from his birthweight. Is this a reason to supplement? The scale, of course, is different, so we are not sure of the actual amount of weight lost. It might even be more. This is not a reason to panic, or even necessarily to supplement. If the baby can start getting milk, the weight loss will quickly be made up. If we do find we need to supplement, expressed milk is preferable to formula.*]

The rest of the physical examination showed no abnormalities. The baby did not latch on to the left side, but only appeared to latch on. It was easy to pull him off the breast even though he was sucking and awake. A hungry baby who is latched on will not slip off the breast easily.

I helped Susan latch him on properly, and the baby took both sides. He drank very well (open mouth wide–pause–close mouth type of sucking for several minutes) on both sides. Susan had less pain with the feeding, but still had significant pain. I taught her how to latch the baby on. She was able to duplicate that. I then suggested she nurse the baby on the first side until he no longer drank (open mouth wide–pause–close mouth type of suck) and then use breast compression to help him continue drinking. Once the baby no longer drinks, the mother should change sides and repeat the process. The baby nursed quite well. The mother realized that the baby had never really breastfed before—in other words, had never actually drank milk at the breast. He was "pretending" to breastfeed on the left side, and couldn't even bother pretending on the right. [*This is probably the most common reason why babies become dehydrated. While it is often described on TV or in newspapers as "dehydration in breastfed babies," that is inaccurate. If the baby had been breastfeeding, he would not have become dehydrated. The problem is that the baby is not feeding at all. The baby may appear to be taking the breast, but he isn't. He doesn't get the milk, gradually becomes sleepier and weaker, and drinks even less at the next feeding. It quickly becomes a vicious cycle.*]

I could not follow the baby up the next day, but offered the mother follow-up with one of our lactation consultants. I did arrange to see the baby on Monday, four days after the initial visit. I phoned the mother the next day and left a message that if the baby was not drinking to get back to me.

At the second visit, the baby was latching on to both sides and drinking very well. The mother still had some soreness, but was improving. The baby's weight was 2.8 kg (6 lb 3 oz). [*This represents an increase of 160 grams—almost 6 ounces—in four days. Again, the scale was different from the first visit. More important, though, was that the way the baby nursed showed he was getting lots of milk.*] He was obviously less jaundiced. [*This improvement is good evidence that the cause of the jaundice was insufficient intake. Many physicians would have told the mother to stop breastfeeding and give the baby formula. Because the baby would have gotten food for the first time in his life—just as he did once he was latched on well at the breast—the bilirubin would have dropped, and the doctor would have been convinced that the problem had been the breastmilk. No, the problem was that the baby was not breastfeeding. Fix that, and the jaundice will improve as well.*]

His bowel movements were now yellow, and he was having many every day, some quite large. He was also urinating much more than before. [*These changes support the observation that the baby is feeding well.*]

At our last visit, the baby was only five weeks old, but he has continued to do well and to gain well on the breast only.

Here, then, is a case of disaster averted. One more day before the mother came to the clinic,

perhaps, and the baby could have become so sleepy from dehydration that a different approach might have had to be taken. It might not have been possible to wake the baby up easily to latch him on properly. I would probably, in that circumstance, have gotten the mother expressing her milk (which was obviously sufficient), and finger-feeding the baby. Once the baby started waking up (maybe the first feeding with finger-feeding, or maybe in a feeding or two), we would work on latching him on. The first rule in these situations is "feed the baby." Getting the baby fed fixes the problem.

Unfortunately, the only approach in too many physicians' repertoires is "supplement with formula." This may be necessary, but nobody can tell without first observing the breastfeeding. And it is quite often possible, especially with a very young baby, to just get him latched on well. The mother and baby will never look back.

Incidentally, this whole problem was a near tragedy that could easily have been prevented on that first day in hospital. Note that the baby's getting water did not fix anything at all. If someone knowledgeable and experienced with helping mothers with breastfeeding had spent just a little time helping the mother with the latching, we would have had one more mother wondering, "How can anyone have problems with breastfeeding?" In this case, the mother and baby were lucky to find appropriate help quickly. Too many do not.

LINDA

Linda's baby was seen at our clinic at 14 days of age, referred by a lactation consultant. The problem was weight loss.

This was the first baby for Linda, age 29. Linda had some high blood pressure and high blood sugars during the pregnancy, but since there had been no special treatment for either of these, presumably they were not serious problems. The labor was at term (39 weeks), and the baby was born after seven hours of labor. The baby weighed 3.61 kg (7 lb 15 oz) and was fine.

The baby was tried at the breast within an hour of birth and apparently breastfed well. [*Note that I say "apparently." Later developments suggest that he was not, in fact, feeding well.*] Linda was with him 24 hours a day, and he was discharged on the second day of life. The baby was given sugar water by cup because he "wasn't urinating." [*My comments from Susan's story about giving water by cup apply here, as well. I guess the water made the baby urinate, but did that fix the real problem? Or prevent the weight loss later on?*]

At the first clinic visit, Linda said the baby was on the breast only. He fed six or seven times a day, one feeding being between midnight and six a.m. He would stay on the breast for an hour. He would frequently fall asleep on the breast, but cry when he was taken off. [*Babies tend to fall asleep at the breast when the flow of milk is slow, not necessarily because they have had enough to eat. This is particularly true in the first few weeks. Just because the baby falls asleep, that doesn't meant the baby has had enough or that the breast is empty. It means the flow of milk has slowed down—or never really got started.*]

According to Linda, her baby was having quite infrequent bowel movements (about every second or third day), and having only three soaked diapers in a day. [*These are definite signs of inadequate intake. The fact that the mother did not know that these signs meant her baby wasn't getting enough milk shows that either she was not taught very well about breastfeeding or that she did not take in the information.*]

On examination, the baby looked reasonably well, and no abnormalities were noted. His weight was 3.23 kg (7 lb 1.5 oz). This repre-

sented a decrease in the weight from birthweight of 380 grams (13.5 oz). [*Again, different scales, so we don't know exactly how much weight was actually lost.*]

The observation of the feeding showed that the baby really was taking the breast poorly. He was doing very little drinking (open mouth wide–pause–close mouth type of sucking). I showed the mother how to latch him on better, and how to use compression, and he breastfed very well.

One week later, Linda brought her baby back to the clinic and told me she thought things were better. [*This does not always mean that the baby is doing better. Sometimes mothers are not able to accurately assess how their babies are doing. But in this case, Linda was right.*] The baby's urine output had increased, and his bowel movements had become larger and more frequent about two days after the visit. [*Once the baby is breastfeeding better, it may take a couple of days before the baby has regular bowel movements.*] The weight, a week after the first visit, was 3.46 kg (7 lb 10 oz), an increase of almost nine ounces in a week. This weight gain was undoubtedly a real weight gain, clear from the drinking the baby was doing on the breast.

The mother was still breastfeeding exclusively when her baby was five months of age, and doing well. [*In most situations in which the baby is not gaining well, or has even lost weight, the problem is not that the mother doesn't produce enough milk—the baby is not getting the milk that's available.*]

MARIA

Maria's baby was first seen at our clinic when he was 15 days old, having been referred by the pediatrician. This was Maria's first pregnancy and first baby, born at 38 weeks' gestation. The labor lasted only two hours, and although the baby was fine at birth, he was not tried on the breast until three or four hours after birth (*three or four hours too late*). At that time, as frequently happens after the initial few hours—when most babies not too drugged by maternal medications are really interested in breastfeeding—this baby was no longer interested. Another opportunity was lost to get breastfeeding started well. [*Babies are often very eager to breastfeed during the first two hours after birth. After this time, they lose interest, and fall sleep, whether they have fed or not. When given the opportunity, newborn babies will even crawl up to the breast and latch on all by themselves. I believe we would see far fewer breastfeeding problems if more babies were allowed to do this. In this case, I can see no excuse—except perhaps the convenience of staff or the rigid following of hospital routines—for not having let this baby breastfeed immediately. The old story that the mother was "too tired" won't even work here—she only had two hours of labor.*]

The baby weighed 3.1 kg (6 lb 13 oz) at birth. The baby and mother roomed in 24 hours a day. No supplements were given. When Maria brought the baby to the clinic, she said that he "breastfed" all the time and would stay on the breast "forever" if she did not take him off. [*Did this baby really breastfeed all the time? No, given his weight loss, he probably wasn't feeding much at all.*] He slept four hours at night, however. [*Sleeping four hours at night in the first two weeks of life is sometimes a signal that things are not going well. Obviously, if the baby is getting plenty of milk and sleeps four, five, or six hours at night, this is fine. However, sometimes these long sleeps at night are clues that the baby is not getting enough to eat.*] The mother had sore nipples.

At the first visit to the clinic, the baby weighed 2.885 kg (6 lb 3 oz). [*Once again, different scales—but we use this information in conjunction with other indicators that tell us the baby is not feeding well.*] The baby was thin and moderately jaundiced. In

fact, the baby was getting some milk and nursing, although his latch was poor.

I showed Maria how to latch the baby on better. This resulted in the feeding being absolutely painless, for the first time ever for this mother. I also taught her how to know the baby was getting milk (open mouth wide–pause–close mouth type of sucking). I taught her how to do the compression. And I taught her to switch the baby from one breast to the other when the baby was no longer drinking on first side.

My assessment was that the baby was drinking well enough that he would not get into trouble over the next week. I made a follow-up appointment for a week later, but offered the parents a follow-up anytime beforehand if they were concerned.

The parents did return five days later because they were worried the baby was not getting enough milk. The baby's weight at this point was 2.9 kg (6 lb 4 oz). [*Only a little more than five days earlier, but we used a different scale. More important, the baby was drinking well enough, and in fact drinking better than he had been five days earlier.*] I reassured the parents and asked them to keep the original appointment.

One week after the initial visit, the baby weighed 2.95 kg (only 70 grams, or a little more than 2 ounces, more than seven days before). [*This pattern of the weight "bottoming out" before starting to rise is common when there has been a delay in fixing the breastfeeding problem. Most important, the baby was continuing to feed better than before.*]

One week later, two weeks after the first visit, the baby weighed 3.13 kg (150 grams, or about 5 ounces, more than seven days before). In addition to the weight gain, the baby was obviously more content, would spend less time on the breast, and was urinating more. The weight gain was not great, but was acceptable, and obviously on the upswing.

One week later, the baby weighed 3.43 kg (300 grams, or just over 10 ounces, more than the week before). The baby was content and fed about every three hours.

A month later, Maria phoned to leave a message that the baby was continuing to gain weight at the rate of about an ounce a day.

When the baby was five months old, Maria called again to say that her baby, on breastfeeding only, now weighed 6.1 kg (13 lb 9 oz). [*It took the baby almost a month to return to his birthweight. But don't forget that when we saw him, at 15 days, he was well below his birthweight and not feeding well. Formula might have caused him to gain weight more quickly, but his mother quite reasonably didn't want to use formula unless it was absolutely necessary. It turned out not to be.*

Note again that this baby also had moderate jaundice because of low milk intake.

This case is typical of many we see at the clinic. It is important to remember that not all babies will begin to improve immediately or as quickly as Susan's baby did (first "real-world experience," see pages 91–93). Because the baby was nursing poorly for two weeks, Maria's milk supply had likely decreased, but fortunately not to the point of no return. Better nursing brought her milk supply up again, so the baby could gain well.]

CELINE

Celine brought Jeremy to the clinic when he was 13 days old. She was 27 years old, and this was her first baby. Her pregnancy was unremarkable, but she commented that she had no breast changes during the pregnancy. [*It is often said, and can be read in some of the information given out to new mothers, that if a mother's breasts do not change during pregnancy, she will not produce enough milk for her baby. This has not been our experience. Although some of the mothers seen at the clinic who were unable to produce enough milk said they saw no changes in their breasts during pregnancy, others had very definite changes and enlargement. Most of the women who said they had no changes in their breasts still produced plenty of milk. Indeed, the first mother we saw in the clinic with the problem of "overproduction" told us she had had no changes in her breasts while pregnant. I remember this still, because at the time I believed "no enlargement, no milk." I also would remind readers that breast changes during a second or later pregnancy tend to be much less noticeable than during a first.*]

The labor and birth were normal. The baby was tried on the breast immediately after birth and apparently latched on well. [*Apparently—but I don't really buy it. A baby who seems to "latch on well" and then refuses the breast when the mother becomes engorged probably never latched on at all, but was only allowing the breast in his mouth. When the engorgement started—and engorgement is usually worse if the baby is not nursing well—the baby found it hard to do what he was doing before, and began actively to refuse the breast.*]

The mother and baby roomed in at the hospital, no supplements were given during the hospital stay, and they left the hospital at 48 hours after birth. The baby's birth weight was 4.09 kg (9 lb).

At the first clinic visit, the baby weighed 4.245 kg (9 lb 5 oz). He had been supplemented from the third day because he was refusing the breast. The mother and baby had been seen at another lactation clinic a few days before, and the mother had been taught finger-feeding in order to help the baby get to the breast. [*See Chapter 10, When the Baby Refuses the Breast.*] For about two days before the baby was seen at our clinic, he had been taking the breast. Nevertheless, Celine was supplementing with 110 to 150 ml (4 to 5 oz) of formula at each feeding. She was also experiencing sore nipples. [*This soreness means that even though the baby has taken the breast, he has not latched on well. Another indicator that he is not feeding well is the large amount of formula supplement he is taking.*]

On examination of the baby, nothing unusual was noted. The baby was latched on poorly, but once the latch was corrected, the baby drank fairly well at the breast. I also showed Celine the breast compression technique and urged her to change sides when the baby no longer drank even with compression. It seemed unlikely that he was taking as much breastmilk as he took formula, so we showed the mother how to use a lactation aid.

My advice was: "Feed on the first side until the baby no longer drinks on his own. Then use breast compression until that no longer seems to work. Then switch sides and repeat the process. If you wish, switch sides again, but do at least both sides before introducing the lactation aid. Then let the baby drink as much as he will take." [*Some mothers will keep the baby on each breast until he falls asleep. This is not necessary, since if the baby is not doing the open mouth wide–pause–close mouth type of sucking, he is not getting much to eat. Waiting until the baby is asleep or almost asleep makes the feedings longer, without necessarily decreasing the amount of supplement the baby will take. Indeed, if the baby is allowed to fall asleep, it may take some time to wake him up enough to take the second side.*

The better the baby is latched on, the less the lactation aid will be needed. And the better the baby is latched on, the easier it is to use the lactation aid. A well-placed tube, with baby well latched on, will give the baby 30 to 60 ml or 1 to 2 ounces in 10 or 20 minutes. If the baby takes an hour to get 30 ml, something is wrong.]

The baby and mother returned to the clinic a week after the first visit. The baby weighed 4.53

kg (10 lb). He was down to taking 110 to 150 ml (4 to 5 oz) of formula over a whole day. Celine did add that he now woke more frequently to feed. However, she was happy about no longer being sore. The baby breastfed very well, and it was obvious he was taking lots of milk, much more than at the first visit. I encouraged the mother to continue working on the latch, the compression and the switching, but having done all that, not to limit the baby's supplementation. The baby would take what he needed.

Here is an excerpt from a letter I received from Celine later:

"Jeremy is just turning four months, the last three of which he has been solely on breastmilk. He now weighs over 16 pounds [7.27 kg]. We are both very well now. I love breastfeeding! I never thought it could be so easy and so rewarding!" [*The lactation aid doesn't always work this well or this quickly. It is even possible that with this mother we could have gotten away without it. However, I felt it was needed, in part because I was not convinced that the mother was going to be able to keep going without it.*

Sometimes it takes several weeks to get off the lactation aid. Some mothers can't get off it at all, since once the milk supply is really down, it can be impossible to bring it back completely. Some mothers can get off the lactation aid when the baby starts to take solids, but even then some can't. The reason: babies like it when the milk flows quickly. Some are so particular that they will only nurse when the lactation aid is in place and providing them with that rapid flow of milk. This is more of a problem when a baby is older (say three or four months) and is obviously aware of whether the tube is in place.]

I also received a call from the mother when the baby was about six months old. The baby was breastfeeding exclusively at the time and gaining well.

RUTH

Ruth's twins were born seven weeks early (33 weeks' gestation). The labor was normal and the babies were born without the mother receiving any medication. The mother had previously nursed two other children (not twins) without problems for about seven months. One twin weighed 2.02 kg (4 lb 7 oz), the other 1.6 kg (3 lb 8 oz). There were no complications of prematurity, the twins did not need help with breathing—not even oxygen—and there were no problems with jaundice. The babies remained in the hospital for five weeks, three weeks in the one they were born in (and where the problems with breastfeeding began), and two weeks in another (where the problems continued).

Ruth's babies received intravenous fluids for the first four days. They got formula from very early on, at first by a tube into their stomachs, and then by bottles that were started within the first week after birth. Breastfeeding apparently was not even attempted until several weeks after the babies' birth. [*These babies were apparently both well, and they were a fair size for being premature. There was no reason not to try them at the breast within a few hours after birth, once it was obvious that they were not running into problems. Of course, it is possible that they would not have taken the breast, but the sooner babies begin, the easier is the learning process. Staff in special care units sometimes argue that a premature baby has to learn to take a bottle before he can breastfeed, and that it is less stressful for a premature baby to bottle-feed than to breastfeed. This is nonsense. Research has produced clear evidence that breastfeeding is less stressful for the premature baby than is bottle-feeding. Furthermore, there is no need to start bottles even if the baby is not taking the breast, since cup-feeding seems to cause fewer problems than does using a bottle. Getting the babies to the breast*

earlier not only helps them learn to feed more quickly, but helps to maintain the mother's supply.

Formula should only have been given to these babies if the mother was not expressing enough. There was no reason to suppose that Ruth could not have provided plenty of milk for her babies. In spite of the rationale that we must supplement breastmilk with formula or fortifier when babies are born prematurely, these babies did not gain weight well.]

At some point, Ruth was started on domperidone. [*This is typical of the medical approach to many problems—don't fix the real problem (poor latch, or, in this case, no latch), just give the mother a drug.*]

The babies were discharged from the hospital essentially being bottle-fed.

At the first visit to our clinic, the babies were almost three months old. The babies took the left breast a little, but were refusing the right side completely. Each feeding consisted of expressed milk, about 30 ml (1 oz), and formula 60 ml (2 oz). At this first visit, the babies weighed 3.35 kg (7 lb 6 oz) and 3.25 kg (7 lb 2 oz). [*Note that this is nowhere near the amount they would have gained if they had still been in their mother's uterus. Achieving that kind of weight gain is the usual reason cited for supplementing premature babies.*]

Neither baby would go near the right breast, arching and screaming rather than latching on. [*I think this is a very clear case of nipple confusion.*] They appeared to take the left side, but in fact, merely allowed the breast into their mouths, which is not the same as latching on. They did not actually breastfeed while at the left breast.

I showed Ruth how to use the lactation aid to give them a supplement at the left breast. With the lactation aid, they did take the right side a little, but not much. They did take more supplement on the left side, but still really didn't have it.

It was important at this stage to increase the

mother's milk supply, so I suggested she take herbs (fenugreek and blessed thistle), and I prescribed domperidone for her, as well.

I asked Ruth to continue using the lactation aid, concentrating on the latch, as well as taking the herbs and medication, and then to return with the babies in a week.

The next week things were much better. The babies were taking the left breast and breastfeeding. The three were managing well with the lactation aid. The babies were still getting some bottles, especially at night, when Ruth felt she needed some relief. The babies weighed 3.49 kg (7 lb 11 oz) and 3.35 kg (7 lb 6 oz). This was a reasonable weight gain for both.

Two weeks after the first visit, the babies were now taking the right breast and were nursing well on the left side. The weights at this visit were lost, or we forgot to weigh them.

Four weeks after the initial visit, the babies weighed 4.02 kg (8 lb 13 oz) and 3.81 kg (8 lb 6 oz). At this point the babies were getting only about 60 ml (2 oz) of supplemental formula a day. The babies nursed very well on both sides. The father, who had not initially been supportive, believing the babies would be fussier when breastfeeding, was now very supportive because he had seen that the one baby who was getting formula during the night was the one who was fussier at night.

By the fifth week after the initial visit, the babies were breastfeeding exclusively and gaining weight appropriately. The babies were still breastfeeding exclusively at six months of age,

when I last saw them. [*The babies progressed from virtually exclusive bottlefeeding, with some breastmilk feeding, to exclusive breastfeeding in five weeks. Keep in mind, these babies had been in the hospital for five weeks. I strongly believe that with a little help and support, Ruth and her babies would have done very well from the start. Ruth's determination made it work in the end, but it should not have been such a struggle.*]

The above case studies are fairly typical and are common in the clinics where I work. Unfortunately, it is not always possible to get results as satisfying as the ones described. On the other hand, it should be pointed out again that so many of the problems we have seen over the years could have been avoided. Even if the mother doesn't produce anything close to the amount of milk the baby needs, the better the start, the more of that milk the baby will get. And the mother can breastfeed for as long as she and her baby want, though supplementation with a lactation aid may be necessary.

Everything said above, which applies to the healthy baby, is also true for the baby who has special problems, such as Trisomy 21, or other congenital or medical problems. Indeed, with rare exceptions, babies with problems don't need less breastmilk (or breastfeeding, which is not the same thing), they need more. Unfortunately, as with the premature twins above, too many health professionals just assume that breastfeeding is not in the cards for the sick baby. Indeed, many believe that formulas are better. This is almost never true.

6

Sore Nipples

Myth: It is normal for breastfeeding to cause sore nipples.

Fact: It is not normal to have sore nipples, although, unfortunately, it is very common. We know it isn't normal because it can usually be prevented or quickly fixed if it does occur. So why do so many women experience sore nipples? As with many other breastfeeding problems, it can almost always be traced back to a poor latch.

Is it normal, though, to have some nipple tenderness during the first few days? This is a question debated by lactation specialists, but one that is, perhaps, not of much importance for the nursing mother. After all, we are talking about some soreness, usually fairly mild, that will last two or three days and then disappear. Some mothers don't experience even this amount of tenderness.

Severe pain, however, is not normal, and any mother who experiences pain that makes her hesitate to put the baby to the breast requires immediate help in getting the baby well latched on. A detailed description of latching on is found in Chapter 4, Getting Off to the Best Start.

Anyone telling a mother that it is normal to have sore nipples for two or three weeks does not know what they are talking about, and should not be advising mothers about breast-feeding. While changing the baby's position and improving the latch will sometimes instantly eliminate the pain, in more difficult cases it may take as long as two weeks to end the sore nipples. That makes it even more important to start solving the problem as soon as possible, to minimize the mother's painful experiences and the possibility of nipple trauma that may take a long time to heal.

Anyone who tells the mother of a three-day-old that, despite her excruciating pain, the "latch looks just fine" is wrong. Though it may not be easy to fix, at this point nipple soreness is almost always due to a poor latch, no matter what it looks like from a distance.

By the way, it does not matter, really, how bad or how "normal" the nipple looks. A mother may have extremely severe pain with normal-looking nipples, and may have minimal, or in some cases no pain at all, even with deep cracks. The problem is the pain, not what the nipples look like. With a crack, there is an increased risk of mastitis, but I do not feel it is much increased, and the complex, difficult treatment required to heal a crack if it does not hurt seems unnecessary to me. And if it doesn't hurt, then time will heal it.

Also, bleeding from a nipple does not make the situation worse. It may seem worse; it looks worse; everyone may worry more. But it is not worse. The problem, again, is the pain, not whether the nipple bleeds or not. If the cause of the nipple pain is eliminated, the bleeding will stop. It is true that the baby may spit up more, as the blood in the milk may irritate his stomach a little, but it will do the baby no harm to swallow some blood. Sometimes, too, the baby who swallows a fair bit of blood will have blood in his bowel movements, but the main concern here is that someone will think it is the baby who is bleeding, which may result in many unnecessary tests.

Some mothers who have had considerable damage to their nipples worry that the nipple will never look normal again. It will. I have seen mothers with damage so bad that it looked as if the nipple was no longer present, but the nipple healed and was normal once the problem was dealt with—though in some cases it took several weeks, even after the pain was gone.

While sore nipples, especially in the early weeks, almost always indicate that the baby is not latched on well, the opposite is not necessarily true. The fact that the mother's nipples are *not* hurting doesn't guarantee that the latch is *good*. Some babies who are not really breastfeeding, but are just allowing the nipple into their mouths, will not cause sore nipples, but are at risk of becoming dehydrated because of the poor latch.

There are a number of factors linked to sore nipples. Most of these cause sore nipples by interfering with a good latch.

Early Use of Artificial Nipples

It is hardly ever necessary to use artificial nipples for the breastfeeding baby. Any artificial nipple, whether on a bottle or a pacifier, encourages the baby to suck with his mouth relatively closed. If the baby comes onto the breast with a relatively closed mouth, he often latches on to the nipple, which is very sensitive and easily damaged. This

is particularly likely to happen during the first few days.

Sometimes, especially during the first few days, the baby gets a supplement because the mother is so sore that she cannot keep the baby at the breast any longer. Or the baby gets a pacifier put into his mouth rather than a supplement. The problem should never be allowed to get to this point. The fact that the mother is having any significant pain during the first days should indicate that someone needs to come and help her with the latch, and quickly. Often pain can be much relieved or even eliminated simply by improving the latch.

Part of the justification for the supplement is that the baby is often spending long periods of time on the breast, and that the long feedings are causing the nipple damage. In fact, long feedings do *not* cause nipple damage. A poor latch causes nipple soreness. Of course, a baby sucking with a poor latch for two hours is going to cause more nipple damage than a baby sucking for one hour with a poor latch. An improved latch will not only decrease the mother's pain, but will help the baby get the milk more effectively, and reduce the amount of time he needs to stay at the breast. For this reason, I find that if mothers use breast compression—which seems to work particularly well during the first few days when there are only small amounts of milk available—their nipple pain may be lessened.

What if fixing the latch and using compression still do not eliminate the nipple pain, and the mother wants to reduce the amount of time the baby is nursing? In that case, I would prefer that the mother give the baby a little sugar water rather than a pacifier or a supplement by bottle. The best way to give that sugar water is with a lactation aid at the breast. Why not a cup- or finger-feeding, or some other technique? Because babies learn to breastfeed by breastfeeding. In the first few days, 10 ml or 15 ml (⅓ oz or ½ oz) of sugar water given by lactation aid will help fill up the baby in a few minutes, so that he won't spend hours at the breast.

Delayed Start to Breastfeeding

I strongly believe that a delay in starting breastfeeding contributes to sore nipples. The mother whose baby begins breastfeeding in the first hour, especially if the baby starts by self-attaching, is much less likely to have sore nipples. The self-attaching baby is placed on the mother's abdomen immediately after birth, without being washed, and allowed to find the breast on his own. This is standard practice in many Scandinavian countries, and the newborn's ability to locate the breast and latch on to the nipple is quite remarkable.

Sometimes a delay in beginning breastfeeding is unavoidable, but most of the time, there is no reason a baby cannot start immediately. I think most pediatricians would agree that drying the baby before he's placed on his mother's abdomen is helpful. A wet baby is more likely to feel cold, and this increases his risk of developing low blood sugar. But that shouldn't delay breastfeeding for more than a few seconds.

Engorgement

Engorgement may herald the onset of sore nipples because when the mother is engorged, the breast becomes hard, the nipple becomes flat, and the baby has difficulty latching on well. He may injure the nipple because he grabs only the end.

The proper approach is to prevent engorgement in the first place. Many women erro-neously believe that engorgement is normal. Although most women will develop obvious breast fullness on the third or fourth day after the baby is born, engorgement to the point of the baby having difficult latching on should not occur. At the risk of sounding like a broken record (an expression from many years back, when records were made from vinyl), the best way to prevent severe engorgement is to get the baby latched on well from the very first day, and to feed him as often as he wants from then on. Remember that some babies in our hospitals do not show cues that they are ready to feed because they are kept warm and snug wrapped in blankets, unable to move their arms, often with a pacifier in their mouths. This, too, contributes to engorgement.

A mother who has had a baby in the hospital should insist on keeping him with her 24 hours a day. Unwrap the baby, keep him in your bed, and don't allow a pacifier to be given. Watch for your baby's subtle signals that he's ready to nurse again—trying to suck on his hands or the blanket, turning his head from side to side as though searching for the breast, making smacking or sucking noises, or whatever cues your individual baby uses to signal you. Responding to these messages and feeding the baby will help prevent engorgement and encourage the development of a good milk supply.

Sucking Problems

There is no doubt that some babies have difficulty sucking correctly or efficiently. And a baby who has a poor suck may cause or contribute to a mother's nipple soreness. Babies with neurologic problems (temporary, as in the case of sedation from drugs, or more long-lasting, such as babies who have been deprived of oxygen before or during birth), or babies with facial or mouth abnormalities (cleft palates, large tongues, or tongue ties) often have real difficulties sucking properly. However, the majority of babies who have sucking problems have them because they were not helped to latch on well and breastfeed.

If a baby goes to the breast and gets milk when he sucks properly, he will learn that this way of sucking gets him what he wants. I would suggest that this might even be one explanation as to why, from the evolutionary point of view, it is helpful that there is less milk in the first days. When the supply is small, a baby has to suck well in order to get milk. If the baby cannot suck well, then he will not get milk, and will not learn to breastfeed. In the old days, if he did not breastfeed, his chances for survival were reduced. In a hunter-gatherer society, babies who could not suck probably had something significant wrong with them (since there was no sedation given to the mother during labor), and in such a society, survival of babies with significant problems was undesirable.

When a baby goes to the breast in the first few days when there is not a lot of milk, he will get milk only if he is latched on well and sucking well. Given a good latch, the baby will get milk when he is sucking well, and the reward of the milk reinforces the baby's correct suck.

Once the milk supply is more abundant, the baby does not have to suck well to get milk. If he can suck incorrectly, or not suck at all, and still get milk, this may encourage him to suck in this incorrect way—which in turn may cause the mother to develop sore nipples. Most babies do, eventually, learn to suck properly (which is probably why most sore nipples improve). But the mother may be pretty uncomfortable along the way!

So, the best way to get a baby to suck correctly is to get him breastfeeding well from the very first day.

If the mother has sore nipples and the baby is not sucking well, then suck training may help the mother with her soreness. The idea is to show the baby how to suck before putting him on the breast. Some lactation specialists have developed elaborate protocols for suck training, but I find that finger-feeding for a minute or two before putting the baby to the breast works very well. Finger-feeding is described in more detail in Chapter 5, but is basically using a small feeding tube held on top of your finger, with the other end in a container of the supplement. You put your finger in the baby's mouth, your nail on the baby's tongue and the tube on top, and let the baby suck.

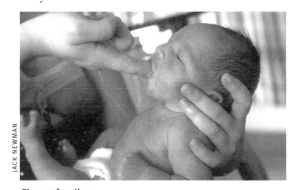

Finger-feeding.

For finger-feeding, expressed milk is always the preferred fluid, but since the baby will be getting very little, sugar water is acceptable as well. Finger-feeding can be slow, but in the case of suck training, this is actually an advantage. The baby will get little to drink if he sucks poorly, but will get more if he sucks correctly. Furthermore, I have noticed that the baby, as he first draws fluid up through the tube, is often sucking poorly, but within seconds of getting flow, he starts sucking much more efficiently.

He wraps his tongue around the mother's or father's finger and begins the backward draw toward the back of his throat, which babies do when they are sucking properly at the breast. Once the baby is doing that, he can be switched over to the breast. Many who promote suck training feel it helps very quickly—and that sore nipples can be cured within 24 hours—but this has not been the experience of mothers to whom I have suggested it. I tend to show suck training less than I once did (though I still use finger-feeding for getting a baby who refuses the breast to latch on), but it can be a useful technique.

There is one problem in evaluating the efficacy of any treatment: in most clinics, it is rare for lactation specialists to use only one technique to help mothers with problems, so it is sometimes difficult to know which, if any, of the various treatments actually helped. It's also quite possible that each intervention helped a little bit, and that all of them together "solved the problem." This question is often complicated by the fact that sore nipples, for example, do improve with time, regardless of what we do. So even if I show the mother finger-feeding (suck training) for sore nipples, I also show her how to latch the baby on better, and often use a nipple ointment (see p. 108), as well as other treatments.

> **Quick Comfort for Sore Nipples**
> You've made arrangements for someone to help you improve your baby's latch—but meanwhile the baby is hungry NOW and your nipples hurt! What can help?
> • You can take over-the-counter pain relievers (such as Tylenol).
> • Use the relaxation or breathing techniques you learned in prenatal classes to help you cope with contractions during labor.
> • Wrap some ice cubes in a face cloth and

> apply to the nipple—this will numb it temporarily.
> • Use breast compression while the baby nurses so the feeding will be shorter.
>
> Remember, these are only temporary measures and don't replace getting the baby properly latched on.

Some Little-Known Causes of Nipple Soreness

Raynaud's Phenomenon

Raynaud's Phenomenon is a well-known symptom of rheumatic diseases, such as rheumatoid arthritis or scleroderma or systemic lupus erythematosis. But most of the time it occurs in people without any of these illnesses. Women are most commonly affected, and usually in their fingers. The phenomenon is triggered by a drop in temperature (as in leaving a warm house to go outside on a cold day). The person's fingers will turn white and often be quite painful; when the fingers are warmed, they will turn pink again.

Raynaud's Phenomenon may also occur in the nipples of nursing mothers. Only one mother I have seen with it had any rheumatic disease, while none of the others had any evidence of these illnesses.

Typically, the pain caused by Raynaud's Phenomenon occurs after the feeding is over, presumably because the outside air is cooler than the inside of the baby's mouth. The nipple, or part of the nipple, starts to turn white, but only after the baby has been off the breast for a few seconds or minutes. Associated with the nipple whiteness is a burning pain that usually continues as long as the nipple is white. The blanching is caused by the vessels in the nipple going into spasm, so that blood does not get into the nipple.

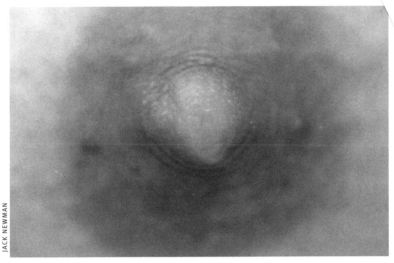

Raynaud's Phenomenon of the nipple. The blanching of the nipple is due to spasm of the blood vessels after the feeding is over. The pain is usually described as burning when the nipple is white, and throbbing after the nipple color returns to normal.

When the vessels open up again, the nipple will turn pink and, frequently, throb with pain. The nipple may then go white again, associated with burning pain, and then return to throbbing. The burning may last seconds or minutes, as may the throbbing, but the pain may last an hour or more.

Raynaud's Phenomenon is almost always secondary to other causes of nipple pain. That is, what seems to happen is that the blood vessels in the nipple become "jumpy" due to trauma caused by a poor latch, for example, or inflammation from a candidal (yeast) infection, or any cause of nipple soreness.

The treatment of Raynaud's Phenomenon is to treat whatever is causing the mother's sore nipples. If the pain during the feeding goes away, Raynaud's Phenomenon will disappear as well, usually within a few days to two weeks.

Occasionally, mothers have no further pain in their nipples, but continue to get Raynaud's Phenomenon. In other cases, women have never had painful nipples at all, yet have Raynaud's Phenomenon. Sometimes, the blanching started during the pregnancy. If the pain is mild, there may be no need to treat. Often the mother is reassured to know what the problem is.

Raynaud's Phenomenon of the nipples is far more common than most lactation specialists or other health professionals think. It rarely needs to be treated, though, since treating the root cause of nipple soreness will almost always eliminate it. However, it is important to know about Raynaud's Phenomenon because the symptoms (burning type of pain that occurs after the feeding is over) can lead to the belief that the cause of this pain is candida (yeast), since candidal infections of the nipple typically cause burning pain, and may continue after the feeding is over (see below). Sometimes, treatment of Raynaud's Phenomenon is necessary.

Sometimes the pain of Raynaud's Phenomenon can be managed by applying heat to the nipple after the feeding is over. Some mothers use hair dryers to warm the nipple; others use cloths soaked with hot water. The problem with this approach is that it is a bit of a nuisance, especially since the time of onset of the blanching is not predictable. It may occur within seconds of the baby's coming off the breast, or it may be delayed several minutes. In some cases, the mothers find that as long as they apply heat, the blanching does not occur, but that as soon as the heat is removed, the blanching occurs.

If these measures do not help, I try medication, particularly if the pain of Raynaud's Phenomenon is severe. Three with which I have some experience are discussed here. Please note that my experience with these treatments is limited, because most of the time the problem disappears when the cause of the sore nipples is dealt with. I see more than a thousand mothers and their babies for breastfeeding problems in a year and communicate with at least another 4,000 by phone or e-mail, but probably treat, or suggest treatment for Raynaud's Phenomenon no more than 10 times in a year. Medication can be useful if the mother continues to experience pain after feedings even though the baby's latch has improved, and her nipples do not hurt during feedings, or if the mother has never experienced pain during the actual feedings, but only afterward.

Vitamin B$_6$

One mother who came to me for help with Raynaud's Phenomenon read something in a book about using Vitamin B$_6$ for this condition. At first I resisted this idea, because I couldn't imagine why it would work, and also because very large doses of B$_6$ have been reported to decrease milk supply. I gave this particular mother nifedipine, and it worked well for her.

Later, another mother came to the clinic with Raynaud's Phenomenon and the nifedipine did not seem to help her at all. So I suggested Vita-

min B$_6$. It worked! We have now used this treatment on many women and it works most of the time. The dose is 100 to 200 mg daily as a single dose for four days, then 25 mg a day from then on. However, if the pain returns on the lower dose, the mother can up it again to 100 to 200 mg daily. These are high doses, but not high enough to decrease the milk supply. Interestingly, several of the women reported that the pain decreased, but not the blanching. I don't know what to make of that. If the pain is due to the blanching and a lack of blood getting to the nipple, why does the pain go but the blanching remain? It really doesn't matter—if the pain is gone, that's good.

Nifedipine, long acting, 30 mg once daily

Many drugs, almost all of them used to treat high blood pressure, have also been used to treat Raynaud's Phenomenon of the fingers. I have had experience only with nifedipine, which works quite well, most of the time.

Nifedipine works often when nitroglycerin doesn't and is less messy. I also think that sometimes the nifedipine has helped with nipple healing, because severe enough Raynaud's Phenomenon can interfere with healing by depriving the nipples of their blood supplies.

As noted above, the dose is one 30-mg tablet of the long-acting form, once a day. Most mothers get relief with this. Side effects are uncommon, although some women experience headache.

I ask a mother to stay on the nifedipine for two weeks and then try going off the medication. Usually the Raynaud's does not return; sometimes it does, though in a less severe form. If the pain returns and treatment still seems necessary, the mother can go on another two weeks of the medication. Usually, this will do the trick, but we did have one mother who needed four, two-week courses before she was pain-free while off the medication.

Nifedipine can be taken during breastfeeding, as can almost all medications. The amount of nifedipine that gets into the milk is very small, partly because it is tightly bound to proteins in the mother's blood, partly because the concentration in the mother's blood is low. Furthermore, much of what the baby gets is not absorbed.

Nitroglycerin paste 2 percent

Nitroglycerin used locally can bring relief, although it does not seem to work if the mother is experiencing any pain at all during the feeding. Here are the steps in using it:

1. For the first 24 hours, the mother should apply the nitroglycerin paste sparingly as soon as the baby comes off the breast.
2. If the nitroglycerin works to eliminate pain during the first 24 hours, the mother should, during the second 24 hours, use it only if the blanching begins. Many mothers find they need it only a few times during the second 24 hours, and then the need diminishes more and more. Most mothers are able to stop the nitroglycerin within a few days to two weeks.
3. If the nitroglycerin does not work during the first 24 hours, it is worth trying for another 24 hours to put the paste on after each feeding. If it hasn't worked in 48 hours, however, it probably won't work.

Other forms of nitroglycerin are available, such as spray. The one mother I remember who tried the spray found that it did not work, but that the paste did.

The paste is a bit messy, but this is a small inconvenience if the pain disappears in 24 to 48 hours. The main problem is that even in the absence of pain during the feeding, nitroglycerin does not work all the time. About 50 percent of the time, mothers get complete relief from it and are able to stop using nitroglycerin within a few days.

There is no concern about the baby getting any of this nitroglycerin, because it is absorbed extremely rapidly—within minutes—into the mother's circulation. Indeed, the mother will know if she's used too much, because she will quickly get a severe headache that usually only lasts a few minutes. Furthermore, even if the baby does manage to swallow some nitroglycerin, it is not absorbed from the stomach, so there is no danger. (People who use nitroglycerin for heart pain put it under the tongue, so that it will be absorbed directly into the bloodstream, something that won't happen if they swallow it.)

While the nitroglycerin paste often worked, the messiness and the side effects, including severe headaches, limit its effectiveness. It is not my first choice for treating this problem, and I hardly ever use it anymore.

Eczema of the Nipples

Eczema of the nipples is not uncommon. It seems to become a problem later on during the mother's nursing experience, typically beginning, at least from the mothers I have seen, around three months after the baby is born. It also seems to be more common in Black and South Asian women.

Eczema needs to be recognized because it can cause severe pain, but it can also, usually, be easily treated. Furthermore, this is another condition that may be confused with a candidal (yeast) infection of the nipples. Just as with a candidal infection, eczema may start after a period of pain-free nursing; the pain is often described as "burning" by the mother, and the nipples may also be itchy. The treatment can be the same, with what I call "all-purpose nipple ointment" (recipe on p. 110), but a simple steroid ointment may be fine for eczema.

I would then treat the mother with 0.05 percent betamethasone ointment (I believe ointments are better on the nipple and areola than are creams), to be applied sparingly after each feeding at first. Once improvement is obvious, usually after a day or two, the mother can start decreasing the frequency of use of the steroid ointment. Most mothers find they cannot stop the ointment completely, but they can keep the problem at bay with infrequent applications (once a day or even less).

The baby may get some of the steroid, but if it is applied after the feeding is over and the baby does not come back to the breast for a couple of hours, the majority of the steroid (not necessarily the greasy stuff in which it is carried) will have been absorbed by the mother. I have never seen problems in babies from this tiny steroid intake, especially since the mother will normally be using the ointment for no more than a few days, at least not at full dose.

Once the problem is under control, the mother can use a lanolin ointment (but not if she is sensitive to lanolin, as many mothers with eczema are), which may decrease the frequency with which the steroid ointment needs to be used. Other general measures for controlling eczema can also decrease the need for the steroid ointment. These include not washing the nipples frequently (a good idea in any case), using soap as little as possible on the area, preventing overheating of the area, exposing the area to sun when possible (without overheating), and avoiding rough or irritating fabrics.

Other Dermatologic Conditions

Dermatologic conditions found in other parts of the body can affect the nipple and areola. For example, psoriasis can cause nipple pain. Patches are found on the areola which are similar to patches found elsewhere. Contact dermatitis is a fairly common condition and may affect women with sore nipples. Contact dermatitis is due to a reaction, usually to medicated ointments or creams applied to the nipple, but may occur because of contact with certain metals (nickel is known for this) or even some other substances (wool, for example). The mother with sore nipples has often used many types of creams and ointments on her nipples and areolas and could often have contact dermatitis. It often looks like eczema.

Nipple Blisters or "Blebs"

Blisters occasionally develop on the end of a mother's nipple. Most commonly, blisters occur during the first few days after the baby's birth, and result from injury of the nipple due to a poor latch. The treatment for these is no different from that for sore nipples due to a poor latch *without* the presence of blisters.

Occasionally, however, the blisters will start to occur several weeks or even several months after the baby is born, apparently out of the blue. There is a relationship between these blisters and blocked ducts (see below), but the relationship is difficult to define. Sometimes mothers develop a blocked duct after a nipple blister appears, and this gives rise to the notion that the blister somehow causes the blocked duct. Furthermore, the blister almost always occurs over a pore that seems to bear a relationship to the location of the blocked duct. For example, a blister on the upper inner side of the nipple is associated with a blocked duct on the upper

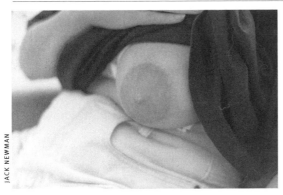

Nipple bleb or blister. It may be small, but it can be very painful. If a bubble is present it can be popped with a sterile needle.

inner side of the breast. However, blisters often appear only after the blocked duct appears; or appear without a blocked duct; or a blocked duct appears without a blister. So, the relationship between the two is certainly not a clear one.

There are some who blame candida (yeast) for these blisters, and I suppose this is possible. Occasionally, it does seem that treatment for candida decreases the recurrence of these blisters, but then, many things get better by themselves, including blisters on nipples.

My hypothesis—which, I admit, does not explain everything—is that blisters occur in areas of previous damage where the milk is not flowing well. Good flow through a duct would prevent the skin from healing over a pore, and thus prevent the formation of a blister. But if the milk is not flowing well, skin may grow over that opening. A plugged duct can diminish the flow through that milk duct, explaining why a blister sometimes appears two or three days after a plugged duct.

In other situations, if a baby is nursing inefficiently (perhaps because of introduction of bottles or pacifiers), he may not "drain" certain areas of the breast well, and create slower flow from certain areas—slow enough that the blister would

form. This might explain why a blister can appear before or about the same time as a blocked duct. And why might one get a blister without a blocked duct? It is probable that the various areas of the breast that are served by a particular duct could interconnect with other areas of the breast served by other ducts; so if the blister appears, the milk would just emerge from a different duct. Finally, a blocked duct can definitely occur without the presence of a blister. This is not too difficult to explain, since any block might occur not at the nipple, but deeper in the breast.

When a blister occurs on a mother's nipple, it can cause severe pain, especially while the baby is nursing. The blister is under tension from milk backed up behind it, and because the baby tends to draw more milk forward, the mother may actually have more pain toward the end of the feeding than early on. Sometimes the nipple hurts when the baby latches, then the pain improves as he nurses, but then the pain increases again as the blister enlarges.

The treatment for a blister is, first of all, to open it up. This can be done by the mother, though apparently this takes courage, similar to that needed to take a bandage off your arm when the hair has grown back! Many mothers can do it, but so can a health professional.

Generally, I do it after the baby has nursed. This gives me an opportunity to help the mother with the latch, which can make a difference to her pain and might prevent further problems. It is noteworthy, however, that it is not always easy to change a baby's latch once he is as old as three months, or sometimes even as young as six weeks. Some babies get into the habit of latching one way; if they get the reward of milk, they will stick with that technique.

I use a sterile needle (a mother at home can flame a sewing needle, and allow it to cool off for a few seconds), to pop the blister. There is no need to dig around, only to open the blister. If there is no "bubble" present, don't attempt to open the blister. It takes a second to do, and usually causes little or no pain. Sometimes a drop of blood will appear, but don't worry about this.

It is worthwhile squeezing the areola just behind the blister once it is opened to express out a toothpaste-like material. It is not always possible to do, but if it is, this action will usually help prevent further blisters from arising.

I also recommend an "all-purpose nipple ointment" (later this page) to prevent infection, and to prevent recurrences. The ointment should be used after each feeding for a week or 10 days. If the blister has not reappeared by this time, it probably won't.

If my hypothesis is correct, once again, a good beginning with a good latch helps prevent these problems.

Another Cause of Late-Onset Nipple Pain: Pregnancy

Many women experience nipple soreness as one of the first signs of pregnancy. One not frequently mentioned cause of late-onset nipple soreness is a new pregnancy.

You don't have to stop breastfeeding if you are pregnant, but many women do find the nipple soreness irritating. Furthermore, because pregnancy often decreases the milk supply, many babies will start pulling at the breast because the flow is too slow. This may aggravate sore nipples.

Treatment is time, as the nipple soreness generally disappears after the first trimester, at least in most women.

You can continue to breastfeed throughout the pregnancy, if you want to and if your older child is still interested, and then go on to nurse both your new baby and your older child, if you want. This is called *tandem nursing* and is increasingly common.

All-Purpose Nipple Ointment

Here is a recipe for an all-purpose nipple ointment. I find it works well for most causes of sore nipples, and is also good for candida (yeast) of the nipples. You will have to ask your doctor to prescribe it for you.

- Mupirocin 2% ointment (15 grams)
- Betamethasone 0.1% ointment (15 grams)
- Miconazole powder is then added so the final concentration of miconazole is 2%.

Compounding pharmacies usually have Miconazole powder, but any pharmacist should be able to get it. If this is not available, Clotrimazole powder (also to a final concentration of 2%) can be used, but I hear from mothers that this is more irritating to the skin. If neither is available, 15 grams of Nystatin ointment can be added instead, but this is less effective.

At one time I used Miconazole cream but found it tended to separate when mixed with the ointments.

If Mupirocin ointment is difficult to find, some other bacterial ointment could be used such as fucidic acid or bacitricin, but these are not as effective.

The pharmacist mixes all the ingredients together to make an ointment of 30 grams (1 ounce). The mother applies it after each feeding, and does not wash or wipe it off. Most of the ingredients are not absorbed by the baby even if he swallows them, and those that are, he will get in such small quantities that there should be no concern. I have used this ointment many times, and there has never been a problem for the baby, except in one or two cases in which the mother stated that the baby seemed to spit up more. It's quite possible, though, that the extra spitting up was due to the baby's getting more milk, since I never prescribe this ointment without also helping the baby latch on better. An improved latch usually leads to the baby getting more milk.

The Mupirocin is an antibiotic. Whatever the cause of a mother's nipple pain, there are almost always bacteria, particularly *Staphylococcus aureus* growing in the abraded or broken skin. Even if nothing is visible, mothers with sore nipples have abraded skin. Whether the bacteria are actually causing infection, or just living happily there, it has been known for some time that antibiotic ointments (without the other stuff in the recipe above) have helped some women with sore nipples. In England, they were prescribing simple antibiotic ointments for nipple soreness when we, on this side of the Atlantic, were saying mothers didn't need nipple ointments or creams for sore nipples—and they were finding some women got significant improvement. It's possible that the bacteria inhibit healing of the mother's sores. Furthermore, getting rid of the bacteria, particularly the *Staphylococcus aureus*, may prevent the bacteria from causing mastitis. Finally, sometimes the presence of bacteria encourages the growth of the candida of the nipple.

The clotrimazole works against candida. The betamethasone is a corticosteroid which decreases inflammation. It is included because much of the pain that occurs with infection, bacterial or fungal or any other cause, is due to inflammation, rather than to the organism itself. Reducing inflammation decreases the pain.

Any of the ingredients may be replaced by others. For example, some might prefer fusidic acid to Mupirocin, or ketoconazole to one of the antifungal agents, or even ketoconazole added to the other two in a resistant case of yeast. Or a different steroid may be used in place of betamethasone. Remember, each ingredient is diluted by the other ingredients, thus decreasing the potency of each. Though 0.1 percent beta-methasone is a fairly strong formulation, within the recipe above, it becomes 0.05 percent, which is less potent.

I believe ointments, which are "stickier," are more healing on nipples than creams, but there is no ointment available containing clotrimazole, miconazole, or ketoconazole.

Treating Sore Nipples

The best treatment is always prevention— getting the baby to latch on well from the beginning. If the mother's nipples are already sore, these are the steps I take to treat the problem:

1. The mother is taught how to help the baby latch on as well as possible. In many cases, this is all that is necessary. I would estimate that 50 percent of all the mothers who come to the clinic for sore nipples get immediate and complete (or almost complete) relief by improving the latch alone. If they come to the clinic before the baby is seven or eight days of age, the rate is significantly higher. Probably another 25 percent get significant improvement, though not painless feeding.

2. If the mother does not get complete improvement, or if I am concerned that she will not manage the latch as well at home as she did in the clinic, I prescribe the all-purpose nipple ointment. Often this helps with healing *while* the mother works on the latch. The mother should use it after all feedings. Once she is pain-free, she can decrease the frequency of application over a week or so, until she is not using it at all. If necessary,

the ointment may be restarted, but the mother should come back for help, because once nipple pain is gone, it should not return. Of course, if the mother manages to get the baby well latched on without pain, the nipple ointment is not necessary.

Lanolin-based ointments do have their proponents, and might be quite good, as many mothers have told me. However, I usually see the mothers only if the lanolin-based ointments have not worked, so it is difficult for me to come to any conclusion. Other ointments (e.g., vitamin E) that mothers have used have not, in my experience, been much good. But again, I don't tend to see mothers for whom these treatments have worked. Don't forget, nipple pain often does get better on its own.

3. I also teach mothers with sore nipples the technique of breast compression. Why? For several reasons. If the baby spends less time on the breast, the mother often experiences more rapid healing of her nipples. If the mother has enough milk, the use of compression often allows her to finish the feeding on just the one side. Not putting the baby to the second side spares that side some trauma, if it is the baby's latching on to the breast that is causing the mother pain. And finally, many mothers complain that the pain of the breastfeeding gets better after a few minutes, but often worsens again as the feeding goes on. This often corresponds to the baby spending most of his time nibbling, rather than actually breastfeeding. If the compression gets the baby drinking again, the pain often decreases.

4. Paper or even cotton breast pads can make the irritation and inflammation to the nipples worse. Wet material rubbing against the

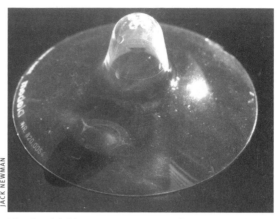

Nipple shield. A poor treatment for sore nipples, I believe. There may be *some* justification in using it for a baby who won't latch on, but even then, only after the mother has developed a good milk supply and nothing else is working.

nipple and areola may cause *maceration* of the area, a rawness caused by the combination of wetness and friction. It is best to keep nipples exposed to the air as much as possible. When this is not possible, breast shells—plastic domes that cover the nipples—can be worn between feedings to protect the mother's nipples from rubbing by clothing or pads. They often help a lot. But they also may cause inconveniences. Some mothers leak more with the breast shells than they would without. If this is only a little more, breast pads may be worn over the shells, but in some cases the mother fills up the shells in minutes, and so they are not useful. In some cases mothers complain of the shell digging into their skin; if the mother does get more pain, it is better not to use the shells. However, these shells usually come with two sizes of hole for letting in the nipple and areola. The smaller hole is for pushing out the nipple so that it is not inverted. This is not the size to use if you are using a breast shell to protect the nipples from clothing or breast pads. The larger one may reduce some of the discomfort and leaking.

5. Nipple shields are mentioned here only to be condemned. Nipple shields are plastic nipples worn over the nipple while the baby is breast-feeding (not between feedings, as is the breast shell discussed in # 4) and are often recommended for two reasons: to help a baby who is refusing the breast to take the breast, or for sore nipples. I believe that for sore nipples, it is a useless and harmful approach and should never be used. The fact that occasionally a mother has gotten relief from using a nipple shield is not an argument for its use. I believe the approaches mentioned earlier would have given the mother quicker and better relief. When a nipple shield is used, the mother runs a real risk of the baby later refusing the breast, and of her milk supply decreasing. However, as a last resort, when the mother has tried everything up to taking the baby off the breast, it can be attempted. If it works, it works, but the mother should really only try the nipple shield while being closely followed by an experienced lactation specialist.

What If Nothing Works?

If nothing else works, time often does. Not always, but often. For some reason, perhaps the fact that the baby grows older and sucks better or more efficiently, by the time her baby is six to eight weeks of age, the mother often does get painless feedings, regardless of what did or didn't help previously. Many "failures," however, are due to a late start with treatment. It is important that if the mother is not starting to experience less pain by the third or fourth day after the baby's birth, she seek help from a competent lactation specialist.

But what if the mother can't keep going until the pain gets better by itself? There are some last-resort options that are still better than stopping breastfeeding altogether.

Take the baby off the breast and feed the baby expressed milk

This is an option I hate to advise, but it may sometimes be necessary. Unfortunately, it is also an option that is suggested too often before the mother has been able to try everything else first. When I hear that a mother was advised to take her four-day-old baby off the breast "so the nipples will heal," I shudder. Surely we haven't tried everything first. Surely, here, too, is a situation where help has come too late, because if the nipples are that sore that early, something should have been done on day one.

Admittedly, sometimes the pain is so bad that there may be no choice. What should be done and how?

First of all, most mothers in this situation find expressing milk less painful than actually having the baby at the breast. But not always. Many mothers are just as efficient at expressing by hand as with an electric pump, but this takes experience, and, at first, many mothers find hand expression slower. If a pump hurts, though, hand expression usually does not.

How should the milk be given? Probably the best way would be with a cup. It is faster than finger-feeding, and less likely to interfere with breastfeeding than a bottle. If the baby is a good finger-feeder, I would suggest that way as the best, but most babies do take their time with finger-feeding. A combined finger-feeding and cup-feeding routine could be tried. However, I am not so high in an ivory tower as to deny that many mothers will opt for the bottle. If the mother must, she must. As long as the mother has a good milk supply, and maintains it by frequent pumping, there is a strong chance to get the baby to retake the breast once the nipples have healed.

How long should the baby be off the breast? At least a couple of days, probably more like three or four days and sometimes longer. We want good healing of the nipples so that when the baby goes back to the breast, the feedings are painless or virtually so. How long to take the baby off the breast is a judgment call, and may depend on the mother's milk supply, how badly her nipples are hurting, how well other treatments such as the ointment are working, how old the baby is, how close to the end of her rope the mother is, and many other factors. It is important to continue the all-purpose nipple ointment if it seems to be helping—three or four times a day at least, or after each expression.

Of course, the baby does not have to be taken off the breast completely. A couple of feedings in the day may make a return to the breast easier. Many mothers find the first morning feedings are less painful, not as long, and generally more pleasant. It might be possible to maintain these feedings, and then have the baby off the breast for the other feedings of the day.

If the mother has only one sore nipple and the other is fine, she should continue feeding the baby on the painless side. If the baby does not seem to be getting enough just from the one side, the mother may give the expressed milk by lactation aid on the painless side, as discussed below.

Another "In-Between" Option

It may be possible to express the milk from one side, and feed the baby only on one breast at each feeding, using a lactation aid to give the expressed milk. In this situation, I would suggest introducing the lactation aid tube fairly early in the feeding (say, after five or ten minutes, depending on the mother's soreness), so that the feeding goes quickly. Many mothers find that if they can keep the baby to one breast at a feeding and be relatively sure the baby will not want to feed for the next three hours, say, they can manage. If a baby feeds one breast at a feeding and goes three hours between feedings, that means the baby only nurses at each breast every six hours. If the mother is unable to express enough, or the baby is already being supplemented, the infant formula can be given through the lactation aid so that the baby feeds on only one breast.

Hypersensitive Nipples

I mention this "entity" to be complete. Once in a while, not even every year, I see a mother who has what seem to be hypersensitive and extremely sore nipples. The mother will often say that she had this problem always, that her nipples hurt during pregnancy, and that breastfeeding was extremely painful right from the first feeding. Nothing has made one bit of difference. I must admit, I don't know what this is or how it happens, and I have no good answer for the problem. In one case I remember, the mother was able to express by pump and feed the baby the breastmilk by bottle. The nipples were still somewhat painful while she pumped, but much less so than when she put the baby to the breast. Nothing we tried over the first three months made any difference. Interestingly, the baby always latched on well, even when he had not been tried on the breast for two or three weeks or even longer. I remember one occasion when we tried the baby on the breast after a month of no breastfeeding, and the baby went on beautifully, but the mother could not tolerate his nursing. The mother gave him breastmilk for about six months.

Candida Albicans

Candida albicans is one of more than 100 different species grouped together in the candida family of fungi. Most are not known to cause illness in humans, but about seven are. *Candida albicans* is the most common cause of illness in this group.

It is said that about 90 percent of all newborns are colonized with this organism within a few hours of birth. *Candida albicans* is generally a pretty benign organism, and rarely causes serious problems unless a person is immunocompromised (unable to mount an effective defense against infections, as in persons with AIDS, or very premature babies with long-standing intravenous lines, for example). As many women know, however, it can cause irritating symptoms in the vagina, and as many mothers know, it may cause thrush in the baby's mouth (seen as white patches inside the baby's cheeks or on his tongue) and sometimes diaper rash. *Candida albicans* likes warm, moist, dark areas. Under normal conditions, though, it lives on or in our bodies in a sort of harmony with us and our other microorganisms.

Candida albicans lives essentially in two forms. One is a yeast form, which can be seen under the microscope as a round cell. This form does not cause problems. It can also be transformed into a hyphal form, when it is stretched out into long filaments or threads—again, seen only under the microscope. This is the form that causes problems.

Antibiotics kill some bacteria, with some antibiotics having a wider spectrum than others. When someone is treated with antibiotics, most of the sensitive organisms are killed or prevented from reproducing. This allows for other, nonsensitive organisms to take advantage of the available nutrients. One organism not sensitive to most antibiotics is *Candida albicans*, so the use of antibiotics gives it a chance to run amok. This is not to say that it is never appropriate to use antibiotics. Indeed, the use of antibiotics can occasionally be lifesaving, and can often decrease the length of illness. But the overgrowth of resistant organisms, including *Candida albicans*, has to be considered as a significant side effect.

Diagnosing *Candida Albicans*

It is now obvious that some mothers get nipple pain due to infection with *Candida albicans* of the nipple. The baby would develop thrush, and the mother would start to get nipple pain at or about the same time. Sharp observers noted that there was often a difference in the symptoms that the mother gave when she described her pain.

- The pain of a poor latch is usually worse when the baby just latches on, and fades as the feeding goes on. Only in the severest cases does the mother have pain throughout the feeding, and even then, the pain still tends to decrease as the feeding goes on.

  In the case of a candidal infection of the nipples, the mother usually describes pain throughout the feeding, often continuing after the feeding is over.

- The pain associated with a poor latch remains limited to the nipple and areola, at least in most cases.

  In the case of a candidal infection of the nipples, the pain may radiate into the mother's back or shoulder. The mother often feels pain in the breast as well.

- The pain of a poor latch is often described as "knifelike" or "stabbing." In the case of a candidal infection, the mother often describes the pain as "burning."

None of these symptoms is absolute, and there may be a combination of factors involved in the mother's nipple pain—she can certainly have both a poor latch *and* a candidal infection.

In addition to the above symptoms, another factor that may be helpful in diagnosing a candidal infection of the nipples is that it frequently begins after a period of pain-free nursing for the mother. By contrast, sore nipples from a poor latch usually develop soon after the baby's birth. This feature alone should be enough to make the mother, or those helping her, think of a candidal infection. However, as mentioned above, other causes of sore nipples may begin after a period of pain-free nursing (eczema, nipple blister).

Other factors may suggest the possibility of a candidal infection. These are as follows:

1. Recent use of antibiotics by the mother and/or the baby. Recent use of antibiotics does not guarantee that a mother's nipple pain is due to a candidal infection, but it is something to keep in mind. Note, however, that in most North American hospitals, mothers who have caesarean sections almost always get a dose of antibiotics during the procedure. Of course, even if neither mother nor baby received antibiotics, the problem could still be candida.

2. The baby has thrush or a diaper rash due to *Candida albicans*. This, again, is only suggestive. A baby does not have to have thrush or a "yeasty" diaper rash for the mother to have sore nipples due to *Candida albicans*. And the fact that the baby does have thrush or a "yeasty" diaper rash does not always mean the mother's nipple soreness is due to *Candida albicans*.

3. The fact that the mother has a vaginal infection with *Candida albicans* does not mean that her nipple pain is due to it. On the other hand, the absence of other sites of infection does not mean that the mother does not have a candidal infection of her nipples.

How does Candida albicans *develop?*

Many mothers who have been diagnosed with a candidal infection of the nipples are concerned about why they got it and where they got it. As mentioned above, almost all humans are colonized with *Candida albicans*, often within hours of birth. There is nothing the mother has done wrong, nothing the mother should have done, or kept cleaner or whatever, to prevent colonization with *Candida albicans*.

Pregnancy itself increases the risk of problems with *Candida albicans*, as many mothers know, as does being on the birth control pill. Diabetes increases the risk as well, and a significant number of women have high blood sugar during pregnancy. As mentioned previously, the use of antibiotics can increase the risk of the mother developing problems with *Candida albicans*.

A poor beginning with breastfeeding can also allow *Candida albicans* to proliferate and invade. It has been shown that growth of *Candida albicans* is enhanced by breakdown of normal skin, and friction and trauma allow the *Candida albicans* to invade. Furthermore, many women have oozing of serum or blood from wounds caused by a poor latch. The conversion of *Candida albicans* from the yeast form to the more aggressive hyphal form occurs rapidly in the presence of human serum.

Thus, even infection of the nipple with *Candida albicans* is promoted by nipple injury caused by a poor latch in the first few days. The prevention of nipple soreness due to *Candida albicans* starts with a good latch from day one.

Treatment of Sore Nipples
Due to *Candida Albicans*

There are many methods of treating a candidal infection of the nipples. One of the problems, however, is that it is becoming more resistant to many of the medications that have been used for years. The following is my approach to the treatment of a candidal infection of the nipples.

Gentian violet

Gentian violet is a fairly old treatment for *Candida albicans*. It has considerable advantages:

- It is not necessary to have a prescription, since it is sold over the counter. This makes it easy to get treatment for a painful condition when your physician is not available.
- It works most of the time. It also works quickly.
- It is an easy way to treat both the baby and the mother at the same time.
- It is inexpensive.

There are, however, some concerns about using gentian violet:

- It is messy, and although it does not stain permanently, clothing may require a few washes to get it out completely.
- On rare occasions, usually when gentian violet has been used improperly, babies have developed ulcers in their mouths. However, stopping the gentian violet has resulted in healing of the ulcers within 24 hours. I must emphasize that this has been a rare problem. I have seen it in only three or four babies out of hundreds for whom I have suggested this treatment.

- Some mothers and physicians are concerned because gentian violet is dissolved in 10 percent alcohol. However, the amount the baby gets is tiny; he is being given a drop or two each day, and most of that is not swallowed.
- Preparations of gentian violet sold in pharmacies usually say that it is toxic. All drugs are toxic. Side effects of gentian violet, in my experience, are extremely uncommon and disappear quickly once the gentian violet is stopped.
- There is also concern that gentian violet may be carcinogenic (inducing the development of cancer). This is based on a study done in mice where the mice were fed huge amounts of gentian violet every day for either approximately half their natural lives or approximately all their natural lives ("approximately," because their lives did not end naturally). Those that were fed the gentian violet for approximately their entire natural lives had a higher incidence of liver cancers than did those that did not get any gentian violet. However, those that were fed the gentian violet for approximately half their natural lives did not have an increase in liver cancers. Furthermore, even the mice who had no gentian violet had a high incidence of liver cancers, which suggests they were bred to develop it. Based on this sort of study, I would have no concern about my baby receiving gentian violet. Indeed, one of mine did get gentian violet, and it cured his thrush, and my wife's problems within a day or two. At the end of the three-day treatment, the level of gentian violet in the bottle did not seem to have gone down— that's how little seems to be needed.

Using gentian violet

1. Gentian violet spreads quickly and goes everywhere, so the baby should be undressed down to his diaper, and the mother from the waist up. Don't use the gentian violet while sitting on your new white plush sofa.

2. Take a clean ear swab, dip it into the gentian violet and paint the inside of the baby's mouth. It will take about a second or two for the gentian violet to spread around the baby's mouth.

3. When the baby's mouth (and lips, not necessary, but inevitable) are purple, the mother should put the baby onto the breast.

4. At the end of the feeding, the baby's mouth

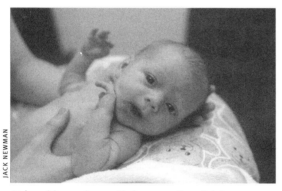

Baby with purple mouth from gentian violet.

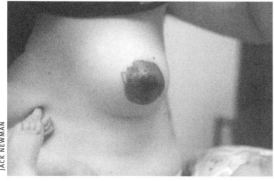

Mother has painted nipple and areola with gentian violet since it did not transfer from baby's mouth when the baby took the breast.

will still be purple, and the mother's nipples and areolas may be purple. If her nipples are not purple, she should paint them with a clean ear swab dipped in gentian violet.

The mother does this once a day for four to seven days. After this time, there should be considerable relief if the mother's problem is due to *Candida albicans*. Indeed, most mothers will have considerable lessening of the pain within a few hours of the first application, if the pain is due to *Candida albicans*. If not, the possibility that the mother's pain is not due to *Candida albicans* should be considered. This statement was truer several years ago when gentian violet treatment rarely failed, but it still has some validity.

5. Don't forget that any artificial nipples that the baby takes, including pacifiers, should also be treated with gentian violet (or boiled) once a day.

Using all-purpose nipple ointment

Due to increasing resistance of *Candida albicans* to many of our treatments, I have suggested recently that mothers combine the gentian violet treatment with the all-purpose nipple ointment referred to on page 110. The mother uses the gentian violet once a day for three or four days. After all the other feedings (except the one during which she used the gentian violet), she applies the all-purpose nipple ointment, sparingly, and does not wash or wipe it off (even just before the next feeding).

The ointment contains more than antifungal agents, as noted earlier. There is a steroid that decreases inflammation. However, like many infections, the pain or other symptoms are more often due to the inflammation that accompanies the infection, rather than the infection per se. This is why I include it, despite the fact that steroids may favor, under certain circumstances, the growth of *Candida albicans*. The antibiotic may help even for a fungal infection, since *Candida albicans* often lives in harmony with certain bacteria, and the presence of these bacteria contributes to the conditions it requires to multiply and cause infection. For this reason, even in cases of definite candidal infection, I prefer the combination rather than, say, clotrimazole or nystatin alone or even combined.

If the mother gets good relief, she should stop the gentian violet after three or four days, and slowly decrease the use of the all-purpose nipple ointment over a week or so. If she does not, she should stop the gentian violet, continue the all-purpose nipple ointment, and check back with her doctor or lactation specialist. If there is partial relief of the pain, gentian violet can be continued up to a week. If it has not worked in that time, it probably won't work at all.

All-purpose nipple ointment could be used alone for *Candida albicans* of the nipple, and can work just as well as gentian violet. However, it does not treat the baby's mouth. Gentian violet is a good treatment for the baby's mouth.

We have been using grapefruit seed extract more and more, not only suggesting that mothers take it by mouth, but also use the liquid form directly on the nipples. Sometimes it can be used alone, but usually we suggest the mother paint a diluted solution (5–15 drops in an ounce of water) directly onto the nipples and areolas, and then use the all purpose nipple ointment, after each feeding, except the feeding the mother uses the gentian violet. We have also found that using grapefruit seed extract orally, either alone or in conjunction with fluconazole, helps with breast pain associated with *Candida albicans*. The oral dose is 250 mg three times a day. It can be continued after fluconazole has been stopped to prevent relapses.

Other treatments

Acidophilus capsules have been used to treat or prevent infections with *Candida albicans*. It is difficult to know, based on anecdotal evidence, how well this works. Some mothers swear by acidophilus, but others have not found it useful. I would not recommend acidophilus as the only treatment for a candidal infection of the nipples or any other area, but it can be used in addition to other treatments.

Vinegar or bicarbonate of soda (baking soda) compresses to the nipple have also been used to treat candidal infection, apparently with some success. The soaks would presumably work by changing the acidity of the milieu in which the fungus is living, and thus interfering with its growth. I have not been overly impressed with how well these work, and, in fact, soaks may wash away essential oils and irritate the skin. Again, many mothers have, apparently, had significant relief—and if it works, it works.

"Yeast diets" may or may not work. I doubt it, but they may. The main problem is that they are so restrictive that they are a real hardship for most people to follow. Most of us would not find it difficult to eliminate alcohol from our diet, but what about sugar, bread, and dairy products?

Elimination of *Candida albicans* from the mother's environment is also neither practical nor of much use. Throwing away frozen milk collected while the mother has her problem with *Candida albicans* seems to me a terrible waste. Although freezing the milk does not kill *Candida albicans*, it is likely, given the antifungal factors in breastmilk, that the fungus will remain in the form that does not cause problems. Also, it is easier to stop wearing breast pads than to boil them daily, or pay for expensive disposable ones. The fact is that *Candida albicans* is with us all the time. It is impossible to get rid of it, and not necessary to try. The main thing is to reestablish a "normal" relationship with it.

To sum up, my usual recommendation for treating *Candida albicans* is as follows:

- Gentian violet, applied once a day for four to seven days. If the pain is gone after four days, stop using the gentian violet. If it is improved, but not completely gone, continue for seven days. If it is not improving at all after four days, stop the gentian violet and call your physician.

PLUS

- All-purpose nipple ointment (as described earlier in this chapter), used until the mother is pain-free, then gradually decreased over a week or so.

If the pain continues, and it is reasonably certain that the problem is *Candida albicans*, I add the following:

- Grapefruit seed extract orally and/or

- Fluconazole 400 mg at first and then 100 mg twice daily until the mother is pain-free for a full week.
- The nipple ointment should be continued and the gentian violet can be repeated. If fluconazole is too expensive, ketoconazole 400 mg loading, then 200 mg twice daily for the same period of time (or grapefruit seed extract can be used). If the Candida is resistant to this treatment, try itraconazole, same dose and time period as fluconazole, although Candida is generally less sensitive to itraconazole than it is to fluconazole. Fluconazole is apparently now available as a generic product (therefore less expensive). Fluconazole should not be used as a first-line treatment or if nystatin alone does not work.
- For deep breast pain, ibuprofen 200 to 400 mg every four hours can be used until the other treatments take effect. The maximum daily dose would be 1200 mg.

Sore nipples can be caused by a variety of things, but they are an eminently preventable problem. A good start and a good latch can prevent sore nipples in most mothers. However, much can be done when sore nipples occur. Get good help.

7

Sore Breasts

Myth: Pain in the breast indicates an infection requiring antibiotics.

Fact: Most pain in the breast is not a bacterial infection and therefore does not require treatment with antibiotics.

Engorgement on the Third or Fourth Day after Birth

You might be saying, "Well, surely, it is normal for the mother to become engorged on about the third or fourth day when the milk 'comes in.' And surely this engorgement hurts."

It is normal for women to feel a change in their breasts—a feeling of fullness that may make their breasts tender and sensitive to touch—within two to four days after baby is born. The amount of fullness is often less with a second, third, or later baby, and may be reduced further if the mother is also nursing a toddler as well as her newborn. It is not normal, however, for women to get such severe engorgement that the breasts are painful, swollen, and red. When breasts become so engorged that the mother is feeling more than discomfort, it is usually due to the fact that breastfeeding has been ineffective up until that time. The breasts should certainly not be so engorged that the baby cannot latch on; this generally means that the baby never latched on well, or at all, in the first place or that the baby was not allowed to nurse frequently enough.

Many lactation specialists do not like the phrase "the milk comes in," even though we tend to use it from force of habit. This phrase implies that there was no milk before, or that there was "only colostrum." "Only colostrum" is another phrase we dislike, because colostrum is no mean fluid. In fact, it is an extraordinary one. Saying that what the mother produces in the first few days is "only colostrum" allows some unhelpful health professionals to convince new mothers that they do not really have to put the baby to the breast at all during the first few days, that there is no harm in the baby not getting colostrum, and that if the mother and baby are separated and the mother can only express a few drops of colostrum (the usual situation), this is not worth the trouble. But it is worth giving the baby a few drops. And if the mother and baby are separated, it *is* worth expressing in the first few days even if only a few drops come out, and even if no colostrum can be expressed, since this breast stimulation will help the mother develop a good milk supply for later. There is enough colostrum during the first few days for the baby's needs, but only if the baby is latched on properly.

Colostrum is chock-full of antibodies, immune-competent white cells and long-chained poly-unsaturated fatty acids. It also has a fair amount of vitamin K, which helps protect the baby against bleeding. The amount of protein in colostrum is quite high, about three times greater than in mature milk, which helps maintain the baby's blood sugar at a time when some are at risk of low blood sugar. Colostrum is a very special fluid. We should sing its praises. But more importantly, we should make sure that, whenever possible, babies get it.

What to Do About Severe Engorgement

If severe engorgement does occur, it is important for the mother and those helping her to remember that it will last only a few days; the worst of it, probably 24 hours. It is also important to remember that the swollen, hard, painful appearance of the breasts does not represent mastitis (breast infection), which can look exactly the same. Mastitis only rarely occurs on both sides at the same time, and it does not often occur three or four days after birth. Fever usually occurs with mastitis, but it can also occur with severe engorgement (milk fever), so the presence of fever does not necessarily mean mastitis. Treatment of engorgement with antibiotics is inappropriate, and may lead to the later development of a candidal infection of the nipples or breast.

Severe engorgement results from more than milk "filling" up the breast. There is also fluid in the tissue, similar to the swelling that occurs in many pregnant women's ankles. This swelling is worse if the mother was given an IV during labor, because of the extra fluid introduced to her system. Engorgement is not only painful for the mother, but causes real problems with breastfeeding. The baby finds it difficult to get a good latch, because the breast is so hard that he can't get much of it in his mouth. This means he can't get much milk out, and the milk ducts may even collapse because of the pressure of the fluid-filled breast tissue. If the breasts continue to be engorged, milk supply will begin to decrease.

Luckily, in most cases, this is temporary, or not significant enough to make a difference to overall breastfeeding success.

Again, it should not be forgotten that severe engorgement can be prevented (see above). However, if it does occur, it should be treated promptly, as follows:

1. The mother may need some medication for pain. She doesn't need to stop breastfeeding because of this medication. Something like ibuprofen, because of its anti-inflammatory effects as well as its pain-relieving effects, is a good choice.
2. The latch needs improvement so the baby can extract milk more easily.
3. The mother should use compression during feedings to get the milk flowing. Once the milk flows, the tension in the breast decreases a little, and this allows milk to flow more rapidly still, improving the situation quite dramatically sometimes. Warm compresses should be used before putting the baby to the breast, or while the baby is nursing, as they may increase the flow of milk. Using the warm compresses is awkward while the baby is nursing, though, and I find compression more effective.
4. Cold compresses or packs after the feeding may decrease the engorgement.
5. Cabbage leaves seem to have a beneficial effect on engorgement, although no one really knows how or why. The cabbage leaves apparently should be of the green variety (not red), and should be placed around the breast after a feeding, three or four times a day, perhaps even after each feeding or each time you express milk. Some have said to keep them in place for about 20 minutes, others until the leaves wilt. As soon as engorgement

is decreasing, the mother should stop the cabbage leaves since some people believe they can decrease the milk supply.

6. The mother should express her milk after the feeding. Some unhelpful medical staff will tell the mother that she should not express her milk because this will increase the milk supply. If expressing increases the milk supply, good. But expressing milk will help decrease the engorgement and pain. Although a lot of the engorgement is not due to milk, getting out the milk will still help relieve the mother's symptoms. Furthermore, if the baby is reluctant to feed on the breast, he can get the expressed milk by cup or finger-feeding (see Chapter 5, Not Enough Milk).

But what if the baby is not taking the breast? The reason the baby refuses to take the engorged breast is that he cannot latch on due to the flattening of the nipple and areola and the hardness of the breast. So, the first thing to try to do is soften up the nipple and areola. This can be done with hand expression, which will soften up this area better than if the mother uses a pump. Once the nipple and areola are less flat and softened up, the baby may take the breast and breastfeed. Breastfeeding, not simply allowing the breast into his mouth, is the important thing.

Lactation consultant Jean Cotterman has developed a technique called Reverse Pressure Softening to help mothers with engorgement. Her description is in the box on this page.

If the baby still does not take the breast, then the breasts should be expressed and the baby fed with alternative methods. Cup-feeding, finger-feeding, or feeding by eyedropper or syringe—all are fine. But do not resort to a bottle.

Remember! Engorgement will get better within a couple of days.

Reverse Pressure Softening
Jean Cotterman RNC, IBCLC

More health care providers are observing that mothers who receive multiple intrapartum IV's [large amounts of IV fluids during labor and delivery] experience delay in expected post-partum fluid shift. Increased edema during the early postpartum period intensifies engorgement, increases subareolar tissue resistance, distorts the nipple, and interferes with comfortable, efficient latching.

I want to share an intervention that has proven very helpful in the first seven to 14 days postpartum. I call it Reverse Pressure Softening. This measure uses gentle positive pressure, and can be performed by the health care provider, and/or taught to the mother herself, if necessary, over the telephone.

Interstitial fluid volume can increase 30% above normal before it appears as edema to the naked eye (Guyton). Consequently, early proactive use of RPS can facilitate increased milk transfer, prevent nipple discomfort and damage, and speed resolution of engorgement.

Conversely, vacuum applied during this period has the potential to cause further accumulation of edema in the tissue within the pump flange area, especially when maximum settings are selected. Such an "extra layer of edema" can effectively bury the sinuses beneath the thickening areolar tissue. When this happens, neither infant tongue action, fingertip expression, nor the pump itself removes milk very successfully.

RPS is best performed immediately before each attempt to latch, for as many feedings as needed. Steady, gentle pressure inward toward the chest wall is exerted for a full 60 seconds or longer, focusing on the areola where it joins the base of the nipple. (A mother can be encouraged to sing a lullaby rather than watch the clock.)

If her fingernails are quite short, she can press with the curved fingertips of both hands simultaneously, with the nails nearly touching the sides of the nipple. The goal is to create a ring of six–eight small "dimples" or pits on the areola at the base of the nipple. If performed by the health care provider, the flats of two thumbs or two fingers can also be used sideways, creating an inch-long depression just above and below the nipple. But this will require another 60 seconds of pressure in opposite quadrants, partially overlapping the first set of pits, to soften the same general area at the base of the nipple.

If swelling is extremely firm, and the multiple fingertip method is being used, one or more three-minute periods of constant reverse pressure may yield better results. (Watching sand flowing through a three-minute egg-timer is one example of a relaxing way for a mother to avoid impatience and clock watching.)

However, if the flats of two thumbs or fingers are being used, a more even distribution of interstitial fluid is obtained by alternating quadrants repeatedly for three or more 60-second applications each.

The effect is threefold:

• Any excess interstitial fluid is temporarily moved inward in the direction of natural lymphatic drainage.

• Longitudinal compression of the sinuses displaces some milk slightly backward into the ducts. Relieving overdistention of the walls of the milk sinuses reduces latch discomfort. Elasticity is freed for drawing the nipple-areolar complex more deeply into the mouth and responding to the stripping action of the tongue.

• The milk ejection reflex is automatically triggered by the steady stimulation of nerves supplying the nipple-areolar complex, propelling milk toward the front of the breast, nearly always within 5 minutes or less.

After application of RPS, any additional fingertip expression necessary to further soften the areola is much easier, more comfortable, and more productive. If engorgement is severe, additional fingertip expression to create a special niche for the chin often permits deeper latching.

Guyton, AC, *Basic Human Physiology: Normal Function and Mechanisms of Disease,* 2nd ed., W. B. Saunders Co., Philadelphia, 1977, p. 321.

Blocked Ducts

A blocked duct is experienced as a hard, painful swelling that may include a significant part of the breast. It may or may not be associated with a milk blister or bleb on the nipple. Luckily, milk flow to the baby is not generally affected, but occasionally it is. A blocked duct will usually improve within 24 to 48 hours, regardless of whether the mother treats it. A blocked duct is not mastitis, and does not require treatment with antibiotics. However, it is not always easy to differentiate a blocked duct from mastitis. Differentiating the two may not be as important as one would think at first glance.

Blocked ducts are common and seem to be mostly, but not exclusively, the problem of the mother who has an abundant supply of milk. It has been suggested that they occur when babies only "half empty" the breast. (The term *half empty* is not really accurate, because the breast is never empty, but it helps sometimes to use the term for explanation.) If this is true, though, it is clear that the best prevention of blocked ducts is getting a good start at breastfeeding, and most importantly, getting as good a latch as possible from as early on as possible.

Treatment of Blocked Ducts

1. Pain should be relieved and the mother should not hesitate to use medication to treat the pain. Any number of medications can be used, including ibuprofen or acetaminophen, though the anti-inflammatory effects of ibuprofen probably make it better in this situation.

2. The baby should continue breastfeeding on the affected side. It is said that the duct unblocks more rapidly if the baby is positioned and latched on in such a way that his chin "points" to the area of blockage (that is, the chin is the part of the baby's face that is closest to the blocked duct). This may be so, but it is not always that practical. A mother with a blocked duct on the top of the breast would have to nurse with the baby lying on his back on a bed, with his feet pointed upward toward the mother's head, and the mother leaning over him on her hands and knees. You can certainly give it a try.

3. While the baby is breastfeeding on the affected side, it can help tremendously for the mother to compress the area of blocked duct. The compression should be steady and the pressure as much as the mother can reasonably tolerate. Sometimes it is worth taking some ibuprofen a couple of hours before an anticipated feed so that more pressure can be applied. I have been able to help a mother get rid of a blocked duct in minutes using this technique. The baby helps the mother by drawing on the breast, and the mother helps as well by putting pressure on the blocked duct.

4. If the mother has a milk blister associated with the blocked duct, it is worth opening it with a sterile needle, and, if possible, squeezing out any toothpastelike material that may come out. Often doing this results in immediate unblocking of the duct. Use the all-purpose nipple ointment after opening the bleb, after each feeding for about a week.

5. Do hot compresses or a heating pad over the area help? Perhaps. Heat should be used before a feeding to help milk flow. If it is soothing, keep using it.

6. Cabbage leaves should not be used for a blocked duct.

What if the above don't work? Well, patience usually does. As mentioned earlier, most blocked ducts settle within about 24 to 48 hours. Occasionally they take a little longer to resolve. However, if there is no relief in about 48 hours, ultrasound treatments may quickly unblock a blocked duct.

Ultrasound treatments do seem to work to unblock a duct, though not always. As well, ultrasound often prevents the blocked ducts from returning. It takes some practice with this technique for the operator to get consistently good results, and many physiotherapists or other ultrasound technicians have perhaps never heard of ultrasound for treating blocked ducts.

Repeated Blocked Ducts?

One cause of repeated blocked ducts may be pressure on one part of the breast.

Check your bra to be sure it isn't too snug in any areas. Nursing bras with a flap that pulls down leaving a "frame" around the rest of the breast are often the worst culprits. You may not need a larger bra, but need a larger cup size (e.g., you might be a D-cup now, rather than a C). Some mothers have also had blocked ducts where the straps of a baby carrier dug into their breasts. Treatment of recurrent blocked ducts is the same as for a single blocked duct.

The dose of the ultrasound is the following: 2 watts/centimeter squared, continuous for five minutes, once a day. Many ultrasound therapists worry because this is a high dose, but I am not aware of any mothers who have had any particular problems after the treatments. Mothers do feel heat when the ultrasound is applied, but that is all. Therapists also worry about using it when infection is present because they feel ultrasound may cause infection to spread. If true it should not be used when mastitis is present.

Usually one treatment is all that is necessary to resolve a blocked duct. Sometimes another treatment may be helpful the next day, but I have not found that more than two treatments has resulted in resolution if two treatments have not done the trick.

Nobody knows for sure how ultrasound helps, but it seems to in some situations.

Recurrent Blocked Ducts

The prevention and treatment of recurrent blocked ducts is the same as for a single blocked duct.

1. Ensure a good latch.
2. "Finish" the first side before offering the second, using compression, if necessary to help finish the first side.
3. Avoid constricting clothing.

I have also found that lecithin occasionally helps, although I don't know how it works.

Lecithin is a phospholipid that is found in many foods. Lecithin is available in capsule or liquid form in health food stores and most pharmacies. Lecithin is not expensive, it is not dangerous to use, it may even be good for the heart, and it does occasionally work for prevention of recurrent blocked ducts. The dose is one tablespoon, three or four times a day, or one to two capsules (1,200 mg each), three or four times a day.

Others have found evening primrose oil helps prevent recurring blocked ducts. The dose is the dose marked on the bottle. I have only occasionally suggested evening primrose oil. It seems to work in a majority of these cases, but a few cases do not constitute proof.

Persistent Blocked Duct

What if the blocked duct does not disappear? What if it lasts a week or two, or longer? Some blocked ducts do get slowly better and may take more than two weeks to disappear, but as long as they are getting smaller, I would not be concerned. However, what if the blocked duct remains without getting smaller? Even if the pain has disappeared, I would doubt that this is a typical blocked duct. What else could it be?

- It could be a milk cyst. Sometimes milk collects within a blocked duct or behind some obstruction to form a lump in the breast. Cysts are not usually painful or tender, but they can be, and probably the presence or absence of pain depends on how quickly they developed. The faster they develop, the more likely they are to be painful.
- I have seen a number of women with a persistent "blocked duct" for weeks and months, who eventually went to surgery for a biopsy, but no abnormality was found.
- I believe any lump that does not disappear, or

is not at least getting smaller after a couple of weeks, should be evaluated by a breastfeeding-friendly surgeon with experience in dealing with breast lumps. Unfortunately, too many surgeons are not breastfeeding-friendly and will tell the mother that nothing can be done until she has weaned the baby. This is untrue. Lots can be done while the mother is still breastfeeding, including the following, if these are necessary:

- ultrasound (for diagnosis, not treatment)
- needle aspiration or needle biopsy
- mammogram
- open biopsy

Even if it is truly necessary to wean on the affected breast (and it is almost never necessary, but some surgeons can be insistent), it is quite possible to continue breastfeeding on the other breast. This will not cause the affected breast to continue producing milk. Many surgeons, even those who are supportive of breastfeeding, don't realize that one breast can be allowed to "dry up" while the mother continues breastfeeding on the other breast.

Mastitis

Mastitis refers to a bacterial infection of part or all of a breast. Mastitis is always associated with a hard, swollen, red, painful area in the breast. Too many women have been diagnosed with mastitis because they have "flulike symptoms" and a fever. Without the changes in the breast, the diagnosis is more likely flu than mastitis. Any cause of fever, a cold, stomach "flu," pneumonia, or hundreds of other illnesses, will give "flulike symptoms," if by this we mean headache, muscle pains, joint pains, fatigue, malaise, chills, and sweats.

It is not always easy to differentiate mastitis from a blocked duct. Many of the criteria used to separate the two are not actually very helpful in making the differentiation. For example, the absence of fever makes the problem more likely a blocked duct, but mastitis may occur without fever. Similarly, if there is enough inflammation around a blocked duct, fever may occur. It is true that the fever associated with mastitis tends to be higher, but again, this is hardly useful, since fevers vary and the temperature obviously depends on when it was taken. It has been said that a blocked duct tends to come on slowly, and mastitis more rapidly, but I think this is false. Overall, mastitis is like a blocked duct, but more so, with the mother having more general symptoms associated with fever, mentioned above. The redness of the breast is often much angrier looking, and the affected area of the breast is frequently hotter.

In any case, it is my feeling that the differentiation of the two is usually not necessary. Both may improve spontaneously, without antibiotics, within 24 to 48 hours. My approach to treating mastitis is as follows:

1. If symptoms are present for more than 24 hours without improvement, the mother should start antibiotics.
2. If the mother has symptoms for less than 24 hours, I will give her a prescription for an antibiotic, but suggest that she wait before starting the medicine.
3. If, over the following eight to 12 hours, her symptoms become worse (more pain, spreading of the redness, enlargement of the hardened area), the mother should start the antibiotics.
4. If, 24 hours later, the symptoms have not

worsened, but also not improved, she should start the antibiotics.

5. If symptoms are starting to decrease, there is no need to start the antibiotics. The symptoms usually continue to resolve and will have disappeared over the next two to five days. Fever will usually be gone within 24 hours, the pain within 24 to 48 hours, the breast hardness within the next couple of days. The redness may remain for a week or longer.

My impression, from our experience in the clinic, is that at least 50 percent of women treated as above never need to start the antibiotics.

The bacterium that causes mastitis is almost always *Staphylococcus aureus*, and if antibiotics are needed, one that is active against this bacterium should be chosen. [Occasionally, *Staphylococcus aureus* is responsive to amoxycillin, or plain penicillin, but in this day and age, this is unusual because of increasing resistance.] Generally, my antibiotic of choice is cephalexin, 500 mg, four times a day for 10 days. Though penicillinase-resistant penicillins are available (e.g., cloxacillin, dicloxacillin, flucloxacillin) and usually quite effective, I have run into several situations when such drugs just did not seem to work, and the mother then responded to cephalexin. Of course, if everyone starts to use cephalexin, it, too, will soon become ineffective. Other possible choices for treatment of mastitis are amoxycillin combined with clavulinic acid, clindamycin, and ciprofloxacin.

A good response to antibiotics is decreasing symptoms within about 24 hours, and in many cases complete resolution of symptoms within about three to five days of starting the antibiotics.

Heat applied to mastitis helps, because heat helps fight off infection. Local heat (heating pad, for example) can help the infection resolve more quickly. Make sure that any local heat is not so hot, or not applied so long, that the skin is damaged. Fever also helps fight infection, and anyone with infection should not treat fever merely because the fever is there. Granted, an adult who has fever often feels terrible, but in this situation treatment of fever is directed to helping the person feel better, not to bringing down the fever. This may seem like splitting hairs, but if someone has a fever and does not feel bad (as is the case frequently with young children), there is no need to bring the fever down.

If the mother does need to treat the symptoms caused by fever, an anti-inflammatory medication is preferable to one that only brings down the fever. Ibuprofen is thus preferable to acetaminophen. Acetylsalicylic acid (ASA, aspirin) can also be used. Though many feel a concern about nursing mothers using ASA, I believe this fear, especially when the ASA is used for only a day or two, is greatly exaggerated.

One benefit of the fever that often goes along with this condition is that it usually makes the mother feel sick enough that she just wants to climb into bed and rest. When you have an infection, rest is good. Tuck the baby into bed with you, of course.

Do I continue breastfeeding?

There is no doubt that continuing breastfeeding is better for the mother (and the baby) when a mother has mastitis. First, the mother will be far more comfortable if her breast is drained. Adding engorgement to mastitis makes the breast more painful still. Expressing milk with a pump or by hand does not make any sense when the baby will do the job much more effectively. Second, the infection is likely to clear up more quickly if the mother continues breastfeeding.

There is absolutely no evidence that the baby is at risk by continuing breastfeeding. After all, breastfeeding mothers and their babies are in such intimate contact, they share a common bacterial flora. The best protection for the baby is to continue breastfeeding. I have now treated many women for mastitis and advised continuation of breastfeeding. In no case has the baby ever gotten ill.

Of course, there are times when the pain of the infection is so bad that the mother just cannot put the baby to the breast. However, if treatment is effective, she should be able to put the baby back to that breast within 12 to 24 hours.

It is also true that frequently a mother can feel so ill with mastitis that she does not have much strength or energy. The best approach is for her to go to bed with her baby, and to continue nursing. Usually, after treatment, she will be feeling better within 24 to 48 hours.

Breast Abscess

An abscess is a pocket of pus formed in an infected area. It is almost always due to delayed or inadequate treatment of an infective process. Believe it or not, abscess formation is actually a protective strategy of the body to localize infection and to keep it from spreading. Without any medical interference, an abscess will eventually work its way toward the skin or some other surface, and then break open so that the pus is discharged. If the pus is discharged out of the skin, this will lead to eventual healing. Of course, either because of their location (e.g., the brain) or because of where they discharge (e.g., into the abdominal cavity), abscesses are not completely benign and can even cause death. Generally, however, a breast abscess, though painful and causing the mother to feel unwell, is not dangerous.

The Typical Story of a Breast Abscess

In some cases, mastitis will proceed to a breast abscess within 24 to 48 hours. This rapid progression is unusual, but I have heard of it occurring at least once. In such a case, I would think that even early use of antibiotics would not have prevented the problem. But most of the time abscesses seem to have developed either because of a long delay in initiating treatment, or because the treatment was ineffective. Almost all the breast abscesses I have seen in nursing mothers can be attributed to these two causes. (You don't have to be a nursing mother to develop a breast abscess. It may occur in nonpregnant, nonbreastfeeding women. It may occur even in newborn babies, regardless of their sex.)

The typical course of a breast abscess is as follows:

1. A nursing mother develops signs and symptoms of mastitis.
2. She is treated, sooner or later, with an antibiotic.
3. Her symptoms improve somewhat but not completely.
4. When the antibiotics are discontinued, the mother often has a worsening of her symptoms, often within 24 to 48 hours.
5. The above cycle is repeated once or many times, until someone makes the diagnosis.

Thus, any mother with mastitis that has not completely resolved within five days or so after starting antibiotics (or, at the very least, is not improving dramatically) should see her physician again to make sure abscess formation has not occurred. If the physcian does not believe an abscess has formed, a change of antibiotics would be reasonable.

How to Diagnose an Abscess

Typically, a mother with a breast abscess will have a lump in her breast that is very tender when squeezed, even gently. There may or may not be redness of the skin, though there usually is. Sometimes the redness can be quite dramatic. On occasion, however, the abscess does not seem tender. I have seen this at least twice, and have aspirated the lump expecting milk to come out, giving a diagnosis of a milk cyst. In both cases I was surprised to pull out pus. Sometimes it is obvious that there is fluid in the lump. Sometimes the abscess is already beginning to move to the skin.

A mother who has the above history and feels a lump in her breast that is quite tender should assume she has an abscess.

The easiest way to diagnose an abscess is to aspirate it with a needle and syringe. This method gives an immediate answer, is more reliable than ultrasound (which can only tell if there is fluid in the lump), is relatively painless (if done correctly), gives a specimen for culture (and thus information for appropriate antibiotics), and gives the mother considerable relief, at least temporarily.

Treatment of an Abscess

Although on occasion a small abscess may resolve with repeated aspirations and the use of appropriate antibiotics, almost always the definitive treatment requires open drainage of the abscess. This means surgery. Antibiotics alone will not cure an abscess. Though repeated aspirations may occasionally work, this process represents frequent visits to the physician or surgeon, sometimes over a fairly prolonged period of time (a couple of weeks)—and even then, there is no guarantee of success. However, more and more breast surgeons are, in fact, successfully treating breast abcesses with repeated aspirations.

Our experience in the clinic shows the following:

- Surgery can be done on an outpatient basis in almost all cases, almost always with local anesthesia. Even if general anesthesia is necessary, there is no reason for the mother to stay in the hospital overnight.
- The mother can almost always continue breastfeeding on the affected side. Mothers from our clinic who have had abscesses drained have nursed up to the moment they go in to surgery, and immediately after the surgery is over, as soon as they are up to it.
- There is about a 7 percent recurrence of abscess reported in the surgical literature. This recurrence rate is not increased by having the surgery under local anesthesia or by continuing breastfeeding.

Surgeons may know about surgery, but generally they do not know a lot about breastfeeding. Thus there are some issues that need to be considered.

- The incision should be done as far away from nipple and areola as practical. If the incision is done near the areola, the mother may not be able to put the baby to the breast either because of pain, or because the baby's sucking will interfere with healing.
- The incision should not be done along the line dividing the areola from the rest of the breast. Many surgeons do this for "aesthetic reasons," but such an incision often interferes with milk production. Furthermore, it makes getting the baby breastfeeding after surgery more difficult.
- Incisions should be "radial" not "circumferential," and as short as possible without interfering with proper drainage of the abscess.

Circumferential incisions are likely to damage more ducts.

• Even if for some reason it is believed that the mother should not breastfeed on the affected side, this is not a reason the mother need stop on the other side. Many surgeons (and other health care professionals, for that matter) believe that if breastfeeding continues on the other side, milk production will continue on the operated side. This is not true. (A mother can "dry up" on one side only, by not feeding on that side.)

I usually continue using antibiotics after the surgery to make sure that the infection does not persist. Surgery cures the abscess, but there may be areas of infection in the breast tissue that could spread.

Should breastfeeding continue on the affected side?

Yes, if at all possible. Sometimes it is stopped, because the incision has to be made so close to the areola that the mother cannot put the baby to the breast. Or sometimes there is such swelling of the breast tissue that the baby cannot latch on. But as soon as the mother can, she should try to put the baby back to the breast. If the mother cannot put the baby to the breast, she should express her milk. If using a pump is painful, expression by hand may be less so. But if both are painful, she might as well put the baby to the breast.

Is an abscess more likely with the next baby?

I don't believe anyone has studied this, but I would guess the answer is no. An abscess occurs when a breast infection is inadequately treated. Breast infections usually occur because of a poor start with breastfeeding. The best treatment is prevention.

Candida Albicans as a Cause of Sore Breasts

While *Candida albicans* is usually thought of as a cause of nipple pain, it can also be a cause of pain in the breast. Breast pain caused by *Candida albicans* can be severe or mild or anything in between. It has the following characteristics:

• The pain usually begins late in the feeding, or after the feeding is over.
• The pain is usually worse in the evenings.
• The pain is generally of a "shooting" nature, or frequently described as "burning."
• The pain may be felt throughout the breast and sometimes in the mother's shoulder or back.
• The pain may last for minutes or hours.
• The pain may begin early on after the baby is born or months later.

Because the pain, which usually responds to treatment for *Candida albicans*, can sometimes occur without any associated nipple pain, it has been suggested that it is due to an infection with *Candida albicans* in the ducts of the breast. This is certainly possible, though it has never been proved.

Treatment for Breast Pain Due to *Candida Albicans*

The treatment for breast pain due to *Candida albicans* is the same as for nipple pain due to *Candida albicans*. Though local treatment (gentian violet, nipple ointment) is less likely to help than for nipple pain, it is worth trying first, especially if the mother has to pay out of her own pocket for oral antifungal agents (they are quite expensive). If, however, the pain is severe or has not responded to local treatments, oral treatment with grapefruit seed extract or fluconazole (as outlined in the section on sore nipples with *Candida albicans*) is indicated. If the mother has nipple pain as well, local treatment should definitely be used. Treatment of the nipple pain alone will often get rid of the breast pain, since in some cases the breast pain is probably "referred" pain—pain experienced in a different part of the body from the actual location of the problem or injury.

Other Causes of Sore Breasts

Raynaud's Phenomenon (see Chapter 6, Sore Nipples) may cause breast pain. The diagnosis is made by observing blanching of the nipples after the feeding is over.

Injuries of the breast (for example, bruising caused by a fall) can be very painful. Breastfeeding should continue if possible, and the pain be treated with ibuprofen or acetaminophen or other pain relievers.

Other Breast and Nipple Conditions

"Rusty Pipe" Syndrome
(bleeding from the nipples)

New mothers may have painless bleeding from the nipples just after the baby is born. This is obviously quite alarming, but it is not dangerous for you or the baby. It is true that swallowing blood may cause the baby to spit up much more, and may also cause him to have black or bloody bowel movements, but again, this is not dangerous, just alarming to see. On occasion, the bleeding may have been noticed during the pregnancy, or it may start much later than immediately after birth. Typically, however, it occurs just after the baby is born. Often the mother is not aware that this is happening, and it only becomes obvious if she is expressing her milk for

some reason, or the baby spits up blood or passes it in his bowel movements.

The best thing is to just keep breastfeeding. The blood usually disappears by about seven days or less after the baby is born.

Nobody knows why this happens, and it is presumed that the increased blood flow to the breast is somehow related.

If the bleeding persists for longer than a week or two, especially if it is occurring on one side only, it is better to see a breastfeeding-friendly, experienced breast surgeon.

Eczema of the Nipple

Rarely, one-sided eczema of the nipple is associated with breast cancer on that side, and is called Paget's disease of the nipple. Any one-sided eczema that does not respond rapidly to a steroid, should be investigated by a breastfeeding-friendly, experienced breast surgeon.

Lumps in the Breast

Most nursing mothers have various areas of the breast that are lumpy. These areas of fullness often migrate around the breast, and though occasionally a little tender, are not painful. It is not always easy to separate them from other lumps that may represent various other entities.

Any lump that is getting smaller is almost certainly nothing to worry about. A lump that is persistent, however, should be investigated. Two or three weeks with a lump that is not getting smaller should be reason for the mother to seek an opinion. Luckily, most lumps in the breast are benign—but it is safer to be sure.

Many, many women will never experience the problems described in this chapter. Nevertheless, it's best to be aware of the symptoms and what can be done about them.

8

Jaundice

Myth: A baby who is jaundiced should be taken off the breast until his bilirubin goes down.

Fact: It is almost never necessary to stop breastfeeding because of jaundice. Not only is it not necessary, but it is not good, because the baby is deprived of breastfeeding. Furthermore, stopping breastfeeding even for a day or two may make breastfeeding more difficult, even impossible, for the mother.

Jaundice is very common in newborn babies. Why is jaundice considered to be such a big problem? Why are so many mothers being told to stop breastfeeding so that the baby's bilirubin will come down? What harm does it do the baby to be jaundiced?

First let's look at what causes jaundice in newborn babies and why it is sometimes a concern.

Physiology of Jaundice

Bilirubin is the pigment in the blood that makes the jaundiced baby look yellow. It is formed in our bodies when our red blood cells die—a normal process. When red blood cells die, the hemoglobin contained in the cell breaks down, and one of the components is bilirubin. This bilirubin is fat soluble and not water soluble. For the body to get rid of it, it needs to be made water soluble. This is one of the jobs of the liver: to take the fat-soluble bilirubin and add a biochemical piece to it to make

it water soluble. Once the bilirubin is water soluble, it leaves the liver and eventually passes into the intestines. Most then leaves the body through bowel movements, but some is reabsorbed into the body after being made fat soluble again by removal of that biochemical piece. This cycle is called the *enterohepatic circulation of bilirubin* (*entero* refers to intestine, and *hepato* to the liver). Water-soluble bilirubin is also called *direct bilirubin* (in the test that's done to measure it, the amount is measured directly) or *conjugated bilirubin* (the process that makes it water soluble is called conjugation). The fat-soluble bilirubin is called *indirect bilirubin* or *unconjugated bilirubin*. All three names (fat soluble, indirect, unconjugated) and (water soluble, direct, conjugated) refer to the same things, but the variety of names can be confusing. You may hear medical personnel use any or all of these terms.

It is interesting that the body does not have to make bilirubin to break down and dispose of the hemoglobin. In fact, it takes more energy to make bilirubin than it would for the body to get rid of the hemoglobin by other routes. For this reason, some scientists have suggested that bilirubin must perform a useful function in the body. It is believed that bilirubin protects the baby against the effects of oxygen free radicals, formed during other metabolic processes, which can injure normal tissue. This will be brought up again when I discuss breastmilk jaundice.

Why do newborn babies develop a visible "yellowness," or jaundice? If you look at the explanation of how bilirubin is metabolized, you can actually figure it out, especially for abnormal situations.

1. Too much bilirubin is being formed

In the normal situation, a newborn baby has more red cells in a single milliliter of blood than does an adult. Furthermore, the cells of the newborn have shorter lifespans, so at any given moment, a baby is breaking down considerably more red cells for his size than an adult. This is part of the explanation of "physiologic" jaundice. *Physiologic* simply means what happens normally in the body.

In an abnormal situation, if more than the average number of red cells are dying, more bilirubin is formed. What might cause an abnormally high number of red blood cells to die?

The classic situation occurs with Rh incompatibility. During pregnancy, a mother with Rh− blood may develop antibodies against her baby's blood cells if the baby's blood cells are Rh+. This occurs because red blood cells can leak across the placenta from the baby to the mother. The mother's immune system recognizes the antigen on the red cells (an antigen is a molecule, usually a protein, that provokes production of an antibody) as something that is not part of the mother's body and starts producing antibodies against it. These antibodies can pass back across the placenta and start destroying the baby's red cells (a process called hemolysis). In severe cases, these babies can be jaundiced from birth, because cells were being destroyed even before the babies were born. So many red cells can be destroyed so quickly that the baby develops severe anemia and may even go into heart failure. In the past, many of these babies developed mental retardation, spasticity, and deafness—some even died. It is

for this reason that so many physicians are frightened of jaundice.

Rh incompatibility often caused such serious problems not only because of the high bilirubin, but because babies who were suffering from this problem also had severe metabolic problems, heart failure, and severe anemia. We are now aware that these factors had more to do with the damage done to the baby than did the high bilirubin alone. There is actually no evidence that a high bilirubin, unless extremely high, has any bad effect on the baby.

The good news is that most physicians who graduated after 1980 have never seen a case of Rh incompatibility. The virtual disappearance of this problem, at least in affluent countries, is one of the great triumphs of modern medicine. A pregnant woman who is Rh− now receives an injection of antibodies, usually around 28 weeks of pregnancy. If there is leakage of Rh+ cells from the baby, these injected antibodies will coat those cells and prevent the production of antibodies by the mother. But the memory of the old days has left many physicians gun-shy about jaundice. This is unfortunate, because it impacts negatively, and unnecessarily, on breastfeeding.

There are other reasons why more cells than usual will break down. Some are similar to the Rh situation. Other antigens on red blood cells can also provoke the mother's immune system to produce antibodies against the baby's red blood cells and cause increased destruction of the cells. When we talk about our blood "type" for example, we are referring to another group of antigens—we call them A, O, AB, or B. Most people are O, which means that they don't have any of this group of antigens on their blood cells. Just as with the Rh factor, if the mother is O and the baby is one of the other blood types, some of the baby's blood cells could get into the mother's bloodstream and cause her to produce antibodies against the baby's blood. This is called ABO incompatibility. It is usually less severe than Rh incompatibility.

There may be more cells breaking down if the baby has a large bruise from a difficult birth or some injury around the time of birth. Sometimes these bruises are obvious, as when they are on the baby's face, but sometimes they can be hidden, as when they are around the kidney. The red cells in the bruise are dead and will break down to form bilirubin.

2. The liver is not able to handle the bilirubin

This may occur in the normal situation. The newborn's liver is relatively immature, and unable to handle all the bilirubin that comes to it for the first few days. This is another reason for babies getting normal physiologic jaundice. Once the liver develops a little more and gets better at making the bilirubin water soluble, the physiologic jaundice decreases. This usually happens after about the third day. The liver in premature babies is even less mature, which is why premature babies often have higher levels of bilirubin than do full-term babies.

Remember that *physiologic* means normal. We expect this type of jaundice to occur, and no treatment is necessary or desirable.

Infants of diabetic mothers also may have higher-than-average levels of bilirubin, because even if born at term, physiologically the infant of the diabetic mother is relatively immature. This may also be part of the cause of higher-than-average levels of jaundice in the baby born with an underactive thyroid. If the baby suffers from lack of oxygen during the birth, his liver may not be able to process as much bilirubin. Sometimes infections of the blood or urine are associated with jaundice in the newborn. Exactly how infection causes higher-than-average bilirubin is

not known, but it may be due to poor fee. There are also some rare genetic diseases which the enzyme necessary for conjugation is absent or decreased. One that is not rare, but is not a big problem, is Gilbert's syndrome. It is not usually noticed in the first days of life, and is not dangerous.

3. There is increased enterohepatic circulation of bilirubin

Remember that once the bilirubin gets to the intestines, some of it is reabsorbed after being unconjugated in the intestinal wall. If the baby is not having many bowel movements, the percentage of bilirubin that gets absorbed is increased, and this may also result in higher-than-average bilirubin.

An increased enterohepatic circulation of bilirubin may occur in babies who have an underactive thyroid, since typically they have few bowel movements, though this would not be the only explanation. Babies who have blockages in their bowels making them unable to have bowel movements, also may have an increased enterohepatic circulation of bilirubin, though jaundice is certainly not their most dramatic symptom.

By far the most common cause of an increased enterohepatic circulation of bilirubin is insufficient intake of breastmilk. I call this "not enough breastmilk" jaundice. The fact of the matter is that some "breastfed" babies are more jaundiced than average in the first few days, not because of the breastmilk they are receiving, as many physicians believe, but because they are *not* receiving breastmilk. Note that I have put "breastfed" in quotes, because these babies are not really breastfed. They are "nothing" fed, or minimally fed, and the fact that they are at the breast frequently, does not change that. A baby can be at the breast but not breastfeeding.

njugated (direct)
(jaundice)

d, or the ducts leading from
blocked, conjugated biliru-
the gut, and spills back into the
blood. This also will cause jaundice. But this is a completely different situation—always abnormal, and quite often serious. The tipoff that this might be a problem is that the baby's urine will probably be brownish, not clear like the typical urine of the well-feeding baby. The brownish color is due to the water-soluble bilirubin's finding a way out of the body through the urine. Fat-soluble bilirubin cannot get into the urine.

Babies with jaundice due to high levels of conjugated (direct, water-soluble) bilirubin need to be investigated as soon as possible, since successful treatments are available for some of the causes, especially if begun early.

What does all this have to do with breastfeeding?

Well, as you see, there is only one reason babies have higher-than-average bilirubin during the first few days that has anything to do with breastfeeding: not breastfeeding well, or even not breastfeeding at all.

It is my strong belief that babies should not be taken off the breast *ever* for the early type of exaggerated jaundice that we frequently see in the first few days. On the contrary, a skilled lactation expert should observe the mother and baby breastfeeding and decide if the baby is breastfeeding well. If the baby is, in fact, breastfeeding well, there is no need for concern: The jaundice will decrease. If the baby is not breastfeeding well, it makes no sense to take the baby off the breast—the baby is not breastfeeding anyway! It is the breastfeeding that needs to be fixed.

If it is not possible to fix the latch or get the baby breastfeeding well, it is important to start expressing the mother's milk for the baby. Colostrum is actually a laxative that makes the baby poop, so it is good for jaundiced babies—the increase in bowel movements will get rid of more bilirubin so that less will be reabsorbed into the baby's body. If it is not possible to get much colostrum, as is frequently the case in the first days (remember, many mothers can get more in the first few days by hand expression than by pump), then techniques to help the baby get on the breast should be instituted, and the baby given the colostrum (plus sugar water, used as a tool to help the baby get going with breastfeeding). The best way to give the baby the expressed colostrum—with or without some added sugar water—is at the breast with a lactation aid. This not only gives the baby the supplement, but helps him learn to breastfeed. Only rarely is it necessary to give formula, though it is difficult to convince many pediatricians of that.

If the high bilirubin is due to ABO incompatibility, or a large bruise, there is still no reason to stop breastfeeding.

It is often said that jaundiced babies do not feed well because they are sleepy. I do not agree. I think they are sleepy because they are not feeding well, not the other way around. You start getting food into these babies and you'll be impressed how quickly they wake up. Only when the bilirubin gets quite high do jaundiced babies become sleepy because of the jaundice. An overly sleepy baby needs to feed, and alternative methods should be used to give the baby some expressed milk, if necessary. Of course, the first approach should always be to get the baby breastfeeding effectively.

Recent studies have come out purporting to show that babies who are jaundiced become less jaundiced more quickly if they are supplemented with formula. These studies are terribly flawed, because no one confirmed that the babies were actually breastfeeding in the first few days. Many of them were not, as shown by the greater weight loss of the exclusively "breastfed" infants.

The point is, however, that it is not the breastfeeding that causes the problem, but the *lack* of breastfeeding. The solution is not to stop breastfeeding, but to fix the breastfeeding so the baby gets breastmilk.

"Breastmilk" Jaundice

This "diagnosis" cannot be made until we are sure the baby is getting substantial and sufficient amounts of breastmilk, usually only by the end of the first week of life. (It is difficult to be 100 percent certain about how much milk the baby is taking in during the first few days, although careful observation of the mother and baby breastfeeding will frequently tell us whether or not the baby is nursing well and swallowing milk.) Again, this is to emphasize that the higher bilirubin in the first few days has nothing to do with breastmilk keeping the bilirubin higher than in formula-fed babies.

However, I don't believe there is such a diagnosis as "breastmilk" jaundice. After more than 25 years of seeing young breastfeeding babies, I would say that the majority of exclusively breastfed, well-gaining babies are a little bit jaundiced, not just for a week or two, but often for three months or more. Usually, it is hardly noticeable, but if you look carefully, it is there. Sometimes there is no jaundice no matter how carefully you look, and sometimes there are babies who are quite yellow. These represent the extremes of the normal, which is slight yellowness. It is true that there is a tendency for those who have had exaggerated physiologic jaundice during the first few days to have more obvious jaundice later, but this is no reason to suppose that jaundice later on is somehow more worrisome.

There is no evidence that what is called "breastmilk" jaundice is bad for the baby. None. On the contrary, bilirubin may be good for the baby, protecting him from potentially damaging chemicals in the body. What we have here is a lack of understanding; that is, too many people do not understand that breastfeeding is the normal physiological method of feeding infants and young children. If most exclusively breastfed, well-gaining babies are jaundiced, then this is normal and not a concern. On the contrary, we should be concerned about babies fed with formula (advertised as being "close to breastmilk") who are *not* jaundiced. What's wrong with them that they are not jaundiced? The breastfed baby should be the model of what to expect, not the artificially fed baby. It is true that jaundice past the first week of life in artificially fed babies may indicate that something is wrong, but the same conclusion cannot be drawn about breastfed babies.

For these reasons, there is no call to take the baby off the breast for 24 or 48 hours "to be sure that it is breastmilk jaundice," and to bring the baby's bilirubin levels down to those of the artificially fed baby. In fact, logically, we should not be worrying the breastfeeding mother at all about her jaundiced baby. We should be saying to the formula-feeding mother, "Your baby's bilirubin is too low. This is probably not dangerous, but just to make sure that it is the formula that is keeping his bilirubin too low, I would like you to put the baby to the breast for a few days, so that his bilirubin moves up into the normal range." That's logical. But it will never happen.

A recent study from Italy found that breastfed babies—those who are really breastfeeding, not just pretending to breastfeed—actually do not have higher bilirubins than formula-fed babies. Many actually had lower levels of bilirubin on day three. Those who lost more weight did have higher bilirubin levels—but then, those babies were not breastfeeding well.

By the way, jaundice of this type tends to be more obvious and to last longer in Chinese, Vietnamese, Black, Native Canadian, and Native American babies, or in any baby whose parents are not both Caucasian.

Is it possible that jaundice at three weeks is a problem?

Yes, it can be. The direct (conjugated) jaundice is always a problem and needs to be investigated. But only rarely does breastfeeding need to be stopped. A few very rare metabolic disorders—galactosemia, for example—may have symptoms of high levels of direct (conjugated) jaundice. Galactosemia is a metabolic disease in which the baby can't metabolize one of the two sugars that make up lactose—the sugar in milk. The sugar stays in the blood and causes serious damage to the baby. If the baby continues to get galactose, it will be fatal. Fortunately, galactosemia is rare, occuring in about 1 out of 60,000 live births, and I personally have seen only one case in 25 years as a pediatrician. It is one of the few true medical reasons to stop breastfeeding. However, there are variants of galactosemia in which the baby has some enzyme activity and is capable of metabolizing the sugar (galactose) and it is possible that the baby can breastfeed in that situation. The baby's blood levels will need to be followed to make sure the baby is capable of keeping the galactose levels within the normal range.

Some medical problems may prolong jaundice. One is glucose-6-phosphatase deficiency, an enzyme deficiency occurring almost exclusively in boys, which may result in breakdown of the red blood cells when the babies are exposed to certain drugs or toxins. Although this deficiency is common (very common in Asia, Africa, and Mediterranean Europe), jaundice hardly ever seems to arise. It is important, though, to know if your baby has the deficiency, if he needs to take certain medications. However, if this is a cause of the jaundice, the mother should not stop breastfeeding.

An underactive thyroid can result in prolonged high levels of jaundice. The baby needs to be treated with thyroid hormone, not taken off breastfeeding. A urine infection occasionally can cause jaundice. Again, the infection needs to be treated but breastfeeding should not be stopped.

The baby also can have more obvious jaundice for the same reason the baby on day three may have higher-than-average bilirubin levels—because he is not feeding well. Interestingly, babies who are not gaining well on breast alone usually do not have the typical jaundice of well-gaining, exclusively breastfeeding babies. Some are jaundiced, though this is not the same thing—it is a result of their not getting enough breastmilk. This is an extension of the jaundice due to "not enough breastmilk" that we discussed with younger babies, and just as in that situation, the solution is not to stop breastfeeding but to get the baby breastfeeding better.

Sometimes a physician will suggest interruption of breastfeeding "to make the diagnosis." I feel this is completely unjustified. These exclusively breastfeeding babies are usually bouncing with health. If there is no reason to suspect an underactive thyroid (fairly rare, in any case, and usually caught by the newborn screening programs), a urinary tract infection, or a liver problem, or these problems have been ruled out, the baby should just be left alone; further tests, including the bilirubins, need not be done. And again, breastfeeding should not be stopped.

9

Colic

Myth: The best treatment for colic is changing the milk the baby gets.

Fact: A lot of things can be done to help the "fussy" baby without switching to formula. These things should always be tried first, both because the benefits of breastmilk are real and important, and because changing to formula frequently doesn't help or even makes things worse.

Fussiness in the breastfeeding baby has become one of the more common reasons for mothers to stop breastfeeding. Formula company advertising has exploited health care professionals' lack of interest and knowledge in breastfeeding to convince them that if the baby is fussy, the best thing to do is switch the baby to one of their "special" formulas. But this strategy is nothing new. In the old days, it used to be said that the baby was "allergic" to the mother's milk, and that switching to formula was the best way to fix the problem. There are still some physicians who use this line, but the reasons have changed. Now they say the baby is "lactose intolerant" or that the baby has "reflux." Both are distortions of the truth. Even if there is *some* truth in these explanations, stopping breastfeeding is not the best way to go. A lot can be done to help the "fussy" baby without switching to formula.

What Is Colic?

Today, any baby who is fussy is called "colicky," and perhaps this is fine, since we don't really know what colic is. The *typical* story of colic is the following: About three weeks after birth, the baby starts becoming fussy, especially in the evenings, often right around 7:00 p.m., and cries inconsolably for hours. Nothing the mother or father does helps with the crying, except temporarily, including feeding, walking, or putting the baby on top of (not in!) the clothes dryer. This whole difficult time continues until the baby is about three months of age, more or less. The baby is usually gaining weight very well, and is otherwise healthy. Any illness in the baby can cause crying. However, the obvious good health and happiness of the colicky baby at other times of the day are reassuring.

Of course, many babies do not fit this typical pattern but have their own patterns of fussiness. Parents who encounter this are so frightened of colic that they often come to see me, saying, "We hope he doesn't have the 'C' word."

So what causes colic? Nobody knows, but theories abound.

Gas

Some doctors used to do X-rays of the baby's abdomen to show parents the intestines full of air in order to prove to them the cause of their baby's fussiness. It was fairly convincing, I would imagine. There's no doubt that a lot of "colicky" babies have gas. They burp and toot all the time. But does the gas cause the crying, or is it really the other way around? A baby who cries a lot will swallow a lot of air. And many babies who pass a lot of gas are not particularly fussy or "colicky." However, getting up the gas is the reason that burping a baby is so important for so many people. But truthfully, I believe that burping is one of those useless rites we go through when we have new babies. Yes, true, some babies spit up less when they are burped after a feeding. But burping doesn't do much to relieve colic.

Gas in the baby's intestinal tract comes mostly from the same source as gas in the intestinal tract of adults; that is, from the digestion of food. Burping won't do anything to decrease that.

Nervous Parents

It is true that colic seems to be more common in first babies. But a colicky baby would make anybody nervous. Hearing a baby cry constantly for several hours without being able to do anything about it makes it difficult to maintain a detached calm.

Colic may simply be less common in second, third, or fourth babies because the parents are more aware of normal behavior in normal babies, and accept more readily that babies do cry sometimes. Sometimes parents have the mistaken idea that new babies only eat and sleep, and when the baby wants to be cuddled and carried around and held and talked to between feedings, they think the baby must have some problem.

More experienced parents have also developed techniques to calm their babies. They are not so worried that the baby might be sick. It's worrying that often drives parents to the doctor or hospital for help—and the doctor may

suggest changing to formula because he feels he should "do something."

And yet it is true that how parents care for their babies may affect whether the baby is colicky or cries a lot. In many developing cultures, colic is almost unknown. There may be many reasons for this. I was surprised, when I first was in Indonesia in 1971, to see girls younger than five years old carrying babies on their hips. Sometimes these babies (often not really babies anymore, but two years old or more) were almost as big as their sisters. The girls obviously knew what they were doing. Mothering was something they learned from a very young age. They learned by the way they were mothered themselves, by watching their mothers, their older sisters, other mothers, and by doing. And boys learned, too. I have friends who never even touched a baby until they had their own in their arms. So are we surprised that many parents are anxious? Taking care of babies is a lot more complicated than driving a car, yet nobody would suggest that somebody get into a car and drive it away if they had never driven before. Actually, most people in affluent societies have seen driving on television and in the movies so much that they would at least have an idea of how to go about doing it. What they see on television or in movies about taking care of babies is, in general, aberrant—a caricature of parenting. And don't forget that your health care professional may have the same background in parenting.

In many developing countries, babies are constantly held by someone—if not the mother, then the aunt, the grandmother, the father, the sister. Someone is always holding the baby. In Bali, Indonesia, they had the delightful custom of having a special dance when the baby turned three months of age. At this age, they put the baby down for the first time. Up until three months of age, the baby was always held by someone and never put down, and the baby never slept alone. The baby also had constant access to the breast. And colic was something they knew nothing about.

You'll notice that there was an extended family, almost always available to hold the baby and carry him around. I remember in Mexico once, waiting a very long time for a meal at a seaside eatery. Behind the restaurant (there were no walls), there was a mother in a hammock. Occasionally she would nurse her baby, but she never got out of her hammock. When the baby cried, someone, I wasn't sure who, would come and get the baby and walk him around. At least three different people, including the father (a man, in any case), did this over the course of the evening. The mother didn't seem nervous at all; in fact, she seemed quite calm. It definitely helps to have a supportive extended family.

Here is a situation that may result in a baby being "colicky" when, in fact, he is not.

MOTHERS' STORIES
CHRISTINE

Christine asked me for information about how to deal with her baby's breastfeeding. Her two-week-old baby was demanding to be fed more than every four hours, and spent an hour or two crying before every feeding. In addition, the breastfeeding was not going well, because he would cry afterward as well. The same thing had happened with her first three babies, whom she stopped breastfeeding after four weeks because she "did not have enough milk and the baby was always crying."

I observed the baby at the breast, and it was obvious that he was getting a fair amount of milk (open mouth wide–pause–close mouth type of sucking). There were also other indications that the baby was getting a lot of milk. He was having two or three substantial yellow bowel movements every day, plus a couple of stains, and the diapers were always heavy with urine. Finally, the scale suggested that he had gained a fair amount of weight.

My suggestion was merely to feed the baby when he seemed ready, before he cried, even if that meant feeding him much more frequently than every four hours.

Two days later, the "colic" was gone, the baby was very peaceful, but the mother was worried about the fact that he nursed 10 times in a day (she kept careful records), sometimes more often. I asked her to hang on, hoping Christine would relax and not worry about the frequency of feeding. (The other children were older and in school most of the day, so time was not as big an issue as it might have been otherwise, with smaller children.)

In fact, two weeks later, the baby had finally established a sort of routine. Every four hours, for goodness' sake! Wouldn't you know it? And he was content and thriving on the breast alone. She nursed this baby for nine months.

A few years ago, the notion that babies should be fed by the clock and only every four hours had pretty well gone the way of foot binding. Of course, mothers may still hear from their doctors that it is good to get a baby on a schedule (although they don't give reasons why schedules are such a good thing), but if your baby wants to feed more often, don't hold back. Go ahead and give him the breast.

We were too complacent in thinking that schedules had disappeared for good.

A program with a pseudoreligious basis has begun to be promoted, the basis of which is "controlling the baby." The parents are to be in charge, not the baby. This meant feeding by the clock, and some bizarre biblical justifications were dredged up to support this approach. It has caught on in the United States and is making inroads into Canada. People who follow this "program" believe they are doing the right thing for their babies, but they are not. Encouraging parents to let a baby cry for an hour, or even 20 minutes or any time at all, just so that you can follow a routine is anti-baby, anti-mother, anti-father, anti-family. It is baby-stupid. These children may be "good" youngsters (if what we mean by good is "controlled"), but I dread to imagine what many of these kids will do when they are teenagers.

Many of these babies do not gain weight well, because by the time they get to the breast they are so tired from crying that they don't latch well and they fall asleep before they eat as much as they need. So the mother decides her milk is insufficient, and eventually breastfeeding is sacrificed to the routine. Surely this can't be what God intended?

Immature Digestive Systems

I guess it is possible that babies' digestive systems are not quite up to digesting food when they are very young. It is known, for example, that there is less lactase (the enzyme that metabolizes the sugar lactose) in the baby's small intestine before about three months of age than after. This is not usually a big problem, except when the baby drinks mostly low-fat milk (see below).

Of course, this does not explain why babies from traditional cultures are rarely ever reported to be colicky. Is there a reason their intestinal tract may be more mature? It is possible, I suppose. There is a compound called epidermal growth factor in colostrum and breastmilk, which hastens the development of the baby's intestines. It is present in particularly high levels in colostrum. In many traditional societies, babies go to the breast from birth and stay there, thus probably getting more colostrum than babies in North America, who are frequently separated from their mothers, given supplements (usually unnecessarily), and so on. Maybe significant amounts of epidermal growth factor, undiluted by other milk, help the intestines to mature. But then, colic appears to be as uncommon in societies where the mothers express and throw away the colostrum (a bad idea, but very rooted in some traditional societies). No, "immature" digestive system does not seem to be the answer.

It has also been suggested that the constant carrying of babies that is practiced in these cultures also reduces colic. Nobody knows why carrying babies might decrease the crying. There are baby-care practices that seem to have no obvious basis in physiology but which may help babies remain content. Some mammals lick their newborns and continue this practice during the early months. This behavior may reassure or comfort the young one, or stimulate certain responses in the skin or brain that are calming. For humans, carrying may do the same.

Overfeeding

This was the traditional physician's diagnosis for colic, and was one of the reasons every-four-hour feedings were adopted—to keep the baby from overfeeding and from getting "colic." For many years we breastfeeding advocates mocked this thinking, but, in fact, we should not have. There is actually something to this, but the answer is not to limit feedings. (See section on Overactive Milk Ejection Reflex.)

What Can Be Done About the "Colicky" Baby?

A baby cannot be called colicky unless he is gaining well on breastfeeding alone. The baby who is not gaining well is probably crying because he is hungry. How often do mothers come to the clinic saying the baby is not gaining well, and in addition, that he is colicky. No, he is hungry, and if the mother gives him more milk (see Chapter 5, Not Enough Milk, as well as Christine's story, in this chapter) he is likely to be *less* colicky.

But sometimes babies can be hungry even if they are getting lots of milk and are gaining weight well. These are the babies who drink inefficiently, who take a long time, and who snack at the breast for long periods of time. If they are taken off the breast, even after a long time, they may cry because they are still hungry. Because they are gaining weight well, they are called "colicky." They can be helped to feed more efficiently if the latch is improved and the mother uses breast compression.

One possible cause is that the baby gets too little high-fat milk. And one easy, and often helpful, solution to colic caused by this is to finish the first side before offering the second. This is the first thing to try when the baby is fussy. Why is this?

Breastmilk gradually increases in fat from the beginning to the end of the feeding, but you must understand that if the baby is not drinking the milk from the breast, then it does not matter how long he is there, he won't get more high-fat milk. Of course, at the beginning of the feeding the baby will get great amounts of milk and will drink fine. But as time goes on, the baby will be doing more and more nibbling at the breast, and less and less feeding. The better the baby's latch, the longer he will be able to take milk from the breast. But once the baby is nibbling, he is hardly getting milk anymore. Keeping him there nibbling for 10 minutes or even 40 minutes will not change very much the amount of high-fat milk the baby gets. The baby is getting milk when there is a noticeable pause in the movement of his chin as he opens his mouth to the maximum during a suck, just before he closes his mouth again. (See pages 58–60 for a full description.)

Typically, especially during the first four to eight weeks after birth, babies tend to fall asleep at the breast once the flow of milk slows down. As they get older, they tend to pull away. Some babies will always just fall asleep, at any age, and others will be pulling away by a week of age, and some will do one thing one feeding and something different the next feeding. The bottom line, though, is that if there is an abundant milk supply, coupled with a less than perfect latch, the baby will drink well only as long as the milk flow is rapid. The better the latch, the longer the baby will drink well, because he can get milk even when the flow is not rapid. He can take the milk out of the breast and not depend on flow alone.

Thus, some babies will no longer be drinking well and will be starting to fall asleep before the milk has a higher concentration of fat. Typically, then, the mother will take the baby off the breast when he sleeps, and since the baby is still hungry, he will wake up and start to cry. The mother will usually offer the other breast. The baby again will drink very well during the rapid flow and fall asleep or pull away. He has drunk two lots of low-fat milk.

Or if, as is happening too often now, the mother is told to feed only on one breast at each feeding, the baby will come off the breast asleep, and then when he wakes up, his mother will give him the same breast again. He will nibble, not drinking well, for a while, then fall asleep again. The mother will end up with a baby who spends very long periods of time on the breast, but who still cries and is fussy. By the way, the concentration of fat in the milk does not change abruptly. Rather, it is a gradual increase as milk is taken out of the breast.

The stomach tends to empty rapidly when it contains food that is low in fat. If the baby's stomach fills up with relatively low-fat milk, the milk empties out of the stomach quickly and gets into the small intestine. In the small intestine are enzymes that metabolize various components of the milk, including lactase (the enzyme that metabolizes breastmilk sugar, lactose). When so much milk gets into the small intestine so quickly, it is possible for there to be too much lactose present for the lactase to break down. When this happens, some of the lactose does not get digested, and that can cause gassiness, and frequent, green, watery, explosive bowel movements. The severity of the symptoms undoubtedly depends on how much lactose is undigested, and this would depend on how much fat is in the milk, the rate of emptying of the stomach and the concentration of undigested lactose in the gut. With time, irritation of the gut might occur, and the baby may pass mucus and blood in the bowel movements. Many specialists in gastrointestinal problems do not believe this or have not heard of this as a possibility, but babies have been "cured" of bowel inflammation simply by following the recommendations to increase the amount of fat in the milk. I believe that incomplete lactose digestion can indeed cause mucus and even blood in the bowel movements. These babies often have quite irritated bottoms, sometimes with sores and bleeding. If the stool can irritate their skin, why not the intestinal lining?

The trick then, is to increase the amount of fat the baby is getting by "finishing" the first side before offering the second. How?

Get the baby to latch on in the best way possible

Unfortunately, by the time I see many of these babies, they are six weeks of age or older. It is not always possible to change the latch of a baby this age who is getting all the milk he wants—he probably sees no reason to change. But it is worth a try. See Chapter 4, Getting Off to the Best Start, and get help from a good lactation consultant.

Be sure you can tell when your baby is actually drinking at the breast

Unfortunately, on the printed page, it is not always easy to describe. Some mothers can hear the baby drink, but there are all sorts of noises that babies can make on the breast that have nothing to do with actually getting milk. A baby who is latched on poorly may make smacking noises as he lets go of the breast and grabs on again. This does not mean he is getting a lot of milk, even though frequently the letting go occurs because the flow of milk is rapid. The best sign that the baby is getting milk is the pause in the movement of the baby's chin that occurs on opening his mouth to the widest point while he sucks. As long as you can see the pause at the widest opening, the baby is getting milk. Don't change sides while he is drinking this way. However, once he starts to nibble, start using "breast compression." See page 72 for another description of how to know whether the baby is getting milk.

Use breast compression

Do not use breast compression while the baby is drinking well. If you do, he may get so much milk so quickly that he will sputter and gag while on the breast, something he may be doing already. However, once the baby is slowing down and mostly nibbling, get your hand around the breast, with your thumb on one side and other fingers on the other, in whichever way is comfortable for you. Close your hand, to compress the breast—not so hard that it hurts, although you would have to squeeze pretty hard for compression to hurt. You don't have to slide your fingers or thumb toward the nipple. In fact, it may be better not to, as that could irritate the skin of the breast. Try not to change the shape of the breast when you compress. If you see the areola or the skin near it wrinkling up, try moving your hand closer to your chest. When you compress, the baby may start to drink. If he does (open mouth wide–pause–close mouth type of sucking), great. Keep the pressure up until he no longer is drinking, and then release. He might have only one or two "drinks," or the drinking may go on for several minutes. It seems that the compression can simulate and stimulate a milk ejection reflex (letdown reflex). If it doesn't work at all to compress the breast, then release and wait for the next opportunity. Young babies often stop sucking when the flow of milk stops, but will restart when they taste milk.

The cycle will be similar to this:

1. The baby was drinking well (not just nibbling), but is now starting to nibble. Start compression. Do this compression when the baby is sucking, but not drinking. Keep steady pressure up until the baby no longer drinks ("pumping" the breast does not work as well, it seems to me).

2. Release compression. Once the baby is nibbling even with the compression applied, release the compression. If you do not, your hand will tire, and it is quite possible that the continued pressure will now interfere with the flow of milk. Indeed, I have seen babies nibbling while the compression is applied, and then start to drink again immediately when the mother releases the pressure. Presumably there was milk backed up behind where the mother had applied pressure. Some babies will stop sucking when the flow of milk stops; others will continue nibbling.

3. If the baby stops sucking, wait for him to start sucking again. Wait for him, and you will work together. He will try to get milk by suckling, and you will be helping him with compression. Repeat the whole process.

4. If the baby continues sucking after you release compression, as many older babies (older than six or eight weeks) will, wait a while. If the baby does not start to actually drink, start the compression. It is also possible for you to wait a little until he stops sucking for a bit, takes a rest, and then starts sucking again. If he does not drink at this point, then start the compression again.

5. Keep the baby on the first side until he no longer drinks, even with the compression. This does not mean that you must immediately take the baby off the breast the first time compression does not help him get more. Wait a little bit. You may have another milk ejection reflex (letdown reflex). The compression may not work now, but may in a few minutes. There is no rush. A few extra minutes with the baby drinking on the first side can make the difference between a "colicky" baby who feeds all the time, and a calmer baby who feeds a little, or even a lot, less frequently. This helps particularly if the baby is also one who spits up a lot.

6. Once the baby comes off the breast on his own, or starts to fall asleep and is obviously

not drinking much, offer the other side. If he has fed really well, he may not want the other side. Do not make yourself a rule about this. Rules and breastfeeding do not work well. Sometimes the baby will be very happy with one side only. Sometimes he won't be. Most likely in the morning he will be satisfied with one breast. Most likely in the evening he won't be. If the baby is hungry, feed him! But finish one side before you offer the other. In fact, if he has finished both sides and still wants to feed, offer the first side again. You may be surprised how much milk is left in the "empty" breast.

Will all this always work and turn a fussy, spitting up, crying baby into the peaceful baby that everyone dreams of? No. Nothing *always* works. But it will work in many situations, and will help in most of the rest. If it does not help at all, there are other ways of increasing the concentration of fat in the milk the baby gets.

Feeding more than one feeding on each breast

This is another little trick that works for some mothers and some babies. The idea is simply to feed the baby at the same breast for two (or in some cases, more) feedings in a row. Obviously you have to have a fairly abundant milk supply, but this should not be a problem for the mother whose baby is colicky. Colickiness in the baby often goes together with a generous milk supply. When it has been a relatively short time since the baby has fed on the breast, the milk tends to have a greater concentration of fat. This occurs because as more milk is removed from the breast, smaller and smaller amounts of milk with a high fat content remain. New milk is always being made, but if the baby is nursing frequently, he is usually removing most of it.

Milk from a breast on which the baby has fed only two hours ago will have a higher fat content than milk from a breast on which the baby has fed four hours ago.

It may not be possible for you to feed the baby twice on one side only. The baby may not get enough this way. Sometimes putting the baby who has come off the breast back to the same side will work, but again, if the baby is not drinking (that open mouth wide–pause–close mouth type of sucking), or if he doesn't seem happy, you may need to give him the other breast.

You may find that if the baby has had two feedings on one side, you will be getting engorged on the other side. There is certainly no harm in expressing for comfort, but try to delay this until close to the next feeding (I know—it can't be predicted). In expressing as close to the feeding as is practical, you will be taking off some of the low-fat milk, which may help to increase your baby's fat intake. I usually suggest expressing until you can see that the milk looks less bluish or watery. Usually 30 ml (1 oz) is plenty—but again, no rules. Don't take off too much though. Your baby will be hungry and expecting rapid flow. Also, you probably do not want to stimulate a further increase in the milk supply.

MOTHERS' STORIES
JANE

Jane brought her one-month-old to the clinic because he was always fussing and would want to breastfeed every hour or less, 24 hours a day. She was extremely frustrated, but was carrying on because she knew breastfeeding was best. She wasn't always sure she could carry on, however.

I examined Joshua, who was obviously a big, healthy baby. Like all exclusively breastfed, well-gaining babies, he was jaundiced (not a sign of illness, but to be expected in healthy, breast-fed babies—see Chapter 8, Jaundice). He weighed 4.5 kg (about 10 lb) while his birth-weight had been 3.3 kg (about 7 lb 4 oz). His urine was normal.

I watched the baby nurse. He went to the breast with an acceptable latch, and drank—or, one could say, almost inhaled—milk for a few minutes, before coming off the breast, crying. The mother put him to the other side and the same thing happened. He actually was still hungry and crying after the second side.

We tried to get a better latch, but it really was difficult. Jane found him too heavy to position in the cross-cradle hold, and Joshua didn't seem to want to change his ways. I taught the mother about compression, but I was not sure it would work because he came off the breast so quickly with so little warning. Nevertheless, it did work a little and the baby was slightly calmer at the breast.

The next week, the baby was a little better, but nothing close to what one would call a contented infant. He had gained 400 g in the week (about 14 oz). I suggested Jane keep Joshua drinking with the compression as much as possible, putting him back to the same side if possible. (Some babies seem to sense that they are being offered the same breast which is not so "full," and struggle and cry, only to take the second, fuller side easily.) If that worked, I suggested Jane try two feedings on each side.

The following week, Joshua had gained another 400 g (14 oz), but was much calmer. He still fed about every hour. Over the next week, Jane started to feed him more frequently on one side and things continued to improve. At the end of the process, she was feeding five times on one side, then five times on the other. Joshua had stretched his feedings out so that he was feeding only five times in 24 hours (by eight weeks of age), so that, essentially, the mother was feeding on one breast one day, and on the other the next day. At first she had to express milk for comfort, but after another couple of weeks she did not have to do even that.

I present this as an extraordinary case. No other mother I have encountered with a colicky, rapidly growing baby had such a dramatic change, nor did any other mother go to so many feedings on one side before offering the other. Feeding on one side only is not so extraordinary. There are plenty of mothers with only one breast who feed a baby just fine and without any supplements. What was extraordinary was how well it all worked. If only it always worked that well!

BARBARA

Barbara brought Elijah to the clinic when he was about four weeks old. He was extremely fussy and was spitting up a lot. He was also feeding quite frequently—at least every two hours and often more. His weight gain was impressive, however, on breastfeeding only. Apparently he was 4.0 kg at birth (8 lb 12 oz), and when he was brought to the clinic his weight was 5.2 kg (11 lb 7 oz).

Elijah was completely normal on examination, and his urine was normal.

I did with Barbara and Elijah exactly as I did with Jane and Joshua. (I chose these two cases because they were at the clinic almost at the same time—a time when biblical names were in vogue in our area.) Barbara came back with Elijah a few times, but nothing seemed to work well, so she switched Elijah to formula. At first, he did better with the formula, but after a few days he started being just as difficult and colicky, so she switched him from milk-based formula to soy formula. This also "helped" for a few days, but then things deteriorated again. Eventually, despite my urging her to at least express her own milk and give it to Elijah in a bottle, Barbara ended up giving Elijah a hydrolyzed formula that seemed to help him, and he was kept on that. I say "seemed to help" because he got better about eight weeks of age, when many babies are starting to get better anyway. Nevertheless, I accept the possibility that it was something about the hydrolyzed formula that helped. But was it worth it? From the financial point of view, it was costing the family $50 to $75 each week just for formula, or about four times what regular formula cost. This was in 1993, and the price has climbed considerably since then. Even regular milk-based formulas are now costing $20 to $30 each week.

Of course, that is not all. The mother and baby both missed an irreplaceable relationship. The baby would have eventually gotten better, regardless of whether treatment suggestions worked. It's true, it's not easy. Is it worth it to continue breastfeeding a fussy baby? I believe it is.

The Overactive Milk Ejection Reflex

A baby whose mother has this "problem" is often very fussy and described as colicky. An overactive milk ejection reflex means that when the mother's milk lets down, the flow is very fast and sometimes quite forceful. This results in difficulties that can be attributed, at least in part, to the baby's getting relatively small amounts of high-fat milk.

The mother usually has an abundant milk supply. The baby goes to the breast, and as the milk flows, he may choke, sputter, gag. Often he will come off the breast and cry, or the mother may take him off the breast to try to calm him or stop him choking. The baby will usually be hungry when he comes off the breast because he will have fed only a very short time. So he will try to latch on again, but the process may repeat itself.

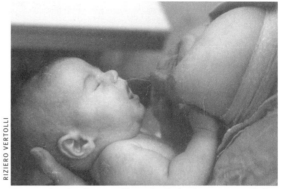

Overactive letdown reflex. The baby has come off the breast because of the force of the milk ejection.

As much as these babies do not like the rapid flow at the beginning, they also hate it when the flow of milk is slow, later in the feeding, and they will often pull off the breast and get upset when the flow slows down. So they are fussy on the breast a lot of the time.

As you can guess, they are probably getting fairly large amounts of relatively low-fat milk.

The best treatment for this is prevention. A good latch from the very first days will help. A baby who is latched on well can control milk flow better, slowing it down when it is too fast, and being able to draw milk from the breast more effectively when the flow slows down. It is possible that the babies learn to latch on poorly because they are constantly being forced off the breast by rapid flow, but I believe the poor latch is the beginning of the problem.

But if you already have this problem, what should you do?

1. Use the same procedures (including, never forget, improving the latch, if possible) as mentioned above to increase the fat intake of

the baby. These will help for the overactive milk ejection reflex by decreasing the milk supply. It takes longer, but often still works.

2. Lie down for nursings. Perhaps because of the effect of gravity, many babies are much calmer when the mother lies down side by side with them to breastfeed. When lying side by side does not help, some mothers and babies are more comfortable with the mother lying on her back and the baby nursing while lying tummy down on top of her. This can be managed if the mother sits at the edge of the bed, latches the baby on, and then lies back onto her pillow. It can also be managed using a reclining chair.

"Foreign" Proteins in Your Milk

When I was a medical student, I was taught that up to about three months of age, a baby's intestine was "leaky" and that babies could absorb whole protein directly from the gut. After about three months of age, the gut "closed" and no longer allowed the whole protein to pass through. Breastfed babies get closure earlier than formula fed babies, at least in part because of an epidermal growth factor present in breastmilk and colostrum. A healthy adult did not absorb whole protein, and proteins had to be broken down in the intestine by various enzymes before the breakdown products (amino acids and amino acids attached together) could be absorbed.

We now know this is not true. At least, it's not true for nursing mothers. It has been well-demonstrated in several studies in Scandinavia, in particular, but also other areas of the world, that various proteins from the mother's diet actually can be absorbed right into her body from her gut and passed on to the baby. The protein in cow's milk (beta lactoglobulin), from

gluten (gliadin), and some other sources have actually been demonstrated to be in the mother's milk.

Often the fact that something like cow's milk protein is getting into the mother's milk is perceived to be a bad thing, both by health professionals and mothers. But there is no reason to assume that because an occasional baby has problems with these proteins, it would be better if they did not appear in the milk. On the contrary, nature rarely does things for nothing. The fact that foreign proteins appear in the milk may actually be important in diminishing the baby's reactions so that he may tolerate these proteins in his diet when he is older.

The proteins are not the only elements that appear in the milk. There are many other things in the milk that prevent the baby from reacting badly to the foreign proteins, while at the same time desensitizing him to those proteins. Desensitization is what allergy shots are all about. Whether they work or not is another question, but the idea is that small amounts of allergens are injected into the body, so that eventually the person develops the right types of antibodies to that allergen, not the type that cause allergic reactions. Cow's milk protein, which appears in breastmilk, for example, appears along with antibodies to cow's milk protein, as well as sensitized white cells (lymphocytes and macrophages), and other immune factors. This makes the situation far different from that which would be implied by the statement "The baby is getting cow's milk protein in your milk." There has been at least one study showing that babies who were colicky did *not* get more cow's milk protein than the ones who were not colicky, but that the concentration of antibody against cow's milk protein in the mother's milk was much lower.

By the way, there is at least one other reason

that proteins and other substances coming out in the milk are not bad. Studies have shown that, in general, breastfed babies accept solid foods better than formula-fed babies. One of the reasons may be that all through their nursing time, from day one, they have been exposed to a variety of tastes. Formula-fed babies are exposed to only one taste (bad, in my opinion).

So, should I stop certain foods if my baby is colicky?

I would first try to get more high-fat milk into the baby. Breastfeeding mothers already have too many restrictions, usually unnecessary restrictions, in our society. However, there is no doubt that occasionally, stopping certain foods may make a tremendous difference in the baby's behavior. My feeling is that it doesn't work most of the time, but it works extremely well in about one baby in 10, somewhat in another one in 10. This is not only because it isn't easy to eliminate all dairy products or all wheat from your diet, but because reactions to food are rarely the cause of colic in breastfed babies.

If you are going to eliminate certain foods from your diet, do only one group of foods at a time. That is, don't eliminate dairy products and wheat and eggs and nuts and peanuts and seafood all at the same time. Furthermore, there will be no lack of people who will let you know that their baby got better when they stopped bananas, beef, broccoli, and so on, and you may soon find yourself restricted to a diet of white rice and water only. Not good.

Start with the most likely group, which is dairy products. Regardless of what the dairy bureau advises, you don't need dairy products when you are breastfeeding. Milk is an easy way to get calcium, but you can get enough calcium without having dairy products. In many parts of the world, dairy products are rarely part of the adult diet. Some mothers are eating and drinking dairy products even if they hate them, because everyone tells them they have to. Some mothers are themselves lactose intolerant, and are suffering abdominal cramps and diarrhea because they think it will help them make milk. It is so unnecessary.

By the way, if you are lactose intolerant, it does not mean your children will be lactose intolerant. It also does not mean that the reason your baby is colicky is that he is not digesting the lactose well. Even adults who are lactose intolerant are not lactose intolerant as babies. True lactose intolerance in babies is very rare. What is often diagnosed as lactose intolerance may be poor lactose digestion, but this is usually due to too much low-fat milk—and that can be fixed.

Remember that the reason you are eliminating foods is to prevent certain proteins from getting into your milk. If you take dairy products out of your diet, it is not to get rid of lactose. Your milk will contain plenty of lactose whether or not you eat dairy products.

You should realize that many of the most common foods that may affect your baby through your milk are extremely difficult to eliminate completely from your diet. It may not be necessary to eliminate them completely to benefit your baby, but milk products and wheat are used in many prepared foods, even in some foods where you would not expect to find them.

If you are going to eliminate a food from your diet, be resolved to do it for at least a week, perhaps 10 days. Some people say even longer, but I doubt that foreign proteins would stick around that long in the mother's blood and milk. If after that time no change has occurred, you could probably go back to that food. If there has been a dramatic difference, I would still, after a few days of tranquillity, reintroduce that food slowly to your diet. The baby may tolerate relatively small amounts of foreign proteins in your milk, and you may be able to find a level of intake that does not seem to bother him.

What if there is a partial response? I would try reintroducing the food to see if it makes a difference. If there is, stop the food again. Should you look for another food? Perhaps, if you feel you must, and if the baby, though better, seems still to be suffering a lot. But be careful what you eliminate from your diet. Women do not have to be terribly careful about what they eat when they breastfeed, but they have to eat something.

More recently, we have begun giving the mother pancreatic enzymes to reduce colic and allergic colitis in her baby. The mother takes one capsule at each meal. This breaks down the protein in her own diet and decreases the baby's reactions. It does not work in every case but has been very helpful for some mothers and babies.

Below I describe a situation I encountered in one of my first patients with the problem of cow's milk protein intolerance in the baby resulting from cow's milk protein in his mother's milk.

MOTHERS' STORIES
BRONWYN

Bronwyn brought Ashley to the clinic when Ashley was six weeks old. Bronwyn said that Ashley cried almost all the time she was awake, which was most of the day and night. She breastfed well, though, and seemed comforted by breastfeeding.

On examination, the baby appeared normal, including slight jaundice, which is also normal in the exclusively breastfeeding, well-gaining baby. She weighed 4 kg (8 lb 12 oz), after a birthweight of 2.7 kg (6 lb 2 oz). The urine examination was normal.

I was not sure what to suggest. I had just started helping mothers with breastfeeding challenges, and this was really the first baby who was brought for this sort of complaint. Not having any other ideas, and having heard of the possibility of milk protein causing such a problem, I suggested Bronwyn go off milk products. Within 24 to 48 hours, Ashley was calm—an almost "perfect" baby.

When the baby was about six months old, Bronwyn called to let me know what had happened. After a few weeks, Bronwyn began to wonder if the change in Ashley was not just a coincidence, especially since Bronwyn was missing her dairy products. So she had a glass of milk. The baby did not start crying spells, but the next day had visible blood in her bowel movements. This lasted part of the day, and then the bowel movements were clear again. Bronwyn reported that she had done this several times over the four or five months since she and Ashley had been at the clinic. As Bronwyn said, "I could turn the blood in her poops on and off like a tap, just by having a glass of milk."

This is a fairly convincing report, but it is not the rule. I don't think it's typical. Such changes in the baby may be more common than I believe, I suppose, since, if the food elimination worked, the mother would not have contacted me. I only rarely get calls or visits at the clinic from mothers who want to tell me everything is just fine.

Other Foods or Supplements

It is best to stop everything but breastfeeding in the colicky baby. Babies usually do not need extra vitamins. Vitamin D deficiency, rickets, though possible in exclusively breastfed babies, is very uncommon. It occurs in babies of mothers who themselves are vitamin D deficient, since their babies do not get enough vitamin D stored up during the pregnancy. Vitamin D deficiency in pregnant women is quite rare in Canada, since women get lots of outside exposure, because they often drink milk (which already has added vitamin D), and because they usually take prenatal vitamins. There is no need for breastfeeding women to give their babies extra vitamin D, except in exceptional circumstances. Women who are likely to be vitamin D deficient are those women who do not get much sun exposure to their skin. Many women who are veiled and dark-skinned and who go out infrequently may be vitamin D deficient, and they and their babies should probably get extra vitamin D. But the majority do not need vitamin D drops. Take your baby outside—it's good for fussiness and good for getting him vitamin D. I am not saying the vitamins cause colic, but several mothers have stated that their baby got better when they stopped the vitamins.

The same can be said for extra iron. The majority of exclusively breastfeeding babies do not need extra iron, at least before they are six months old. Medicinal iron can cause constipation and fussiness. Some babies born prematurely do need extra iron, but sometimes it is possible to eliminate the iron, or at least decrease the dose. Try taking the baby off the iron to see if that decreases his fussiness.

If your baby was born very prematurely, check with your pediatrician before stopping iron supplements. However, even a very premature baby can do without extra iron for a week or two.

What If None of These Approaches Works?

Colic almost always disappears, no matter what you do or don't do, by the time the baby is three or four months old. Eventually it will get better no matter what. Stick with the breastfeeding.

Based on the experiences of many of our patients, you won't be sorry.

But I can't take another day, let alone several more weeks.

Okay, you can't continue as you are going. Then try the following "last resorts." At least your baby will still get breastmilk.

1. *Use a nipple shield*. Nipple shields have been used for many breastfeeding problems, often unnecessarily and often to the detriment of the breastfeeding relationship. But in the situation of the overactive letdown, they can work. The old types are actually better for this than the more "modern" ones. The reason for this is that the old types act more like a bottle. The space fills with milk, and the baby drinks as if he were sucking from a bottle. You see, in most cases colic is not a question of the baby being "allergic" to your milk, but rather a question of how the milk is being delivered. The reason some babies get better when they are put on the bottle with formula usually has nothing to do with the fact that it is formula in the bottle, but rather that the baby is being fed by bottle. Indeed, see our next "last resort."

2. *Give your milk by bottle*. If the nipple shield does not work (some mothers find them awkward to use, and some babies don't like them), then give your milk by bottle. The steady, fairly rapid flow of the bottle makes feeding easier. The baby can still choke on a bottle nipple, but since the flow is steady, choking occurs less frequently. Better your milk than formula.

3. *Use lactase drops*. What if you feed the baby your milk with a bottle, and the baby still is fussy and shows symptoms of lactose intol-

erance? You can buy a commercial preparation of lactase to add to your milk. Just follow instructions on the container. It takes a few hours to work, so you cannot use your milk right away, but you will then have lactose-free breastmilk. (Incidentally, breastmilk can stand out at room temperature for several hours, at least six or eight hours, without being refrigerated. It is, after all, antibacterial, and is not likely to "spoil.")

Soothing a colicky baby

Some things to try:
• Walk around with your baby in a carrier or sling—this seems to work best if you do it throughout the day, when your baby is happy or sleeping rather than waiting until he gets fussy.
• Massage your baby's tummy, using a little baby oil or cornstarch to prevent friction on his skin. Massage from just under your baby's ribs down toward his legs, then go to the top again and repeat.
• Take the baby for a ride in the car (in his car seat).
• Rock with the baby in a rocking chair.
• Hold the baby, tummy-down, with his tummy along your forearm and his face supported by your hand, and move him gently in this position.
• Try putting your baby in a wind-up baby swing, with rolled-up towels to support him in a comfortable position if necessary.
• Have a leisurely, warm bath with the baby.

Recent Marketing "Advances" in Infant Feeding

The formula companies—always alert to finding ways of helping physicians help mothers stop breastfeeding—have been particularly ingenious in finding products to deal with colic, "reflux," and "lactose intolerance."

Lactose-Free Formulas

This is the "treatment" for the baby who has colic and watery, green, explosive bowel movements. Until recently, the only easily available lactose-free formulas were soy milk formulas, but concerns about their safety have been raised, and the formula companies now make cow's milk formulas with no lactose. They have marketed these formulas so well that many physicians will simply recommend them for fussy babies, even before trying some of the techniques discussed above.

This feeble approach to dealing with the colicky baby is a result of physicians' poor training in infant feeding, and their dependence, once they are in practice, on formula company representatives to keep them "up to date." Of course, the formula company rep does nothing of the sort. He or she keeps the physician up to date on the company's latest products. The formula company reps often quote an article by Michael Woolridge and Chloe Fisher in the medical journal *Lancet* from a few years ago to justify their suggesting lactose-free formula. But Woolridge and Fisher do not mention using formulas free of lactose. Here is what they said:

> Low-fat feeds result in rapid gastric emptying, fat being a potent inhibitor of gastric emptying. Hence a baby on low-fat milk feeds will require frequent feeding, which may further stimulate milk production. Lactose intake may also contribute to the baby's symptoms. Lactose is present at an invariant concentration in milk, so high volume feeds represent high lactose feeds. Rapid gastric emptying will cause a high lactose load to be presented in a short time to the jejunum and ileum. In a proportion of babies this load may be more than can be

handled by the lactase available in the intestinal brush border. If excess lactose enters the colon, there may be increased fermentation, with resulting colic, flatus, and the production of loose, acid stools. These symptoms: a) failure to thrive, b) colic and irritability (crying as if in pain, windy), and c) watery diarrhea, are diagnostic of lactose malabsorption, and typify "overfeeding" in its traditional sense.

Our view is that infants should be encouraged to finish suckling from the first breast first—in other words, to come off the breast spontaneously before being offered the second breast should the baby still show signs of hunger. No restrictions should be placed on the length of time spent feeding on a breast and there should be no enforced change from the first to the second breast. For a proportion of mothers, especially those whose milk supply is over-abundant, this practice may mean that one breast will suffice at each feed. If the contralateral breast is offered first at the next feed, milk production should stabilise at a lower level than if both breasts were offered at every feed and there will be no long term imbalance in production. One vital caveat is that if the baby is to be allowed to feed to satiety on the breast, all efforts should be made to ensure that the baby is correctly positioned on the breast. Otherwise, the breast will not be drained effectively.

This is just a more technical way of describing the situation in which the baby is getting lots of low-fat milk, and the solutions the authors recommend are the same as described earlier in this chapter. The treatment is to fix the problem, not to change to a formula.

Formula with Added Rice

This product is more recent even than the lactose-free formulas. Some babies are colicky, and rather than having frequent, watery, green bowel movements, they actually spit up a lot. The diagnosis is "reflux." The answer? Another formula, of course. And it might work. Just as with "lactose intolerance," I have seen babies whose mothers have said, "When he takes breastmilk from a bottle, he doesn't spit up as much, but when he takes it directly from the breast, he is a fountain." The fact is, again, the method of delivery is often the issue.

Attention to how the baby is latched on, to "finishing the first side before offering the second," to compression—all will help with the baby who spits up a lot and who is also colicky. If the baby only spits up a lot, this is a laundry problem, not a medical problem, and physicians should be reassuring the mother that her milk is the best for her baby and to carry on. Unfortunately, all too often they go for the "special" formula.

And after all is said and done, time will cure the problem.

Reflux Esophagitis

This was the hot new diagnosis of the 1990s. Of course, reflux esophagitis exists. Not only may the baby spit up a lot, but he may have pain (and therefore crying) from irritation of the tube (esophagus) leading from the mouth to the stomach. Nothing better demonstrates how the bottle-feeding mentality negatively influences breastfeeding than the physician's usual approach to dealing with "reflux." Here is how most physicians would treat a formula-fed baby with reflux.

• Offer small, frequent feedings. If that doesn't work then,

- Add cereal to the bottle. If that doesn't work then,
- Prescribe medication.

Thus, when faced with a breastfeeding baby exhibiting spitting up and fussiness, most physicians will often use the model of the formula-feeding baby, because that is what they know. So, the first suggestion is to make the feedings short and frequent. If that doesn't work, the mother may be advised to express her milk, put it into a bottle, and thicken it with cereal.

Most physicians will not watch a mother breastfeed her baby, but if they did, they would notice, perhaps, that it is extremely uncommon for babies to spit up while they are on the breast. It does happen that a baby will spit up while still latched on to the breast, but even I, who watch thousands of feedings every year, only see a baby spit up on the breast once a year or less.

By applying the bottle-feeding model to breastfeeding, we give breastfeeding mothers the worst possible advice with regard to dealing with reflux. The feedings should not be short (whatever that means). The baby should be on the breast for as long as he'll hold on to it, even if he is not drinking. While he sucks, there are small waves of muscle contraction in the esophagus (tube from mouth to stomach) in the direction of the stomach, which likely explains why the baby does not spit up while on the breast. When the baby is getting very little milk at the end of the feeding, little is coming in from up top, and the stomach is emptying. So when he finally comes off the breast he will spit up less or not at all. It's simple, but requires an understanding of breastfeeding.

It's Not Working

You've tried everything that has been mentioned, your baby is still breastfeeding, which is good, but he is still colicky. What now? First, you should know that colicky breastfed babies tend to be very intelligent. This may be because they get so much attention and handling and care, or it may just be that smart babies are often colicky. (Of course, this doesn't mean that your noncolicky baby won't be intelligent.) It is, though, partly due to the breastmilk.

But the colicky time will pass. One day, your baby will no longer be colicky. It may happen between one day and the next, or the change may be gradual, but someday it will happen. It may even happen when he turns three months old, as it did with our first, and as the books say it's supposed to.

Lie down with your baby and nurse him while lying down. This can be especially helpful in the evening when babies sometimes want to suck and suck and suck, and cry if they don't. If you lie down with your baby, you may fall asleep. You won't know, then, how long he has been on the breast. An eight-hour uninterrupted sleep will be only a memory for a while. Nap and rest when you can. You can face the difficult moments better when you are well rested.

Use whatever family you have to help you—not to feed the baby, but to walk the baby, do housework for you so you can have a few minutes to yourself.

A glass of wine or beer may help also, and it will do no harm. It might help you sleep when you lie down with the baby. You may be calmer when he cries. If the rest of the family has a glass as well, they will also calm down.

One thing having children does is change your perception of time. With a new baby, a 24-hour day can seem like an eternity, even if he's not colicky. But the weeks and months fly by. Before you turn around, he'll be six months old, six years old, 20 years old. This time will never, ever be back, either. Enjoy what you can of it, even if it is difficult. Take pleasure in your baby's smile, even if he graces you with it only as you feel ready to throw him out the window. I don't know how babies know, but they smile just as you have gotten to the end of your rope. It's a survival mechanism, that smile.

Know that by giving the baby this time, by struggling to stay awake in the night to calm him, by holding and comforting and singing to him, you are doing the right thing. Put him to the breast and comfort him. That way, at least, you can fall asleep. Nobody else will do this. You can't pay a babysitter to do what you are doing. The payoff comes later. When you see how charming your previously colicky baby becomes, you can say, "I did that."

10

When the Baby
Refuses the Breast

Myth: If a baby is unable to take the breast during the first few days after birth, he will never take the breast and it is not worth continuing to try.

Fact: It is not unusual for a baby who has at first refused the breast to begin nursing later. It is definitely worth continuing to try. When the mother has a generous supply of milk, the baby will almost always eventually take the breast on his own by the age of four to eight weeks.

When a baby cannot take the breast, it can be disheartening and frustrating for the mother and everyone around her. Many women—already feeling quite emotional in those early postpartum days—are devastated. It often feels personal, as though the baby is rejecting *her*. It can be helpful for the mother in this situation to know that this is not her fault and that it is almost always just a temporary problem. Her baby will learn to breastfeed, given some time and patience.

It is not clear why some babies cannot seem to take the breast, but usually a combination of factors comes into play. Probably no single factor mentioned below would be *the* cause of the baby's refusing the breast, but when two or three or more factors are added together, the cumulative effect is that the baby finds it impossible to latch on.

It is interesting that when babies are born after labors with few interventions, they rarely have problems latching on. I do not remember ever hearing of this as a problem when I worked in Africa—although, dealing with 1,500 deliveries a month, I was not able to be current on all the babies that were born.

Babies "latch on" where they get a good flow of milk. Thus, if a baby goes to the breast and the milk flows slowly, or not at all, he may not latch on. (Many babies will latch on, but not well; they are unable to get much milk, so they nibble for a while and then fall asleep. This is probably the situation, unfortunately, for most babies during the first days until the mother's milk becomes abundant.) The baby may struggle and fight, or he may just go limp and seem to sleep, or even do both at one attempted feeding, or sleep at one attempted feeding and struggle at another. In all these cases, the baby has not really latched on. When the baby struggles and cries at the breast, it is obvious to everyone that he has not latched on. However, when the baby only nibbles or sleeps at the breast, it may not be obvious to the inexperienced helper or to the mother, and in that case, the baby may be at risk for serious weight loss (see Chapter 5, Not Enough Milk).

Mothers do have enough milk for their babies in the first few days. But the baby must latch on well in order to get that milk.

Why the Baby's Not Latching On

1. The baby is not put to the breast early

When a baby is allowed to follow his instincts and find the breast and latch on immediately after birth, the chances of his later being unable to latch on are much reduced. Studies in Scandinavian countries, where babies are routinely placed on their mothers' abdomens after birth and allowed to find her breasts and self-attach, report that it takes, on average, about an hour for the baby to latch on to the breast. Some will, of course, latch on almost immediately after birth; other babies take much longer; and a few never do self-attach.

While it is better than nothing for mother and baby to have a few minutes together after birth to begin breastfeeding, in many cases this is simply not long enough to allow the baby to latch on. If the baby does begin to breastfeed, he should be allowed to nurse until he lets go on his own or falls asleep, rather than being taken away because some arbitrary time limit has been reached.

When the baby is taken away without breastfeeding soon after birth, and returned hours later, he may then refuse the breast. Sometimes these babies just ignore the breast when held in position to feed, as though they don't know what to do with it. Others shake their heads back and forth as though searching for something but not able to recognize the breast even when it is right there.

On the other hand, we don't want babies being pushed at the breast when they are not ready for it. This causes aversion to the breast and more problems with breastfeeding.

2. Maternal medications during labor

There is no doubt that narcotics given to the mother during labor interfere with the baby's being able to self-attach or to latch on. Narcotics given to the mother during labor enter the baby through the placenta and may depress his nervous system. Occasionally, this depression is so profound that babies need to be given another medication (a narcotic antagonist) at birth to stimulate their breathing. If something as vital as breathing can be depressed by a narcotic, it is easy to see how narcotics may also interfere with the coordination a baby needs to latch on and suckle well. Some narcotics are better than others, but it is interesting that probably the worst narcotic from the point of view of breastfeeding is also one of the ones most commonly used in labor—meperidine (Demerol). It is a problem because it stays in the baby's body for a long time and may affect the baby for many days. Other narcotics have similar actions, but do not stay in the baby's body for as long a time. Not all babies whose mothers received narcotics during labor are unable to take the breast, but add in a few more interfering factors, and there may be problems.

Does epidural or spinal anesthesia cause problems? This question has not been definitely answered, and there are studies that claim to prove both sides. One of the issues not often addressed is that of other factors being added in. It is quite possible that this type of anesthesia causes only minimal interference with breastfeeding—that there is a definite effect, but it is very small. If breastfeeding support in hospital is good and hospital routines are conducive to initiating breastfeeding, then overall there may be no issue. However, if breastfeeding support in hospital is poor and hospital routines are not conducive to initiating breastfeeding (an altogether too common situation), the small effect of epidural or spinal anesthesia may be enough to tip the scale for many mothers and babies.

Many studies also do not take into account how long the mother has had the epidural. It may make no difference to breastfeeding if the mother has an epidural for a couple of hours only at the end of the labor, say, but could make a difference if she had the epidural in place for 24 hours. It is indisputable, however, that drugs from epidural or spinal anesthesia do get into the mother's bloodstream, and thus do get into the baby, though usually only in very low concentrations.

3. Separations of mother and baby

Babies learn to breastfeed by breastfeeding. They should therefore be given every opportunity to take the breast in the first few days. Separation of the mother and baby results in missed opportunities for feeding. Of course, there are situations when mothers and babies, because of illness of one or the other or both, cannot be together, but these situations are not common.

Many hospitals explain that they take the baby away from the mother so she can rest and recover from labor, but there is no evidence that mothers who are separated from their babies are better rested. On the contrary, most mothers are more rested and less stressed when they are with their babies. Most mothers have eagerly awaited this baby for too many months to want the baby to be taken somewhere else. The pleasure most mothers have in holding and stroking their new babies and putting their babies to the breast makes the fatigue they had during labor almost magically disappear.

Mothers and babies who are together from birth learn how to sleep in the same rhythm. Thus, when the baby starts waking for a feed, the mother is also starting to wake up naturally. This is not as tiring for the mother as being awakened from a deep sleep, as she often is if the baby is elsewhere when he wakes up.

The baby shows long before he starts crying that he is ready to feed. His breathing may change, for example. It is interesting how moth-ers can often sleep through all sorts of noises, yet wake up with the baby's change from regular deep breathing to rapid shallow breaths. Or the baby may start to stretch. The mother, being in light sleep, will awaken, her milk will start to flow, and the calm and not-too-hungry baby will be content to nurse. A baby who has been crying for some time before being tried on the breast may refuse to take the breast even if he is ravenous. Mothers and babies should be encouraged to sleep side by side in hospital. This is a great way for mothers to rest while the baby nurses. Breastfeeding should be relaxing, not tiring. And the baby is more likely to take the breast and be patient at the breast if he is not starving.

4. Early use of artificial nipples

Only in extremely rare situations do artificial nipples need to be used, even if supplementation is truly necessary (which it would not be, most of the time, if mothers got good help with latching early). The alternatives are not ideal, but they are better than using artificial nipples.

Unfortunately, many babies are given either pacifiers or bottles of formula or sugar water within the first few days of birth. This can seriously interfere with the baby's breastfeeding.

The worst case seems to be when the baby does not latch on in the first hours after birth, or seems to resist or refuse the breast, and is then taken away to the nursery and given a bottle or two. When he gets hungry again, and is brought back to his mother, he fusses at the breast, searching for that firm rubber nipple that gave him milk last time. Since that feeding frequently goes badly, too, the baby is often given another bottle; soon he is convinced that milk comes from artificial nipples and he resists the breast even more.

If the baby is fussy all the time, and neither improving the latch nor compression help, and the mother cannot be encouraged just to keep the baby at the breast longer, then giving the baby a supplement of expressed milk (first choice) or sugar water using a lactation aid is preferable, in my opinion, to giving the baby a pacifier or a bottle. I want to emphasize that fixing the breastfeeding technique must come before giving a supplement, because in too many hospitals, giving the supplement is the first step. Even if given by lactation aid at the breast, this is wrong. The latch should be fixed before any supplements are suggested. But if the baby is still frantic, I find that often after just 5 ml or 10 ml of sugar water, the baby will calm right down. Of course, if expressed breastmilk is available, it is preferable to sugar water.

Mothers should be encouraged to start expressing as soon as there is any possibility of feeding the baby other than at the breast. If no one suggests this to you, you suggest it. Ask to be shown how to hand-express colostrum.

5. Problems of the nipples and breast

Mothers often believe that the main reason the baby will not latch on is that they have flat nipples, or inverted nipples or other anatomic problems of their breasts. Women are often encouraged to believe that they just do not have the "right equipment" to nourish their babies. There is no doubt that a nipple that protrudes is easier for the baby to latch on to. But the baby has to latch on to the breast, not just the nipple, so even inverted nipples can work just fine. Remember, too, that mothers and babies change with time, and a breast that is difficult for a baby on day two, may be just fine on day seven or day fifteen. A proper latch always helps, since, with a proper latch, a baby gets more milk; if a baby gets more milk, he is likely to stay where he gets it.

Inverted nipples

An inverted nipple is one that sinks down into the breast rather than protruding. Inverted nipples can make it more difficult for the baby to get on to the breast, but not impossible. In some cases, as the baby comes on to the breast and applies pressure with his mouth, the breast tissue seems to move away from him, slipping away so he cannot grasp the breast. Mothers have more problems if the nipple is not only inverted, but also seems to have a ring of firm tissue around it, making it more difficult for the baby to grasp.

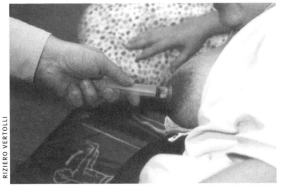

RIZIERO VERTOLLI

Using a nipple "everter" or "extractor" to pull out a flat or inverted nipple before the baby is tried on the breast. Easy to make.

Inverted nipples can sometimes be pulled out (everted) using a device shown in the photo. These devices are available in most breastfeeding clinics. There are also commercial gadgets that can be used during the pregnancy to pull out the nipple.

Inverted nipples usually become "uninverted," or at least less inverted, as the baby starts to latch on, as the days go on, but also within a single feeding. The baby's suckling will help the nipple to protrude.

Flat nipples

Flat nipples (nipples that don't protrude, but also are not inverted) may also make latching on more difficult (especially in conjunction with inappropriate interference), but far less so than inverted nipples. A good beginning and good latching technique are usually all that are necessary.

Large or very long nipples

Very large nipples can be more of a problem than inverted or flat nipples. They may result in no problems at all, but a very large or very long nipple can make it difficult for the baby to take the breast properly to get milk. To breastfeed, the baby needs to take not only the nipple into his mouth, but a good portion of the breast as well, so that he can compress the milk ducts and extract the milk. When the nipples are very large, the baby's mouth is filled up with nipple, and he can't get much of the breast. In such a case, it sometimes takes several weeks to get the baby latching on well, but this problem definitely improves as the baby grows. However, if the mother's milk supply is abundant, the baby will get milk even if his latch is not very good.

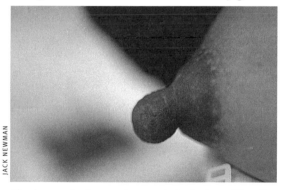

The large nipple may be an obstacle to getting the baby to latch on properly, but with time and patience it can be done.

Engorged breasts

Engorgement on the third or fourth day after the baby's birth may result in a baby not being able to latch on. I do not believe that babies latch on just fine until "the milk comes in" and then refuse the breast because of engorgement. I believe that the baby never really latched on at all, though he did allow the breast into his mouth and made some sucking motions. But when it becomes more difficult for the baby to latch on because of the engorgement, the fact that the baby was not latching on before now becomes painfully obvious. Prevention is the best treatment here, which means getting a good latch from very early on.

If engorgement is making the breast so hard that the baby can't compress it to latch on, it may help to express or pump some milk to soften the area around the nipple and make latching on a bit easier. Good positioning and latching technique will often get the baby to latch on in spite of engorgement. See also the sidebar entitled "Reverse Pressure Softening" by Jean Cotterman under Sore Breasts/Severe Engorgement.

Very large breasts

Sometimes women with very large breasts have difficulties latching their babies on because they find it awkward to get the baby positioned and to support their breasts while feeding. As well, some women with very large breasts also have flat nipples, adding a further complication.

The problem of handling large breasts can be alleviated by using a sling (made from any reasonably soft material) that holds up the breast in the same way as a sling helps hold up an arm in a cast. Using a sling under her breast allows the mother to use one hand to direct the nipple and areola correctly, rather than using that hand to hold up the breast. Women with very large breasts sometimes find that lying down with the baby makes it easier for them to handle their breasts, and easier for the baby to take the breast.

6. Baby problems that make latching on more difficult

Some babies cannot latch on because they have

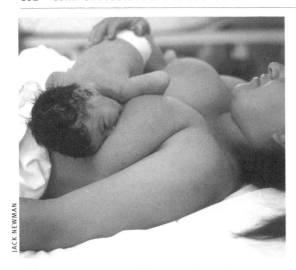

JACK NEWMAN

This baby was just born. He crawled toward the breast and latched on all by himself, after a quick right turn. His mother has large, pendulous breasts with flat nipples. But the baby latched.

medical problems that make it more difficult, or in some cases impossible. In many situations, however, even with anatomical problems, babies can latch on if given time, and if the mothers are given guidance. It is not possible to discuss the entire range of problems that may interfere with the baby's latching on, because these are legion (though, luckily, none is common). The mother should not accept, however, that breastfeeding is just not possible. In many cases, mothers whose babies have these problems have not even tried, because they were always told that breastfeeding was impossible and that it was not worth wasting time trying to get the baby onto the breast. In some situations, breastfeeding may turn out to be impossible, but it is always worth trying.

Even if it turns out to be impossible to breastfeed, you can still provide your baby with breastmilk. If you keep up your milk supply, maybe the baby will latch on a few weeks later or even a few months later, depending on the causes of his breastfeeding problems.

Neurologically depressed babies

Some babies are temporarily depressed, neurologically speaking, usually from the mother's receiving medication during the labor. Other babies have longer-lasting problems. Examples are babies with Trisomy 21 (Down syndrome), or babies who were deprived of oxygen during labor or during the pregnancy, or babies with anatomical abnormalities of the brain. Even in these cases, however, some will latch on right away, despite their problems, and others take more time. Most will latch on eventually. Don't get discouraged. Time, patience, encouragement, and skilled help can work wonders. And it is worth it. Babies with medical problems need breastmilk (and breastfeeding) more, not less.

In fact, my experience with babies with Trisomy 21 is that they can usually latch on and breastfeed well. At first they tend to be very floppy, and many have large tongues (or small mouths) that can interfere with their taking the breast. As in all such cases, making sure that the mother develops a good milk supply is the key to getting the baby latched on. This usually means she should pump or express her milk frequently if the baby is not taking the breast well.

Babies who have been deprived of oxygen during birth can have very serious medical problems. Their neurological injury, and often the treatment for the injury, may interfere with breastfeeding and their latching on. However, these babies also improve, in general, and again, time, patience, encouragement, and skilled help are key.

Anatomic abnormalities of the mouth or oral cavity

Babies may be born with abnormalities of the mouth or oral cavity. The most common of these abnormalities are a cleft palate, cleft lip, or a combination of the two. Babies with cleft lip alone, or cleft lip with an indentation of the gum line, usually should have few problems breastfeeding. A cleft lip may be overcome, if it is causing problems, by positioning the baby in such a way that the mother's breast fills in the cleft. Tape may also be used to close the cleft, if necessary.

A cleft palate is more problematic. With our current level of expertise and knowledge, it is true that many babies will not be able to latch on. However, if no attempt is made to get the baby breastfeeding, then the baby will definitely not take the breast. Unfortunately, many cleft palate programs assume that breastfeeding is impossible and discourage the mother from trying, in the belief that she will undoubtedly be disappointed. I believe this is a bad approach. Many mothers wonder later about the loss of breastfeeding and grieve that they had not at least tried. What exactly is the harm in trying?

In fact, if more mothers did try to breastfeed their babies with cleft palates, maybe more would succeed. Over the past 10 years, we have learned a great deal about helping normal babies breastfeed. Experience with helping mothers get babies latched on has resulted in a group of lactation specialists who can help the mother get almost any normal baby to take the breast. A few years ago, many women simply gave up breastfeeding when they ran into challenges, but now we have skilled people who can help them. If we made attempts with babies with cleft palates, and got more experience, maybe more of the babies with cleft palates would also be able to breastfeed.

Some cleft palate programs encourage the use of an obturator, a plastic mouth piece that fills the cleft. These have apparently been used with almost all cleft palate babies in Switzerland, and we hear reports of success with breastfeeding.

Cleft palates may be complete, running right to the front of the mouth, in which case they are pretty obvious. Or they may be partial, involving only the soft palate or part of the soft palate. If they are partial, they may not be obvious at first glance. All babies who refuse to latch on, or make an unusual amount of noise when they are trying to suckle at the breast, should be examined to see if they have a cleft of the soft palate only. Sometimes these are easier to feel than to see.

Tongue tie

A tongue tie is not included among the abnormalities because, strictly speaking, it is not really an abnormality in the sense that a cleft palate is an abnormality. But a tongue tie can be an impediment to successful breastfeeding.

Under the tongue we all have a whitish vertical strip of tissue called the *frenulum*, which attaches to the floor of our mouths at one end and to the tongue at the other. When the frenulum is tight, it can prevent the baby from getting his tongue well forward to cup under the breast and extract the milk. If the baby cannot get milk well from the breast, he may refuse to take the breast, not out of orneriness, but out of frustration. I do not believe that a mild or moderate tongue tie alone prevents a baby from latching on, but if this condition is combined with other factors, such as early introduction of bottles, or poor positioning at the breast, even mild tongue ties could certainly result in inability to take the breast. Finally, if the tongue does not protrude well, the mother can get sore nipples from the baby's tongue striking the nipple.

Many physicians are adamant that tongue tie could not possibly cause problems for breastfeeding and that release of tongue tie is completely unnecessary. Parents are often caught between the physician who says that snipping the

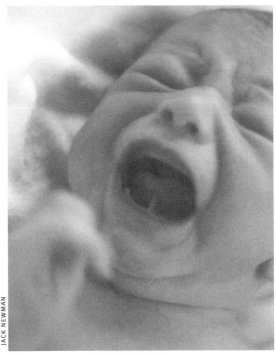

JACK NEWMAN

A tight frenulum (tongue tie) prevents the baby's tongue from wrapping around the areola.

frenulum is pointless, and lactation specialists who are urging the parents to have it done.

Snipping the frenulum used to be a common procedure in newborns. In some areas it was actually routine for every newborn to have his frenulum snipped at birth. First the umbilical cord, then the frenulum. However, over the years, evidence showed that a tight frenulum probably did not interfere with speech development, for example, unless the tongue tie was really severe. These studies were being done however, when breastfeeding was also decreasing in frequency, and the question of whether a tongue tie might interfere with breastfeeding was probably not even considered. Whatever the reason, doctors stopped doing releases of tongue tie.

Our clinic experience, though, suggests that snipping the frenulum can make a difference to the mother's comfort during breastfeeding, to the ease with which the baby gets milk, and in helping babies who are not latching on to latch on. It is an extremely simple procedure. The actual snipping of the frenulum takes less than a second and rarely causes the baby pain. The babies do usually cry because they are being held down, but it is helpful for me for the baby to cry, because he opens his mouth, making the whole procedure quick and easy. Since the frenulum is bloodless, there is rarely more than a drop or two of blood in the baby's mouth after the procedure, if it is done properly. Bleeding almost always stops as soon as the baby goes to the breast.

Does it do any good to clip the frenulum? Sometimes it makes a difference. Sometimes it does not. Most of the time, because I do more to help this baby breastfeed than just cutting the frenulum, I am never sure if it makes a difference. If this procedure were complicated or dangerous, I would not do it. But since it is not complicated, and as long as certain precautions are taken (cut only what is bloodless), not dangerous, I don't hesitate to do it.

Suctioning at birth

Although suctioning the baby's nose and throat and even his stomach is routine in many hospitals, this procedure is not necessary for a normal baby who is not having any problems. In some circumstances, it is necessary and helps the baby to breathe properly. But a healthy, full-term baby who is breathing fine at birth does not need to be suctioned. There is concern that suction may actually cause some babies to stop breathing. I have seen this happen several times. And there is evidence that suctioning of the stomach may result in the babies' sucking and nursing less well. It may not be surprising that vigorous suction can interfere with the baby's desire to take the breast. These procedures may cause irritation to the mouth and throat, but even more probable, the abnormal stimulation may disorganize the baby's suckle by sending very strong and unusual signals to the brain.

How to Help
When Baby Refuses the Breast

Just a reminder that the best treatment is prevention. Avoid narcotics during labor, if possible. The baby should be allowed the opportunity and time to crawl up to the breast and "self-attach." Suctioning at birth should be avoided unless it is medically necessary, which it usually is not.

The First 24 Hours

Most babies do not really have to feed in the first 24 hours or so. Yes, we have stressed repeatedly that it is important for the baby to have the opportunity to begin breastfeeding as soon as possible after birth. But if the baby, for whatever reason, is not feeding during that time, it is not a reason to panic and bring in bottles of formula or start finger-feeding.

In fact, up until the 1970s many hospitals had routines that included the provision that babies were not to be fed at all for the first 24 hours. My most poignant memory of obstetrics training as a final-year medical student in Toronto (1969), aside from one Italian woman who sang opera beautifully when she was having labor pains, was what an incredible racket came from the nursery. The babies were crying and crying because they were not supposed to be fed during this time. That was the rule: nothing for 24 hours. As mentioned elsewhere, this approach was based on the observations of many nurses that babies fed formula during the first day or so were often cranky, spit up frequently, or had diarrhea. Now that formulas are more like breastmilk, from the

point of view of concentration of ingredients, this is less of a problem, and so everyone goes bananas if the baby has not fed for four hours. But trying to force a baby who may not be ready to take the breast may result in the baby's resisting, crying, and developing an aversion to the breast. If hospital staff become really worried because the baby has not fed for six hours, the baby will often be started on supplements, probably given by bottle. This may further undermine the baby's willingness and ability to take the breast.

If, however, it seems necessary to get the baby feeding, finger-feeding is a good way to wake a sleepy baby, and it avoids a bottle. A baby usually will start sucking if something is put in his mouth, even when he is quite sleepy. If he also gets some fluid, he will often wake up and be ready to feed. It is not necessary to use the finger-feeding very long—only a minute or so sometimes, until the baby wakes up. In this situation it is not necessary to use formula. The fluid used, of course, should be expressed milk (colostrum) whenever possible. Expressing should begin as soon as it has been deemed necessary to feed the baby, for whatever reason. Even a few drops of breastmilk (colostrum) are worth giving to the baby, and can be mixed with sugar water to be given easily. (You need a certain volume of liquid to get it through the plastic tube.) If no milk can be easily expressed, then sugar water is fine in this situation. We are trying to get the baby awake and feeding, not necessarily trying to get a lot of calories into him.

Don't be discouraged if you aren't able to express much milk. Remember that in the first few days many women can express more by hand than they can even with the best industrial-size pump. Remember, too, that not being able to express any milk means nothing as far as your current or future milk supply is concerned.

So colostrum is preferable, because of the antibodies and active white cells and other benefits. Sugar water is preferred over formula for a couple of reasons. One is that giving the baby formula in this situation suggests to the mother that formula is good and necessary, and that it will save your hungry baby. It is also possible that a single feeding of formula, at this early age, may set off a chain of events that leads to the baby later developing diabetes or allergies or other problems.

If the formula is necessary, fine, we give it. But it is rarely necessary in the first 24 or even 48 hours.

Some babies will not wake up when finger-fed, but if they feed, they have at least gotten some fluids and some calories. They will probably wake up more after this. Some babies, as they go longer and longer without fluids, will get sleepier, rather than more upset. This is the danger when babies are only seeming to latch on when they go home. They seem to be breastfeeding but are not, and the mother may interpret the increasing sleepiness as a sign that the baby is satisfied and full of milk. It is not. It is very important for the mother to be able to tell if the baby is actually getting milk at the breast.

The intense pressure to start feeding comes, essentially, from the fact that new mothers and babies are often leaving the hospital within 24 to 36 hours of a normal birth. I find this quite understandable. It is difficult for both the staff and the new parents to be faced with a 24-hour-old baby about to go home who has never fed in his whole life. Given the scarcity of resources in many communities for follow-up of new mothers and their babies, the problem is not only difficult, but potentially serious for the health of the baby.

Once the baby is alert and interested in eating, finger-feeding should be stopped, and the baby then tried on the breast (using the best positioning possible). He may take it. If he does, fine. If not, pushing him to take it will not work—he will either go limp, or go ballistic. You want the baby's experience at the breast to be calm and pleasant. If he gets upset, comfort him and calm him down before trying again.

Sometimes it will be helpful to use a lactation aid at the breast to help the baby latch on and stay at the breast. Again, expressed breastmilk is the best to use, followed by breastmilk diluted in sugar water, followed by sugar water—at least in the first 24 hours or so. This requires help and some skill, as the tube needs to be held in place along the mother's breast as the baby latches on. If the baby sucks a couple of times, he will get something and may stay latched on. This technique, as well as other techniques to help latch on a reluctant baby, will be discussed later when we deal with getting the older baby onto the breast.

The baby can get all the fluids he needs, and all the calories he needs (if the mother is using colostrum), with just finger-feeding in the first 24 to 48 hours. Finger-feeding can be slow, but in the first couple of days, babies don't need a lot of fluid or calories, and finger-feeding will be adequate to the task.

24 to 72 Hours After Birth

Many babies who don't latch on in the first 24 hours will do so during the second or third day, usually because the milk flow is increasing. Again, good positioning, as good a latch as possible, and getting milk into the baby, encourages the baby to take the breast.

As during the first 24 hours, if there is urgency to get the baby onto the breast, the same techniques can be used as were used during the first 24 hours: good positioning and latching, lactation aid, and finger-feeding.

After 72 Hours

Once the baby is getting older than three days, his caloric requirements increase significantly. If the mother is able to express her own milk to provide all the baby requires, this is great. In some cases, banked milk may be available. But if the mother is not yet able to express enough for the baby's requirements, it may be necessary to add formula. Seventy-two hours is not a "line in the sand," but most babies will do fine with some expressed milk and some sugar water for the first two to three days of life. However, significant amounts of sugar water for more than the first two or three days are not good for the baby. It is for this reason that expressing of milk should begin early, so that the mother develops a good milk supply, and so that colostrum will be available for feeding. Colostrum not only gives the baby immunity and nutrition, but helps the baby evacuate his meconium, significantly reducing his risk of developing jaundice.

So the baby is three days old, now, and still not latching on? First of all, don't despair. Keep working at it. Babies change, develop, and learn. Breast tissue changes and becomes more flexible; nipples elongate or become "uninverted." Although some lactation experts might recommend a nipple shield at this point, I feel strongly that this is not the right way to go. A nipple shield looks like a regular nipple used on a bottle, but is usually made of thinner material. When they are used, the mother fits the nipple shield over her own nipple, and puts the baby to the breast.

Nipple shields can be tried later, if other approaches have not worked, but not now. Using a nipple shield in the first week after the baby was born is, I believe, a way of saying, "I don't know what else to do." You are not giving you and your baby enough time.

A Few Principles

1. A baby will usually latch on if he gets what he wants. What does he want? MILK. This is why it is so important that the baby come to the breast just so, with the lower lip as far away from the nipple as possible. Or, to put it another way, the part of the baby's face that touches the breast first is his chin. When the baby comes to the breast like that, he gets his gums under the milk sinuses, and if he starts sucking he will start to get some milk. The mother should help the baby get milk by compressing the breast as the baby comes on to the breast, so that he will get some flow as soon as he gets his mouth around the breast. Some mothers express a little milk before the baby comes to the breast, so that there is a drop or two on the nipple. This sometimes encourages the baby to suck.

2. An angry baby will often not latch on, no matter how hungry he is. Sometimes mothers believe that if the baby is really hungry, he is likely to take the breast better. This is almost always untrue. The hungrier, or the more upset the baby, the less likely he is to take the breast. It is also not true that if the baby is very hungry he will take his "less favorite side." If the baby seems to prefer one side over the other, try first with the easier side, not the harder one. Or if the baby does not have a preferred side, but you seem to have more milk on one side than the other, start where you seem to have more milk.

3. If you bring the baby to the breast, and he doesn't latch on, it is better to let the baby come off the breast, and start all over. If you hold him against the breast, hoping he'll latch on, he's more likely to get angry or to go limp. This won't help him latch on. It's much better to take the baby off the breast and try

again—even if you do this six or seven times in a row—than to keep him at the breast.

How do you know a baby is not latched on? A baby who does not suck is not latched on, even if he has the breast in his mouth. Or if the baby slips off the breast, he is not latched on. Even if you are not sure if the baby has taken the breast or not, if the baby is not actually sucking, you are better to take the baby off the breast and start again. If the baby does make sucking motions, then compress the breast to give him some milk flow, and he may start drinking. If he drinks, great.

4. You and the baby need lots of skin-to-skin contact. Even if you cannot get the baby to latch on right away, skin-to-skin contact helps. Take the baby into bed with you. The baby should have only a diaper on, and you should be undressed from the waist up. This close contact may encourage the baby to latch on.

More About Latching On

If the baby does not latch on within the first three or four days, it is important to get help from someone who is experienced. Often, with skilled help, the baby will latch on. And sometimes, a baby latches on just once and there is no looking back. He gets it and that's it—he's a breastfeeding superstar. It's not always that easy, of course, but it happens often enough that it is worth the effort. I encourage mothers to seek out that help by the time the baby is four days old, because the sooner the baby gets on the breast, the more likely it is that he will continue latching on. I see too many mothers with three-week-old babies who are not latching on. This is too long to wait to ask for help.

If the baby is not going to take the breast, there is no point in struggling for half an hour or more.

Take a rest after a few minutes. Try the other side—he might take it. But if he does not quickly take the second side, go to finger-feeding.

The purposes of finger-feeding in this situation are:

• to calm the baby down. As previously mentioned, an angry or upset baby is not likely to take the breast.
• to get the baby sucking as he would on the breast. Finger-feeding has to be done correctly for this to work. That is why you need help from someone with experience.

When the baby is finger-feeding well, you should be able to feel his tongue cupped around your finger and drawing backward. After you have had the baby feeding like this for a minute

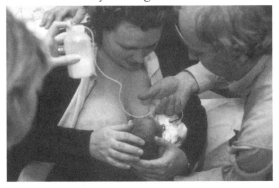

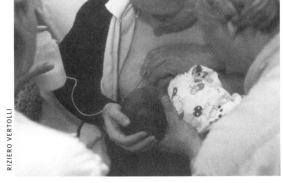

Finger-feeding is being used to calm the baby before trying him on the breast (top). Then, an attempt is made to latch him on with the lactation aid, so that he gets good milk flow when he starts to suck.

or two, try again at the breast. Of course, if you are worn out from trying or from frustration, let him go longer with the finger-feeding, until you feel up to trying again.

If the baby has not latched on with this feeding, you can finish the feeding with finger-feeding, or with cup-feeding. The main disadvantage of finger-feeding is that it is slow. And like all alternative methods of feeding, the baby might get to like it too much. The chances are less than with the bottle, since finger-feeding is frequently slow and the sucking motions the baby must do are different, but some babies do get "finger-feeding spoiled."

It is sometimes easier, if you have a helper, to have the baby latch on to the breast when the lactation aid (the same tube and container of milk you used for finger-feeding) is lined up along the breast with the end just at the end of the nipple. The tube will probably be full, as you may have just finger-fed the baby. The baby will get a faster flow of milk through the tube as he attempts to suck, and may remain at the breast nursing. There should be no difference in how the baby is positioned or moved toward the breast when the lactation aid is being used. As far as everyone, including the baby, is concerned, this is just a breast that has more flow than it had before.

Sometimes it is easier to get the baby to take the breast when you and he are lying down, side by side. Why is that, when most mothers find that feeding lying on their sides is more difficult, at first? I'm not sure, but if it works, great.

I have seen an Australian video that shows a one-week-old baby latching on for the first time while in a bath with his mother. The baby is lying on the mother, skin to skin, both are immersed in warm water, and the baby just latches on, all by himself. Others have also had success with mothers and babies bathing together.

Don't wear yourself out trying one thing after another, though. Do what you can, and don't get discouraged.

> "The child, offered the mother's breast,
> Will not in the beginning grab it;
> But soon it clings to it with zest."
> —Goethe, *Faust*

Artificial Nipples

If at all possible, at this stage, try to avoid using bottles or pacifiers. It is quite easy to use a cup to feed even a very young or small baby, but, like many skills in life, it is necessary to learn how. And babies learn most easily by being shown. Not all health professionals are even aware that a newborn baby can cup-feed, so they cannot teach you. Still, if you must give a bottle, go ahead, but try to do it as little as possible. Keeping up your milk supply is more important than avoiding a bottle.

If the Baby Still Doesn't Take the Breast

There comes a time when it is more important to maintain the milk supply than to avoid artificial nipples. For some mothers this time comes within a few days of birth. For others, the finger-feeding is no problem, and they can keep it up for weeks. The main problem is that finger-feeding is usually slow, though some babies can manage to do it as rapidly as if they were drinking from a bottle. Nevertheless, even when finger-feeding is not a burden for the new parents, there comes a time to say, "We've tried this long enough, let's try something new."

In my own practice, I find it is worth changing the approach if the techniques above do not work by the time the baby is about two weeks of age. No timetable need be followed, and if the baby is close to latching on, it is not necessarily even advisable. Generally, however, I will then suggest to the mother that she express her milk and give it by bottle or use a nipple shield. A nipple shield is not always the solution, because a nipple shield is not always easy to use, but if it does work, it is easier for the mother than expressing the milk into a bottle and giving the bottle.

Remember, when the mother has an abundant milk supply, the baby will almost always latch on when he is between four and eight weeks of age. There are exceptions, but most will do so. Be patient. It's difficult, but it will pay off. One day at a time.

I usually see the mother a week later, after she has used the nipple shield and/or the bottle, and try again. Often the baby will then start latching on. Indeed, it would appear that around the two- or three-week mark, any change in what we try seems to make a difference. It is almost as if the baby thinks, "Oh, there's more than one way to get this stuff!"

So if a mother has been trying another approach—if, for example, she arrives at the clinic bottle-feeding her two-week-old baby—I will ask her to try finger-feeding. Then we put the baby to the breast. It is gratifying how many babies do latch on after a few days of finger-feeding (just before the feeding), and, indeed, sometimes after one single session.

Keeping Up Your Milk Supply

This is essential. As mentioned several times before, with an abundant milk supply available to him, the baby will almost always eventually latch on, no matter how he is fed.

If your milk supply is not abundant, it is, of course, more difficult. But most babies will still

latch on, if the mother has good help. Even if you find you must supplement with artificial baby milk at first, once the baby latches on, you probably will find that your milk supply increases in response to the baby's suckling, so that you may eventually not have to use supplements.

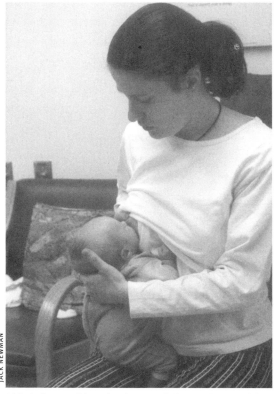

JACK NEWMAN

This baby would not latch on until the mother tried this position. Why did this work? Can't say. Until then, nothing we could do could make that baby take the breast. After he started latching like this, he started taking the breast in the more usual positions.

Even if the mother has an abundant supply, I sometimes suggest fenugreek and blessed thistle, and sometimes even domperidone, to increase her supply and rate of milk flow if the baby is not latching on. The greater the flow rate, the more likely the baby is to take the breast and stay there.

If the Baby Never Takes the Breast

This is unfortunate. But *your* milk in the bottle is still better than formula in the bottle.

It might also be possible to continue breastfeeding with a nipple shield if this has worked, and I am aware of a few mothers who have used one for many months without problem. It is not the best solution, but it is better than expressing and giving the expressed milk in a bottle, because it takes less time. In fact, if you tried the nipple shield earlier and it didn't work, you could try it again; the baby might now be willing to accept it.

And never say never. I am aware of a few mothers whose babies did not take the breast for four months or longer but eventually *did*—including one who took the breast for the first time when he was nine months old! I have even been e-mailed by a mother who pumped and gave her milk by bottle, and when the child was 26 months old he latched on and breastfed. Maybe more babies would begin breastfeeding after several months if their mothers kept up their milk supplies.

Keep offering the baby the breast, particularly when the baby is not ravenous, and when he is content. Keep him near you, skin to skin, whenever you can. Sleep with the baby next to you, with your breasts available to him. You never know, he may latch on in the middle of the night.

Finally, if your first did not latch on, do not assume that what happened with the first is likely to happen with the second. Breasts change, not only during the period immediately after birth, but also with the years and with new pregnancies. The factors that caused the problem with your first baby may not be present with later babies. So if you were not able to get your first to latch on, get information before the birth of the new baby. Have your baby where it is known that the staff have experience with helping mothers breastfeed and will be sympathetic to your desire to breastfeed. And get help early from an experienced lactation specialist if it looks as if the baby is not taking the breast well.

The "Nursing Strike"

Some mothers and babies run into a problem, which for want of a better expression has been called a "nursing strike." A baby, who up until then has been nursing relatively well, suddenly stops taking the breast. Even though obviously hungry, the baby will cry, scream, and push away if the mother tries to put him to the breast. Often, the more the mother tries, the more upset the baby gets. This "nursing strike" occurs typically around three months of age, and also around eight months of age, though there is some variability. It is not a common problem, but it is a most distressing one for the mother and the baby, as well as the rest of the family.

The nursing strike may occur suddenly without prior warning, or gradually worsen over a few days. Typically the baby does not actually refuse to nurse all the time. He may take the breast when he is sleepy, either going into a sleep or coming out of a sleep, and he may nurse well at night. But though the baby is obviously hungry, when he is alert during the day, he may adamantly fight the breast. Many prefer sucking their hands and not drinking. The great majority of these babies nurse well enough during the night or when they are sleepy to continue to gain weight. Perhaps they don't gain as rapidly as previously, but the weight gain usually remains at least adequate and sometimes much more than adequate. These were almost always rapidly growing babies from the beginning, and the slowdown in weight gain may be only relative to what the mother was used to, and still quite good. Some babies I have followed with this problem have gained weight nursing only three or four times in 24 hours.

The nursing strike may last for only a short period of time, or it may go on for weeks. The majority of nursing strikes do *not* go on for weeks, but gradually get better over a few days to a week or two. Some stop as suddenly as they start.

This problem seems to relate to the mother's abundant milk supply. I believe the baby probably was not latching on well from the beginning, but since I rarely see these mothers and babies before the nursing strike begins, I am only guessing here. Many mothers say they and their babies had problems with an "overactive letdown reflex" (see Chapter 9, Colic). Their babies would go to the breast, and when the letdown occurred, the baby would sputter, choke, and sometimes pull off the breast, crying from getting milk too quickly. This problem of the overactive letdown reflex then seems to get better for a few weeks, and then *boom*, the baby is on strike.

This nursing strike is not caused by an ear infection, or thrush in the mouth—thrush rarely bothers the baby.

The nursing strike should be distinguished from the problem caused by the decreased milk supply some mothers experience around three months after birth. In some cases the decreased supply is due to the birth control pill. In others, there is no obvious reason. In this case, the baby wants to go to the breast, but quickly becomes frustrated and begins to pull. In other words, the baby goes to the breast, obviously wants to nurse, but pulls off and cries because he is not getting milk well. Note, however, that occasionally babies on a nursing strike will go to the breast for very short periods of time—just long enough to take the edge off their hunger—and then pull away. It may not be easy to distinguish this behavior from that of the baby who is pulling off because the milk is not coming. This is another reason to learn how to know the baby is getting milk (the open mouth wide–pause–close mouth type of sucking that tells you the baby is getting milk). If the baby pulls off while just nibbling on the breast, it is because he is frustrated, not because he is on a nursing strike.

Why might your milk supply be down?

1. You have gone on the birth control pill. If you have, it's best to stop it.
2. You are pregnant.
3. You have been trying to stretch out the feedings, or "train" the baby to sleep through the night. If this is the case, better to feed the baby when he is hungry or when he is sucking his hand.
4. You are using bottles more than occasionally. Even when the milk supply is well established, frequent bottles teach baby a poor latch at a time when he expects rapid flow. With slow flow, the baby may pull away from the breast, further decreasing time at the breast, and further decreasing breastmilk supply.
5. An emotional "shock" can, occasionally, decrease the milk supply.
6. Sometimes an illness, particularly when associated with fever, can decrease the milk supply. So can mastitis. Usually, however, this does not occur with illness, luckily.
7. You are doing too much. Remember, you don't have to be supermother. Let the housework go. Sleep when your baby sleeps. Let the baby nurse while you sleep.
8. Some medications may decrease milk supply. Medications to look out for include antihistamines (e.g., Benadryl), pseudephedrine (e.g., Sudafed), and perhaps diuretics (drugs taken to increase urine output).

9. Some combination of the factors listed above.
10. Sometimes the milk supply decreases, particularly around three months, for no obvious reason.

One more reason requires a little more explanation. In the first few weeks, babies tend to fall asleep at the breast when the flow of milk is slow (this slowing of the flow occurs more rapidly if the baby is not well latched on). The baby will suck and sleep and suck, without getting large quantities at this point, but the mother may have a letdown reflex (milk ejection reflex) from time to time and the baby will drink more. When the mother's supply is abundant, the baby usually gains fine, though he may spend long periods on the breast despite the mother's abundant supply. However, by the time babies are six or eight weeks of age, younger sometimes (or some just always fall asleep when flow is slow), many babies start to pull away from the breast when the flow slows down, often within a few minutes of starting nursing. The mother will then likely put the baby to the other side, but then the baby will do the same thing. He may be hungry still, but may refuse the breast and suck his hand. He won't get those extra letdowns, which give him a few extra gushes of milk that he would have if he had stayed on the breast. So he drinks less, and the supply also decreases because he drinks less, and the baby then gets slower flow earlier in the feeding (because there is less milk) and you see what may happen. It doesn't always happen this way, and many babies may gain even if they do spend only a short period of time on the breast, but the baby may still pull off and suck his hand because he wants more sucking.

The way to prevent this is to get a good latch from the very first. However, many mothers are being told the latch is good even if it isn't. A better latch can help, sometimes even at a late date. Using compression will often keep a baby drinking (see protocol for "not enough milk"). Sometimes domperidone will increase the milk supply significantly. Do not use it if you are pregnant, however.

Why does a nursing strike happen?

No idea. I have never heard an explanation that I found convincing. And I have never come up with a hypothesis that I feel even comes close to explaining why.

Some babies do go on a complete nursing strike that can be traced to a specific event. For example, one mother had a 10-month-old baby boy who was nursing well. He was teething, and during one feeding he bit her hard, catching her by surprise. She cried out loudly and took him off the breast, and he started to cry. Her startled reaction had clearly upset him, and when she tried to nurse him again some time later, he refused and cried again. This was a complete nursing strike—he wouldn't nurse at all—but after three days she managed to get him to nurse in his sleep, and then he went right back to his previous pattern of breastfeeding.

What to Do

Remember that the nursing strike will usually get better spontaneously. Remember, too, that if the baby is breastfeeding well even three or four times in a 24-hour period, he will probably get enough milk to keep healthy. Six wet diapers in 24 hours is a good indication that the baby is not getting dehydrated. The diapers do not have to be soaking to prove the baby is maintaining hydration, though if they are not soaked, he may not be getting enough to gain weight well. However, should the baby become unusually sleepy, you should get help to make sure he is all right.

It is futile to try to force the baby to take the

breast when he does not want to. Do not try. The baby will get angrier, and chances are you will not get him to the breast in any case. Let him suck his hand if that is what he wants to do.

Try the baby on the breast when he is sleepy. This will often work. If he drinks at the breast, that's good. When he starts nibbling, use gentle compression to keep the flow going.

Take the baby into bed with you at night—him in a diaper only and you undressed from the waist up. Skin-to-skin contact may encourage him to take the breast. Do not try to get through the night without feedings.

Sometimes the baby will take the breast if you walk around with him in your arms, in breast-feeding position, until he gets a little sleepy, then try him on the breast. If you are using a pacifier, let him suck on the pacifier until he is calm and a little sleepy and then try him at the breast.

This is not the time to start a bottle or continue with the bottle. Your baby will almost always get enough with breastfeeding only, whatever little he seems to be doing. If you are truly concerned about his intake, give him your expressed milk with a spoon, eyedropper, or cup.

This can be a trying time for everyone. Remember, though, that there is a light at the end of the tunnel. Soon your baby will be back to nursing again.

The approach for the baby on a nursing strike at eight months of age is similar. There is more leeway because most eight-month-old babies are eating solid foods as well, and your milk can be mixed in with the solids even if the baby refuses to take the milk directly from you. Nursing strikes at this age usually do not last as long as they do when the baby starts at three months of age.

MOTHERS' STORIES
ANNA

Anna brought her baby, Samuel, to the breast-feeding clinic when he was nine days old. He was not taking the breast at all at that time.

Samuel was born after an uneventful pregnancy. The labor began just a few days before the due date, and was essentially also uneventful. Samuel's birthweight was 3.5 kg (7 lb 11 oz). Samuel was grunting at birth and was kept in the special care unit for a few hours until the grunting disappeared. He was treated with antibiotics for two days.

Anna first tried Samuel at the breast a few hours after he was born, but he would not latch on. She was instructed on how to finger-feed, which she did using sugar water. [*The mother should have been encouraged to start expressing her milk as soon as it was decided the baby needed to be fed. Unfortunately, this was not suggested. Any colostrum could have been added to the sugar water—even a few drops would have been good for the baby.*]

When I first saw Anna and Samuel, the mother was feeding some formula, but mostly expressed breastmilk. The baby was sometimes being finger-fed, sometimes bottle-fed. Samuel's weight at this point was 3.55 kg (7 lb 13 oz). [*The weight seems good, but nothing can be decided simply based on the weight, as the baby was weighed on a different scale from the hospital scale.*]

Anna has very large breasts, and the nipples are flat and difficult to grasp. Nevertheless, with my help, we were able to get the baby to latch on by carefully positioning him at the breast and waiting until his mouth was open wide before moving him onto the breast. Samuel fed well, and once he was no longer drinking at the breast, I introduced the lactation aid with the mother's expressed milk in order to keep Samuel breast-feeding.

Anna went home with the following plan:

1. She would "prepare" Samuel to take the breast with finger-feeding. Only a minute or two of finger-feeding is necessary. Then she would try him on the breast, compressing the breast to get a jet of milk as he came onto the breast.
2. If Samuel took the breast, fine. If he took the breast but did not actually drink, she would use breast compression and/or the lactation aid to keep him nursing. I had shown her the kind of sucking to watch for, to know if he was drinking well.
3. Return in one or two days if he was still not latching.

Anna and Samuel returned the next day. Anna could not manage to get Samuel to take the breast. [*This is not surprising. Samuel was able to take the breast when two extra experienced hands were there to help the mother. I had given this mother and her baby a lot of new information and techniques, and it is not easy to take it all in at one sitting.*] At the clinic, once again, the baby took the breast, but required the lactation aid still to keep breast-feeding. At this visit, the baby weighed 3.57 kg (7 lb 13.5 oz). Anna was encouraged to keep up the previous approach.

The next visit was six days later. Samuel weighed 3.69 kg (8 lb 2 oz). For the past couple of days, he had been taking the left breast well, and was taking the right breast a little. The mother had developed soreness of the nipples, which was treated with the usual measures (improve the latch, apply all-purpose nipple ointment).

Over the next few days, the baby took the right side better and better. By the time the baby was three weeks old, he was nursing very well.

The mother returned to the clinic to learn how to breastfeed lying down, which she had not managed on her own. [*I think she came primarily to show off her beautiful baby.*] He weighed 4.66 kg (10 lb 4 oz), breastfeeding exclusively.

When Samuel was 10 weeks old, Anna brought him again. For the past few days he had been nursing less and less well. And now he was refusing the breast most of the time. Nevertheless, he nursed well during the night, and sometimes, if Anna could try him at the breast when he was half asleep, he would also nurse. The pattern was obviously that of a nursing strike, although it was happening a little earlier than the typical time, which is at about three months of age. [*Nursing strikes are not common among the babies who were refusing the breast early on. At least not in my experience.*] Anna followed our advice, which was to feed him when he was ready, and not try to force him to the breast, which would have been a futile exercise.

Samuel's nursing strike lasted only a couple of days, and then he was back at it. Anna ran into other problems, including a candidal infection of the nipples and breast, which required five weeks of fluconazole, but she was eventually rid of it.

Anna nursed Samuel until he was over two years of age, and happily nursed her second baby as well.

CATHERINE

Catherine brought Roger to our clinic when he was 37 days old. He was refusing the breast. Roger had not been tried on the breast until two hours after birth, despite the fact that he was well and the mother was well. [*Two hours too late. I am not saying he definitely would have taken the breast had he been tried immediately after birth, but he might have. We will never know. Most babies are ready and willing in the first two hours, and some will self-attach.*] When he was finally tried on the breast, he refused to latch on.

The mother and baby were rooming in together. The baby was finger-feeding using formula. [*Hospital staff should have encouraged Catherine to start expressing her milk as soon as it was decided the baby had to be fed. Even if she got drops only, this could have been used, dissolved in sugar water, and she would have understood that her breast-milk is very important. As it is, she got the message that formula is very important. Formula is not necessary during the first day or two, except under extraordinary circumstances.*]

Catherine was seen at another breastfeeding clinic, and no one was able to help her get the baby to latch on. She tried a nipple shield, but it did not work well. [*The nipple shield is not always easy to use. It should not be used except by lactation specialists who have experience with its use. The nipple shield can be a useful tool, but unfortunately, as with all tools, if it is not used correctly, it can do more harm than good. Starting a nipple shield on day two or three—not done in this particular situation—is poor practice, in my opinion. It does not give time a chance to work.*]

Catherine was expressing her milk and feeding Roger her own milk almost exclusively, but because of difficulties expressing enough, she was also giving a little formula. [*A perfect example of how the pump does not get milk out of the breast as well as a baby who is nursing well does, and why pumping is not a good way of knowing how much you can produce. Roger was able to be breastfed exclusively once he was on the breast.*]

When I tried to help Roger to take the breast, he went ballistic. There was no way to get him even near the breast. Even holding him in a breast-feeding position made him angry. There was obviously nothing to do on that particular day.

I told Catherine that she should not be discouraged, since many babies take the breast between the ages of four and six weeks. [*This was really going out on a limb. After all, the baby was almost six weeks old already. I would have been smarter to say between four and eight weeks of age.*] I was not completely confident because it had been a long time since I had seen a baby this resistant to taking the breast.

Nevertheless, I suggested Catherine try him on the breast when he was content, and not try to push him to take the breast.

Not long after, I received this e-mail:

"My almost eight-week-old, non-latching baby, FINALLY got on today for an HOUR!!! AND he has fed again, AND he is comfortable on the breast and sucking and swallowing vigorously.

"It is great to have him on after all that work.

"Yesterday I told him that if he would latch on I would breastfeed him until he is two or three. Of course he can't understand . . . but . . . who knows? It is so exciting. So, now you know a baby older than six weeks who has gotten on." [*Actually, I had seen a few babies older than six weeks who started taking the breast after months of not latching, but they were definitely the exceptions. If the mother's supply is good, the baby will usually latch on all by himself between four and eight weeks of age.*]

The message? Keep your milk supply up. Keep at it, but be gentle with your baby. Get good help. Chances are that it will work.

11

Breastfeeding While on Medication

Myth: A mother who is taking medication must stop breastfeeding until the medication is out of her system.

Fact: This is almost never true. Breastfeeding and breastmilk are very important to the health of the mother and baby. Even if the baby gets some of the drug his mother is taking through her milk, breastfeeding is not more hazardous than giving infant formula.

Even today, despite all that we have learned about the risks of formula-feeding, many physicians are telling mothers that they must stop breastfeeding when they are taking various medications. In fact, it is not only unnecessary for mothers to stop breastfeeding, but definitely more harmful than continuing breastfeeding in all but a tiny minority of cases.

The question is not whether the baby will get any of the drug that the mother is taking. He usually will get some of the drug through the milk, though there are exceptions—there are some drugs that don't get into the milk at all. The question is: Is breastmilk that contains tiny amounts of medication more hazardous for the baby and the mother than infant formula? The answer is almost always no. Infant formula is almost always more hazardous for the mother and baby than is breastmilk with a tiny amount of medication.

To explore this question further, let us look at the formula manufacturers' claims that their products are "closest to breastmilk." In the first place, this claim is misleading, since the various formulas cannot all be "closest to breastmilk," so someone is not telling the truth. In the second place, "closest" does not mean "close." Toronto is closer to Halifax than Winnipeg is, but that hardly means Torontonians live just around the corner from Haligonians. And in any case, since we don't really know exactly what is in breastmilk, we don't even know how to get "close."

Serious research on the composition of breastmilk has not been going on for very long. Only in the last generation has human milk been studied intensively, and what is obvious is that there is no one standard "breastmilk." Every woman has somewhat different milk—"designer milk" made for her baby, not some "theoretical" baby that infant formula is made for. Let's look at how breastmilk varies.

How Breastmilk Varies

From woman to woman

This should not be surprising. Almost all our bodily fluids vary from person to person, with exact amounts of any individual component being impossible to state. Quantities of almost anything measured in blood, for example, are given as a range, not an exact number. Anything within that range is considered normal. The differences in the concentration of various components in the milk from woman to woman may not have any significance at all for the baby's growth and development, but which woman's milk is the formula company going to copy?

According to the mother's diet

Again, this is not earth-shaking news. The mother's diet does influence the concentration of various components of her milk. For example, a mother who is a vegetarian has different amounts of various fatty acids (the building blocks of fats) in her milk than a woman who eats meat. A woman who eats a lot of fish will have different fatty acids in her milk than either of the first two mothers. And other things mothers eat add components to the milk that are not usually considered a "normal" part of the milk. When women eat garlic, as another example, the milk tastes and smells different. But why would we consider that garlic (or rather, components of garlic) is not a "normal" part of breastmilk, if garlic is a normal part of the mother's diet? Since it is possible that garlic helps prevent atherosclerosis and may have some immune-boosting qualities, maybe formula companies should be adding garlic to their modified cow's milk.

It is often said that these dietary additions to the milk, such as garlic, are bad for the baby. But, in fact, they are not, except in rare cases. Babies who are breastfed usually accept solids better than do artificially fed babies, presumably because they have been exposed to a variety of tastes throughout their breastfeeding experience. When they start eating solids, they are already used to these tastes. Formula, on the other hand, always tastes the same.

The appearance in the milk of things the mother eats can also decrease the risk of allergy in the breastfed baby. Thus, the appearance of cow's milk protein in the milk is not necessarily bad, as many people think. Though cow's milk protein in the milk might cause some babies to be colicky, most are not affected this way. What it may do, and this is only a hypothesis, is desensitize the baby to cow's milk protein, much as allergy shots are supposed to desensitize the person receiving them to the various allergens. By appearing in the milk only in tiny quantities and accompanied by antibodies and special white cells, the cow's milk protein (and this may also apply to other proteins) might actually allow the baby or child to tolerate cow's milk better later on.

On the other hand, the total amount of food the mother eats does not matter as much. Even women who are eating very little seem to produce good milk, though the quantity may decrease a little. This decrease, though, is not usually significant enough to result in insufficient production.

There are some foods or herbs that may increase or decrease the amount of milk a mother has, but there is no research to back up what may only be a myth. Parsley and sage may decrease the supply. Fenugreek may increase it.

During a feeding

Breastmilk changes during a feeding. The best-known change is in the fat content. As the baby takes milk from the breast, the concentration of fat increases. At the beginning of the feeding, the milk may contain 1 percent fat, but by the end it is 5 percent or more, and the overall average amount the baby gets is about 4 percent. We don't know why this should be, but it may serve as a sort of appetite control for the baby.

During the day

Breastmilk composition varies widely throughout the day. For example, there is more lactose in breastmilk in the late afternoon than in the early morning. The amount of fat is highest in the morning and lowest in the late afternoon. The amount of protein is lowest in the early morning and highest in the evening.

We don't know why this happens or whether this benefits mother and baby. But these variations may be more significant than we know. So which milk would the formula companies copy? The milk produced at 6 a.m.? At 6 p.m.? At midnight?

During the entire nursing period

It is obvious that the milk of the first three or four days—which we call colostrum—is different from the milk that comes later. Colostrum is different in color from more mature milk. It is also stickier and thicker. It is wonderful stuff, and it is too bad that the majority of breastfeeding babies in North America don't get any, or don't get much. It is loaded with many, many white blood cells. There are up to 5 million white cells in each milliliter of colostrum, and the average is about 1 million. One million white cells in each milliliter is 100 times more than in your blood. And it is jam-packed with antibodies. It is also a laxative, which is important for clearing out the baby's intestines, reducing the level of jaundice, and preparing the baby to digest breastmilk.

After three or four days, breastmilk changes and becomes "transitional milk." The milk becomes whiter, but has a slightly golden color, indicating that there is still some colostrum mixed in. After about a week or two, the milk could be called "mature milk" and is a bluish-white color at the beginning of the feeding, and white later in the feeding.

But milk continues to change in ways that are not obvious to the eye. For example, the number of white cells in breastmilk decreases over the first few months, but even six months after the baby is born, the mother's milk will have an average of 100,000 cells in each milliliter of milk, or 10 times more than you would have in your blood (actually 10 to 20 times more, since the range of normal for the number of white cells in your blood is 5,000 to 10,000/ml, depending on the lab). Many of the other immune factors also decrease in concentration, but some actually increase.

Lysozyme, one such immune factor that attacks the cell walls of bacteria and kills them, is present in the milk in greater concentrations after the first year than before. It should be noted that a *decrease* in immune factors does not mean an absence or insignificant amount. After all, formulas have no immune factors at all (except for nucleotides, which are not really of much significance), yet when we talk about the immune factors in breastmilk decreasing, people seem to think this is a serious concern. Yet nobody worries about the virtually total absence of immune factors in formula.

It has been shown that an exclusively breastfeeding five-month-old baby who is gaining weight well is not getting that much more milk than an exclusively breastfeeding one-month-old baby who is gaining weight well. He generally takes only about 10 percent to 20 percent more milk, even though he may weigh twice as much as the one-month-old. In other words, the five-month-old is getting only about 60 to 70 calories per kg per day, whereas the formula-fed baby of the same age is getting 90 to 100 calories per kg per day. Why is it that formula is needed in such large amounts, relatively speaking? The requirements of the appropriate constituents of breastmilk are somehow better and more efficiently used than the substitute constituents found in artificial baby milks. (Could this be one of the reasons why studies find formula-fed babies more likely to grow up to be overweight as adults? Perhaps they have gotten used to eating larger amounts of food in order to get the nutrients they need.)

Anyone who says there is no value in breastmilk after six months (unfortunately this seems to include many physicians, and even pediatricians) doesn't understand that the milk is different, but certainly hasn't changed to white-colored water. Breastmilk is still valuable from the nutritional and immunologic points of view, and, let us not forget, breastfeeding still has bonding, psychological, and emotional benefits.

Depending on the baby's gestational age

A baby who is born prematurely has different needs from those of a baby born at term, depending on how much he is premature. Interestingly, the milk of the mother whose baby is born prematurely is different from that of the mother whose baby is born at term. A premature baby needs more protein and more sodium than a baby born at term. Well, milk of the mother who delivers prematurely has more protein and more sodium. A premature baby is at greater risk of developing infection. Well, milk of the mother who delivers prematurely has more white cells and antibodies. The baby born prematurely has missed out on some of the iron he would have stored during the pregnancy. Well, milk of the mother who delivers prematurely has more iron. The baby born prematurely has missed out on some of the long-chained polyunsaturated fatty acids that are important to the development of his brain and vision. Well, milk of the mother who delivers prematurely has more of these fatty acids.

Other variables

There is evidence that if the mother offers one breast twice in a row to the baby, the milk of that breast will be different the second time than if she had offered the other breast for the second feeding. Specifically, the second feeding on the same breast will have a higher concentration of fat.

If the mother breastfeeds for the normal period of time—that is, three or four years—the milk will vary with her menstrual period. Many mothers claim the supply is down during the bleeding phase, but the components of the breastmilk change also. On average, a woman who breastfeeds a baby longer than a year will get back her period about 13 or 14 months after the baby's birth.

There is also evidence that milk is different if the mother has had several previous pregnancies than if this is her first pregnancy.

Why Is All This Important?

It is important because when we start to talk about whether it is safe to continue breastfeeding while a mother is taking various medications, there is more to the issue than "Will the drug appear in the milk?" The reason so many physicians are nonchalant about telling mothers they must stop breastfeeding is that they assume breastfeeding and formula-feeding are about the same. But formula cannot ever be close to breastmilk, because there is no such thing as a single, uniform breastmilk that the formula companies can copy. "We just add or subtract x amount of protein, y amount of fat, z amount of sugar, and there you have it: instant breastmilk." The fact that so many people believe the advertising is a monument to how marketing can make us believe that big is small and black is white.

There's more. How do we know that milk expressed for analysis is the same as milk the baby gets when he is breastfeeding? In fact, there is evidence that expressed milk is *not* the same as the milk the baby gets. A lot of the early research used "dripped" milk to get samples. The mother would feed the baby on one side, while the dripped milk from the other side was collected for analysis. This "sample" of breastmilk is not representative of what the baby gets. All the research based on dripped milk is inaccurate.

Is formula really that different?

It is. And it is not just a question of which of the many variations of breastmilk should be used as the standard for creating the "best" infant formula. Even assuming that the published standards of what breastmilk contains are precise, what is called "formula" is only an approximation of breastmilk.

Just for starters, breastmilk and any formula smell different, look different, and taste different. So even grossly (and "grossly" is a very good word to use here, because I think most formulas look and smell gross!), they are not similar. As an example of how we don't really understand breastmilk, just contemplate this. Both breastmilk and formulas contain about the same amount of sugar. Yet breastmilk tastes a lot sweeter. Formula is not even close. (In fact, to my palate, it doesn't taste sweet at all.)

But let's get down to molecules. Essentially, our diets contain proteins, carbohydrates, fats, trace amounts of metals such as iron, zinc, and chromium, and vitamins. Unfortunately, our diets now also contain toxins.

Proteins and fats, important components of our diet, are made up of building blocks that determine the character of those proteins and fats. Thus fats are made up of fatty acids, and proteins of amino acids. The fatty acids and the amino acids that the baby gets in his milk are far more important from the nutritional point of view than the exact amount of protein or fat.

"Fats" is virtually a four-letter word in today's society. But you cannot live without *some* fat. Both breastmilk and artificial baby milks contain about the same amount of fat, although obviously breast milk changes throughout the feeding and from one feeding to another, while formula is always the same. But the fatty acids that make up fats in breastmilk are present in very different amounts from those in any formula.

One of the major deficiencies of infant formulas is the absence of docosahexaenoic acid (DHA), one of the long-chained polyunsaturated fatty acids (PUFA). This fatty acid is completely absent from any formula available in North America, yet it is important for the development of the baby's vision and brain. It is also a component of virtually every cell in the body. Eventually the formula companies, under pressure from consumers and with an eye to profits, will start adding some PUFAs to their milks, but it is more than a question of just throwing in a few of these fatty acids. They have to be added in a certain proportion—but which? The problem is that they are not absorbed the same way from breastmilk and from formula, so manufacturers cannot just take the proportions of PUFAs found in breastmilk.

In fact, formulas with added PUFA's have just come out in the United States, and soon will likely be available in Canada. Interestingly, studies seem to show no benefit for the babies when formulas with and without PUFA's are compared. In other words, you can't just throw in some PUFA's and say, "more like breastmilk," again. Formulas do need to be improved, and it's good the companies are doing research and trying to improve them. But even if the added PUFA's do eventually have benefit for the babies, one improvement does not make the formulas "almost like breastmilk."

Breastmilk also contains more cholesterol than do artificial baby milks. A good point for formulas? Not necessarily. Studies on apes show that if they don't get cholesterol in the first few months, their bodies don't handle it well later on. It is as if you need cholesterol in the first few months in order to protect yourself from it later.

Just as the building blocks of fat are different, so are the building blocks of proteins. Proteins are made up of amino acids. Though the amount of protein in formula is approximately that of breastmilk, many of the amino acids are present in quite different amounts. For example, infant formulas contain much more phenylalanine and tyrosine than breastmilk. In elevated amounts, these can depress the central nervous system of premature babies, and possibly newborn full-term babies as well, so this is not necessarily a good thing. For many years taurine was not added to infant formulas. Then, when it was decided that taurine might be a necessary amino acid, the manufacturers added it, and with great fanfare an advertising campaign emphasized the improvement of the new stuff, not the inadequacy of the older stuff. And this still goes on. When the docosahexaenoic acid is added, you can bet there will be a lot of hoopla about it, forgetting that up until then, artificially fed babies were not getting any DHA after their births.

This is not meant to be a treatise on the biochemistry of breastmilk and infant formulas. It is meant as an "eye opener," so that people can understand that what they are buying when they buy infant formula is not a perfect copy of what the mother produces in the breast. It is not really very close to breastmilk.

What's missing from infant formulas?

Lots. There are no antibodies in infant formulas. No lysozyme, no epidermal growth factor, no white cells, no oligosaccharides to help fight infection. No lots of things. In fact, there are dozens of components in breastmilk, all with their own functions, which are not present in infant formulas. What functions? We don't always know. Some components have multiple functions. For example, lactoferrin is probably responsible for the fact that so much of the iron in breastmilk is absorbed by the baby. But it also denies iron to bacteria, which need it to multiply, and thus decreases their rate of growth. It works together with white cells and antibodies to kill bacteria more effectively. And maybe it has more functions as well. We are only beginning to discover the wonders of breastmilk.

Do all these differences really matter?

They do. Yes, I know, you have met many people who were raised on formula and are "all right." You yourself never tasted your mother's milk, perhaps, and yet you are "all right." Wonderful. Humans are very adaptable, and can manage to survive and do well despite all sorts of trauma and stresses in their lives. Abused children grow up with many difficulties, yet can overcome these difficult beginnings to be lovely adults and live good lives. Babies born prematurely are at risk for all sorts of health problems, yet many grow up to be healthy children or adults. Modern medicine can treat and cure many illnesses. Yet surely, we should not then discard breastfeeding as a better start just because most babies fed artificially are "all right."

Research is accumulating to show that children who were breastfed have higher intelligence quotients and achieve better results at school than those who were not breastfed.

Furthermore, the effect is greater if the baby was breastfed longer. This does not mean that a child who has the potential IQ of a genius will drop to the average IQ if not breastfed. The average difference in most studies is about 8 IQ points, so a person with a potential IQ of 140 will still be very bright, even if he didn't breastfeed at all. But there is still a significant difference.

And there is some evidence, though no definite proof yet, that children who are breastfed have a lower risk of developing juvenile diabetes, and more recent evidence that they have a lower risk of developing adult-type diabetes. There is some weak evidence that the breastfed baby is at lower risk of developing Crohn's disease (a chronic inflammatory disease of the gut). There is good evidence that breastfed babies have fewer and less severe infections of the lungs, of the middle ear (otitis media), and of the digestive system. Breastfed babies, especially if nursed longer than a year, have fewer problems with malocclusion and thus breastfeeding may save you a bundle in orthodontic costs. There is some evidence that allergies are fewer and less severe in breastfed babies. And there are other illnesses, for which some evidence is available—weak evidence, for example, that breastfeeding protects against multiple sclerosis.

Many parents have come to accept the problems of formula-feeding as normal. For example, many baby books will tell you that it is normal for a baby to have five or six ear infections in the first two years. This may be normal for a formula-fed baby, but—at least in my experience—it would be unusual for a breastfed baby. So when a parent has a child with repeated ear infections, she doesn't think that this is a problem possibly connected to lack of breastfeeding, she thinks it's normal and her child is doing just fine. Those repeated ear infections not only cause the child pain, but can affect the child's hearing at an age when he is learning to talk, causing speech delays and difficulties.

Don't forget that breastfeeding is a two-person arrangement. The mother also derives benefits from breastfeeding. The breastfeeding woman is likely to have less osteoporosis than the woman who did not breastfeed. There is some evidence for a decrease in the incidence of breast cancer, ovarian cancer, and cancer of the uterus. None of this is conclusively proven, but the studies are intriguing. For most breastfeeding women, weight loss after pregnancy is more rapid and more complete.

These are some of the issues involved. There are more, but it is not within the scope of this book to discuss at length the risks of artificial feeding.

What's this got to do with my taking medication while breastfeeding?

It has everything to do with it. The essential question in all this is: Does a small amount of medication in the mother's milk make breastfeeding riskier than not breastfeeding? The answer, after all the above is considered, is almost always no. Breastfeeding with a small amount of medication in the milk is not riskier than feeding the baby formula, except in a few specific situations. It is almost always less risky. There are safer and less safe drugs for mothers who are breastfeeding, but the majority are still safe. There are health risks for both the mother and the baby when the mother does not breastfeed. This may not just be a question of taking the baby off the breast for a week or ten days. It may be a question of permanent weaning, since off the breast for a week often means, in practice, off the breast forever.

Why is breastfeeding while on medication not usually a problem?

Because only small amounts of any medication get into the milk. So small are the amounts that the risk to the baby is minimal. Many people believe that the baby gets a dose of medication comparable to that which the mother gets. This is only rarely true. In fact, the baby almost always gets only tiny amounts. As a rule of thumb, about 1 percent of the total of what the mother takes gets into the milk. There are some medications that come out in greater quantities than that. Others come out in even smaller quantities.

Let us take, as an example, the quite often used antibiotic amoxicillin. A fairly typical dose for an adult would be about 500 mg three times a day. If 1 percent of the total maternal dose in a day gets to the baby through the milk, then he will get about 15 mg spread over the day. This is hardly enough to worry one bacterium. A 5-kg baby (11 lb) who is treated for an ear infection would get 200 mg in a day, more than 10 times more than he would get through the milk. In fact, the amount of amoxicillin that gets into the milk amounts to 0.7 percent of the total dose the mother takes, so that in the above case the baby would actually be getting only about 12 mg of amoxicillin in a 24-hour period.

Why does so little get into the milk?

Any drug you take is diluted throughout your body. Because of this dilution in various tissues, the concentration of drugs in the blood is often measured in micrograms (millionths of a gram) or even nanograms (billionths of a gram) in each milliliter, even though the amount of drug you take is usually measured in milligrams (thousandths of a gram), or occasionally even in grams. Many drugs are distributed in the body in such a way that very little is in the blood. One

example is paroxetine (Paxil), a drug used for depression. Less than 1 percent of all the drug the mother has in her body is actually in her blood, the rest being located in other tissue such as fat or brain. Thus, very little of this particular medication can get into the milk.

An easy example to illustrate the above is alcohol, probably the most commonly used drug in the world. Alcohol is one drug said by some to require a mother to stop breastfeeding (two hours for every ounce of alcohol taken is a typical recommendation). I disagree completely, because the occasional use of alcohol is not going to give the baby significant amounts. Whisky is 40 percent alcohol. Wine is 9 to 12 percent alcohol. Beer is 3 to 5 percent alcohol. Even de-alcoholized beer is 0.6 percent alcohol. In various jurisdictions, however, you are considered too drunk to drive if you have 0.05 to 0.1 percent alcohol in your blood. Now alcohol is one drug that is at the same level in the milk as in the mother's blood. If the mother has 0.08 percent alcohol in her blood, her milk will have 0.08 percent alcohol. This is nothing! And I strongly believe telling mothers to interrupt breastfeeding after a drink or two reflects little more than the emergence once again of puritanical attitudes in late-20th-century North American society.

Some drugs are used topically—on the skin, or in the vagina, the nose, or eyes. Even when large amounts are used, it is unlikely that absorption of most drugs from these sites will be sufficient to produce more than trace amounts in the mother's blood.

What, in addition to the concentration of the drug in the mother's blood, determines how much gets into the milk?

One of the most important factors is the amount of any drug that is attached to proteins in the mother's blood, since only the drug that is unattached to protein is available to get into the milk. Some drugs are attached to proteins almost completely. Ibuprofen (a nonsteroidal anti-inflammatory drug) is over 99 percent bound to protein. Thus, only less than 1 percent of the amount found in the mother's blood is available to get into the milk. The result is that though mothers may take a dose of 400 mg every six hours, the milk contains less than 1 mg in a liter. Most babies do not drink a liter of breastmilk in a day. If we treated a baby with ibuprofen, we would generally give 5 to 10 mg per kg of his weight, so that a 5-kg baby would get 25 to 50 mg every six hours. Thus, the amount a baby would get from the milk in 24 hours when the mother is taking full doses every six hours, is less than 1 percent that we would give him. In the case of the antidepressant mentioned earlier (paroxetine), it is 95 percent protein bound, so that of the already small amount in the blood, 95 percent is not available for transfer into the milk.

Another important factor is the size of the drug. Although most drugs are small enough to get into the milk, some are not. Examples of drugs too large to get into the milk are the following: insulin (for treating diabetes), interferon (for treating multiple sclerosis and some other chronic illnesses), and heparin and low-molecular-weight heparin (for preventing blood clots). There are others, but they are not commonly used. Proteins and most hormones (such as chorionic gonadotropin) used for various treatments are too large to get into the milk.

But that is not all that needs to be taken into consideration. What will the baby really get even if he does get some in the milk? Many mothers have been told they must stop breastfeeding for drugs such as gentamicin (an antibiotic). Would it cause a problem for the baby? Well, gentamicin is given by injection. And it is given by injection because it does not get absorbed from the gut. Thus, the mother gets it by injection into the muscle or by intravenous, but the baby gets it in the milk, orally—and therefore doesn't absorb it. Thus, though gentamicin is a relatively toxic medication and can cause serious problems with the kidney and hearing if the blood levels rise too high, the blood levels of gentamicin will not rise in the baby at all, because the drug is not absorbed from his gut. This fairly simple principle is surprisingly unappreciated by many health professionals.

It is possible that this antibiotic will kill some bacteria in the baby's gut and thus change the sorts of bacteria that are found there. But giving formula will also change the bacteria found in the baby's gut. Why is it fine to change the bacteria in the gut with formula, but not with an antibiotic? (Actually, it is less likely to be changed by the tiny amounts of antibiotic—though possible—than by formula.) It is true that the baby might become allergic to the antibiotic in his mother's milk. But the baby might also become allergic to the cow's milk or soy milk protein in the formula. In fact, allergies to these milk proteins are much more inconvenient and restricting than are allergies to antibiotics.

Following are just a few drugs that are little absorbed from the gut (some are absorbed more than gentamicin). I have mentioned only a few of the many medications mothers might be given. It should be noted that when given orally, the dose of the drug has been adjusted to account for low oral availability. Nevertheless, that concerns the mother, not the baby. Because of dilution of any drug in her body, the amount that gets into the milk is generally very small, and of that small amount, only a *very* small percentage is absorbed by the baby. An interesting drug is omeprazole, a drug used to decrease acid secretion of the stomach. It is poorly absorbed by the gut, and, in fact, destroyed by the acid of the stomach. What the mother takes is specially coated omeprazole, to protect the drug from the acid, but what the baby gets is no longer protected. Thus, oral absorption by the mother is not bad, but oral absorption by the baby is poor.

The names of the drugs below are the generic names. The trade name is often better known by the mother, but some drugs can have several trade names.

Anti-infectious Agents (antibiotics, antiviral agents, antifungal agents)

- **Amikacin** This drug is in the same family as gentamicin, and essentially none of the antibiotics in this family is absorbed from the gut in any significant amount. Other examples are kanamycin, tobramycin, and netilmicin.
- **Carbenecillin** This is a penicillin, but unlike most penicillins that are well absorbed, this one is absorbed in small amounts only (less than 10 percent).
- **Cefazolin** Many drugs of this family are poorly absorbed. Others are very well absorbed. Others that are very poorly absorbed are cefepime, cefoperazone, cefotaxime, cefotetan, cefoxitin, ceftazidime, ceftriaxone, cephalothin, cephapirin. There are others, such as cephalexin, ceftibuten, and cefaclor, which are well absorbed, and others, such as cefuroxime and cefpodoxime, which are in the middle range. However, there are other reasons cephalosporins (the name of this family) should not interrupt breastfeeding.
- **Clotrimazole** This is an antifungal agent used as a topical treatment for candida. Several other members of this family of drugs are not absorbed at all from the gut, but some, such as fluconazole, ketoconazole, and itraconazole, are.
- **Furazolidone** An antibiotic generally used for giardia lamblia. Very low absorption from the gut.
- **Mebendazole** This is a drug used for worms. Almost none is absorbed by the mother, and almost none of the tiny amount that might get into the milk is absorbed by the baby.
- **Methicillin** Another penicillin-like drug, which is not absorbed from the gut.
- **Vancomycin** Used for methicillin-resistant *Staphylococcus aureus*, this drug is absorbed in tiny quantities from the gut. Of the tiny amount that appears in the milk, only a tiny amount will be absorbed by the baby.

Antiallergic Agents

- **Cromolyn** Less than 1 percent of the total dose is absorbed from the gut. Thus, even if the mother takes it by nasal spray, the amount that appears in her blood is small, the amount in the milk is small, and the baby will absorb almost none.
- **Epinephrine** Though not strictly an antiallergic medication, this drug is sometimes carried by highly allergic people who might develop a life-threatening allergic reaction before help is available. It is given by injection and rapidly destroyed in the stomach. None is absorbed from the gut, except, perhaps, by very premature babies.

Antiasthmatic Drugs

- **Ipratropium** Used by inhalation, this drug is absorbed in tiny quantities from the gut.
- **Zafirlukast** A member of a new class of anti-

asthmatic medication, this drug has very low absorption from the gut.

Drugs for Blood Pressure Control

- **Esmolol** Virtually none is absorbed from the gut. Its half life is also extremely short (see below).
- **Magnesium sulphate** This is used particularly for high blood pressure around delivery. For many years mothers were told, and, unfortunately, are still being told in some places, that they cannot breastfeed while on this medication. The absorption from the baby's intestines, though not zero, is quite low, and only a small amount gets into the milk in the first place.
- **Nisoldipine** A calcium channel blocker, only 5 percent of which is absorbed from the gut.

Contrast Media

- **Gadopentetate** This is the injection you receive when you have an MRI (magnetic resonance imaging) scan. Unfortunately, radiologists have been telling mothers that they must stop breastfeeding for 24 hours when they get this injection. But the oral absorption (what the baby will get) is 0.8 percent of the tiny amount that will get into the milk.
- **Radiopaque iodine-containing agents** Almost no oral absorption occurs with any of these compounds. They are not a reason to interrupt breastfeeding, regardless of what mothers are told by the radiologist. If you are to have an intravenous pyelogram, a CT (computed tomography) scan, also known as a CAT scan, or other test using radiopaque contrast media, you are likely to be told that you cannot breastfeed for 24 to 48 hours afterward. Because of the poor oral absorption of these drugs (and

other reasons), this advice is misguided. In fact, the iodine-containing contrast medium does not even get into the milk.

Antidiarrheal agents

- **Loperamide** Almost none is absorbed.

This list does not exhaust the drugs that are very poorly absorbed from the gut. If you are receiving a drug by injection, it is quite possible (though not necessarily so) that the drug is poorly absorbed from the gut.

Some Other Guidelines for Using Drugs While Breastfeeding

Is this drug or test really necessary?

Unfortunately, many tests are done and many drugs prescribed without really being necessary. Many physicians, unfortunately, believe that something "needs to be done" when a patient comes to them with a medical complaint. Many drugs and tests are prescribed because it is easier to do the test or give the drug than to speak to the patient about the complaint. Most fevers are not caused by illnesses that require antibiotics. The majority of illnesses causing vomiting and diarrhea do not require medicines.

An example of how tests may interfere with breastfeeding, and how it is often not necessary to do tests, follows. Around three to six months after her baby is born, a mother might find herself with symptoms of an overactive thyroid. These symptoms include irritability, inability to sleep, excessive weight loss, jitteriness, nervousness, or sometimes excessive fatigue. A blood test is done, and the mother is found to have hyperthyroidism. Now, the question comes up: Is this hyperthyroidism due to postpartum thyroiditis, an inflammation of the thyroid, or to

Graves' disease, a more chronic, more serious problem? The usual way of distinguishing these two entities is to do a thyroid scan with radioactive iodine. Radioactive iodine is something the baby should not get, so the mother is faced with stopping breastfeeding after the test. But is the test really necessary? The answer is no.

In the first place, a woman presenting with hyperthyroidism three to six months after the birth of a baby almost always has postpartum thyroiditis, not Graves' disease. Second, postpartum thyroiditis improves all by itself over six to ten weeks. These two causes of an overactive thyroid also show differences in the blood tests used to diagnose hyperthyroidism.

It is not necessary to do the thyroid scan. The mother can be treated with propranalol (a drug compatible with breastfeeding), and her symptoms and blood tests followed. If, as is likely, she has postpartum thyroiditis, her blood tests will start to get better over the next few weeks. If she has Graves' disease, they won't. In that case, she can start taking propylthiruracil (PTU) to treat her illness—and she does not have to stop breastfeeding, because this drug is compatible with breastfeeding.

It is amazing what can be done if we consider breastfeeding important and look for a way to preserve it. Unfortunately, for too many health professionals, breastfeeding is not valued, so they do not even consider alternatives to the "usual routine."

Is the drug used for babies?

A drug that is used for babies should be fine for a mother to use while breastfeeding. Here is a true story. This is what the mother told me on the phone (paraphrased):

"I am confused. I went to the doctor a few days ago for a cold and he gave me amoxycillin. Since I was breastfeeding my three-month-old, he told me I had to stop because the baby would get some of the medicine. I did stop. Today, the baby has a cold. I took him to the doctor, and the doctor prescribed amoxycillin."

What's wrong here? Everything!

1. The mother went to the doctor for a cold. The old adage says: if you treat a cold, it lasts a week, and if you don't, it lasts seven days. It's still true. Why do people go to doctors for a cold?

2. Treating a cold with amoxycillin is an example of the abuse of antibiotics, and one reason we may soon have no safe antibiotics for some bacteria, or no antibiotics at all for certain infections. Colds are caused by viruses, and antibiotics do not kill viruses.

3. The mother was told she could not breastfeed while on amoxycillin. Given the risks of not breastfeeding for both mother and baby, plus the fact that so little amoxycillin gets into the milk, this is irresponsible advice on the part of the physician.

4. The baby got a cold. It is quite possible that the baby would not have gotten the cold if the mother had been advised to continue breastfeeding. There is no guarantee, of course, but the baby's risk of getting sick increased once he was no longer breastfeeding and not getting the antibodies and other immune factors in the milk.

5. The mother took the baby to the doctor for a cold. Okay, mothers are more worried about their babies than about themselves. An experienced grandmother would have been of more help than the doctor.

6. The baby got amoxycillin for a cold! This was

not only unnecessary, but risky, since the drug can give the baby diarrhea.

7. Doctors give advice, not commandments. But this mother was told she must stop breastfeeding. Unless there is a "life or limb" threatening situation involved, the mother should have been given information with which she could make an informed choice about continuing or stopping breastfeeding. Of course, the doctor would have had to be informed himself, which he clearly was not.

Babies getting drugs through breastmilk are getting only a tiny percentage of the amount they would get if they were being treated directly. It is extremely rare to have to stop breastfeeding for a drug that is used for babies.

Is the drug safe during pregnancy?

It is not always true that a drug safe during pregnancy is safe during breastfeeding. When the baby is inside her, the pregnant woman is helping the baby get rid of the drug she is taking, so dangerous accumulations of the drug do not usually occur in the baby. Buildup of drugs in the baby during breastfeeding is sometimes a concern, especially when the drug has a long half-life (discussed in more detail later), but this is rarely the problem.

For example, doctors may be concerned about the effect of a drug on the baby's developing brain. This is the reason so many women are told they cannot breastfeed while on antidepressants, even though they have been taking these drugs while pregnant.

A mother taking a drug that may have an effect on the central nervous system is exposing her baby's developing nervous system much more during pregnancy than during lactation. The baby's brain is at a much earlier and more sensitive stage of development during pregnancy.

Furthermore, the baby will generally be exposed to higher levels of a drug during pregnancy than during breastfeeding, since he will have blood levels comparable to the mother's (very few drugs do not pass through the placenta). Thus, if such a drug is safe during pregnancy, it is safe, generally, during breastfeeding.

Making Decisions About Medication During Breastfeeding

Most drugs are safe during breastfeeding, but some are safer than others. Information available to your physician or pharmacist can help them choose the drug least likely to cause problems. Some of this information has already been mentioned: drugs that are not passed into the milk, and drugs that are not absorbed from the gut are safe for breastfeeding; drugs that are highly attached to protein in your blood are safer than those that are not.

Drugs that stay in the body for a short period of time (short half-life) would be preferred to drugs that stay in the body for a long time (long half-life). A half-life is a measure of how long it takes for half the drug to disappear from the body. It takes about five half-lives for a drug to disappear virtually completely from the body once you stop taking a drug. Or, it takes about five half-lives for a steady blood level to be achieved once you have started taking a drug.

For example: Many nonsteroidal anti-inflammatory medications are essentially the same from the point of view of pain relief, side effects in the mother, and relief of inflammation. Many are highly protein-bound (higher than 99 percent protein bound), so the amount of any of these drugs that gets into the milk is small, which is also good. However, some have longer half-lives than others. Ibuprofen has a short half-life, about two hours, whereas naproxen has a long half-life, about 12 to 15 hours. So we know that both of these medications are safe and unlikely to appear in the mother's milk in large amounts (because both are highly protein-bound). However, ibuprofen is the better choice because of its shorter half-life.

You should not assume that your doctor or even your pharmacist knows much about drugs and breastfeeding, or that they are concerned with helping you continue to breastfeed. Often the information they may use to decide if a drug is acceptable during breastfeeding comes from the drug manufacturer itself, found in a book called the *Compendium of Pharmaceuticals and Specialities* (*CPS*) in Canada, and the *Physician's Desk Reference* (*PDR*) in the United States. The manufacturer is concerned about its own medical legal liability, not the importance to the mother and baby of breastfeeding. There is hardly a single drug among the thousands discussed in the *CPS* or *PDR* that is said to be acceptable for breastfeeding mothers. The *CPS* does have a section in the front, in the lilac-colored pages, which has a much more reasoned discussion of drugs and breastfeeding. Unfortunately, physicians and pharmacists rarely consult this section. The American Academy of Pediatrics, every few years, puts out a guideline for the use of drugs during breastfeeding. It is very conservative in its approach to drugs and breastfeeding, yet it calls many drugs "compatible with breastfeeding" that are not "allowed" according the *CPS* or *PDR*. However, physicians and pharmacists seldom refer to this guideline, either.

A textbook by pharmacologist Dr. Thomas Hale has been available for several years now. Called *Medications and Mothers' Milk*, it provides a good approach to drugs and breastfeeding, even offering alternatives to drugs that may be a problem. In addition, it is revised every year or two to include new drugs and new information. However, physicians and pharmacists rarely refer to this resource.

If you receive a prescription from your physician and are told immediately that you cannot breastfeed, you should first suspect your physician's commitment and understanding of breastfeeding. A physician who is supportive of breastfeeding will make an effort to use a medication that does not cause problems for the breastfeeding mother and her baby. In this day and age, it is extremely unusual that only one medication can treat the mother's problem. If the drug prescribed is truly a problem, another can usually be found that will be adequate and yet not be unsafe. Even if the physician goes to the trouble of consulting the *CPS* or *PDR*, this still does not mean, as mentioned above, that the drug cannot be used, because according to these two books, almost every drug known to man is potentially a problem. If the physician consults with a pharmacist or the company itself, it does not mean that he is getting good information. The pharmacist may still consult the *CPS* or *PDR*, and the company pharmacist will always maintain the company's stance as written in their official information.

The breastfeeding-friendly physician will not only look to more reliable sources of information, he will also look for ways of getting around the difficulty of a drug that may concern him. With a little thought, it is usually possible to find a way to continue breastfeeding. A few true examples from our clinic may be helpful.

MOTHERS' STORIES
CYNTHIA

Some women are prone to bladder infections. Women who have a lot of these infections and who have frequently been prescribed antibiotics to treat them, may find that only one or two antibiotics work for them.

Cynthia came to the clinic wanting desperately to continue breastfeeding her two-month-old baby Justin. Cynthia had a history of bladder infections and had definite symptoms of a urinary tract infection, well known to her after many years of them. She had had a midstream urine sample sent for culture a few days before, which grew a bacterium resistant to everything that it was tested for except ciprofloxacin and gentamicin. She had been put on amoxycillin while waiting for the results of the culture, but this was not effective. She was now told that she would have to stop breastfeeding because the only oral drug available to her was ciprofloxacin, which was definitely contraindicated during breastfeeding. What to do?

What we did not know at the time of this case was that, in fact, ciprofloxacin is *not* contraindicated during breastfeeding. It was said to be because work in beagle puppies showed that they developed joint damage when they (not their mothers breastfeeding while taking it, incidentally) were treated with this drug. However, more recent studies, done with children who have been on large doses of ciprofloxacin, sometimes for years, has shown no evidence at all of joint damage. Humans are not beagles.

At the time Cynthia came to the clinic, the drug had been around for so little time that it would have been foolhardy to say it was okay to breastfeed while taking it, even though other members of this family of antibiotics were compatible with continued breastfeeding. Just because two drugs are in the same family does not mean they act in the same way in all situations.

So we were left with a dilemma. The answer was provided by Cynthia herself, who said that we should teach her to give herself injections and she would treat herself with gentamicin (because gentamicin has to be given by injection). After all, we teach diabetics to give themselves injections; she could learn as well. Why not? And that's what happened. So this seemingly insoluble problem was solved because everyone believed breastfeeding was important and took a little time to find a solution.

LAURA

Warfarin, a drug that helps prevent blood clotting, is the most commonly used such drug at the present time. And it is contraindicated during pregnancy. Incidentally, the situation in pregnancy is not the same as the situation during breastfeeding. Though a drug that is safe during pregnancy is generally safe during breastfeeding, as described above, a drug that is *not* safe during pregnancy can still be safe during breastfeeding. Warfarin is one such drug. Tetracycline is another (more on tetracycline later). Women who require anticoagulation (prevention of clotting) during pregnancy are treated with heparin or low-molecular-weight heparin, which has to be given by injection. Once they have given birth, the majority are put on an oral preparation, because nobody likes getting injections.

Laura called our clinic because she was pregnant and getting heparin for a blood clot in her leg. She was to go on warfarin when the baby was born, and had been warned that she could not breastfeed if she was taking this drug. She really wanted to breastfeed, as she had nursed her first for 18 months and had found it a wonderful fulfilling experience. We told her that warfarin would not be a problem, and she was thrilled to hear this. Her physician, however, was not so thrilled, and stated in no uncertain terms that he was not going to risk the baby's life by "allowing" her to breastfeed while taking warfarin. (My usual good taste and discretion will prevent me from saying what I think of that approach.)

The mother felt she could not offend the

physician or change physicians, since, though he had never been very supportive of breastfeeding, he was a friend of her family. Furthermore, Laura was, undoubtedly, not sure whom to believe. Why would we necessarily be right just because we told her what she wanted to hear?

The problem is not insoluble. Warfarin inhibits the action of vitamin K, which is involved in the production of several clotting factors. But the inhibition works both ways. Vitamin K inhibits the action of warfarin. So, the solution was to give the baby vitamin K every so often, as long as the mother was nursing and on the warfarin. The question came up: How much vitamin K? Every baby in our jurisdiction gets an injection at birth and does not usually need any more of it. And since even with the warfarin the baby did not need extra vitamin K, the answer as to how much to give was not clear. We finally settled, with even the family doctor's consent, on half a milligram by mouth once a month. Needless to say, the baby was fine.

It would, of course, have been possible to continue heparin after the birth of the baby, but frequent injections are a pain, especially if necessary for several months.

Looking after a baby when you're sick

You're feeling terrible—with a bad cold, stomach "flu," or some other illness. All you want to do is lie in bed and sleep. How can you deal with a nursing baby at the same time?

It isn't easy, but millions of mothers around the world have done it. And breastfeeding actually makes it easier.

If you have a small, not-yet-mobile baby, just bring the baby into bed with you. Pile diapers and wipes on a chair beside the bed and make sure you have any drinks or snacks that you can consume close by as well. You can nurse and rest together.

A mobile baby can be more challenging. One mother put her mattress on the floor, closed and latched the bedroom door, and rested on the mattress while her baby crawled around the room (previously babyproofed) and crawled back to her every time she wanted to nurse. A box of special toys and perhaps some of baby's favorite solid foods can help keep him busy while Mom relaxes.

If you're very lucky, you may be able to get someone to come over and help with the baby, bringing him back to you when he needs to nurse.

"Problem" Drugs That Are Safe

Medication for Infection

Tetracycline

Tetracycline is a drug commonly said to be a problem for the breastfeeding baby. This is based on the fact that it is not used for children, at least under the age of eight years. The reason? It is taken up in the teeth and causes permanent, disfiguring discoloration and weakness of the enamel of the adult teeth. For this to happen, children had to be on large doses over quite a long period of time, yet tetracyclines have not been used for many years in young children. Tetracycline is much less used these days than it was 20 or 30 years ago, but the memory that it is bad for children's teeth seems to have made it an automatic no-no for breastfeeding mothers. In fact, tetracycline is not a problem for the nursing mother or baby, and breastfeeding may and should continue. Why?

• The amount that gets into the milk is tiny, and extremely unlikely to cause the baby to eventually develop discolored teeth. Not only that, but courses of antibiotics tend to be shorter than many years ago. It was the prolonged use and large doses of tetracycline that caused the problems with teeth.

- Everyone who has studied pharmacology, even at the most elementary level, has been taught that tetracycline should not be given with milk, because it attaches to calcium and does not get absorbed from the intestines. How does the breastfeeding baby get the tetracycline? With milk.

Some of the newer tetracyclines are less well-bound to calcium and thus may get absorbed by the baby in small amounts. Although these are not likely to be a problem, it might be better to use an alternative medication. Fortunately, a number of alternatives are available.

Metronidazole (Flagyl)

This particular drug may be responsible for more mothers stopping breastfeeding than any other. And yet its use is not a reason to stop breastfeeding.

Here is what the *Compendium of Pharmaceuticals and Specialities* (*CPS*) says about metronidazole in its lilac pages. "Without more direct evidence of the harmful effects of short-term use in humans it seems overly conservative to withhold the drug or discontinue breastfeeding in patients . . . for (whom) metronidazole may be the treatment of choice." Actually, given the risks of not breastfeeding, I would say that the "conservative approach" is to encourage continued breastfeeding.

Ciprofloxacin

This antibiotic has already been discussed with regard to the fact that there's absolutely no evidence that it causes joint damage in humans.

There are newer antibiotics in this group that are also compatible with breastfeeding.

Prednisone

Prednisone is a steroid given for a number of conditions, including asthma and lupus. Prednisone treatment has frequently been cited as a reason for a breastfeeding mother to stop breastfeeding, but it should not be a problem, even with long-term use. This is true of all steroids, whether given by intravenous injection, intramuscular injection, topically to the skin, or by enema. Once again, the baby will not get doses comparable to what the mother gets. He will get only tiny amounts. Dr. Hale, in his book *Medications and Mothers' Milk*, notes that even with a very high dose such as 120 mg/day, the baby would get only about 47 micrograms of prednisone (and its active breakdown product prednisolone) in 24 hours. This intake by the baby would be insignificant.

In many cases now, steroids can be taken by inhalation for illnesses such as asthma (probably the most common reason for using steroids these days). Inhaled steroids stay primarily in the lungs, and only a small amount is absorbed into the body. Thus, the baby would get even less than if the mother took the steroid by mouth or other route.

Antidepressants

Probably the main reason for telling mothers that they must stop breastfeeding when they are taking antidepressant medications is that we are unsure what effect the drug may have on the baby's developing brain. And this is true. We do not know for sure what sort of long-term effects even small amounts of these drugs might have. On the other hand, we *do* know that there are definite effects of not breastfeeding on the child's developing brain. Study after study that has looked at the question shows an advantage for IQ and development for the breastfed baby over the artificially fed one. One study published in 1998 showed that children who were breastfed did better in school than those who were not breastfed, and that the longer the child was breastfed, and the more exclusively, the better the child did in school. This study is particularly interesting because it was started when the children were born, and the children were followed until they graduated from high school. Social and economic factors were taken into account. So the issue is this: Is it better for a mother who needs treatment to stop or not start breastfeeding when we know artificial feeding has a detrimental effect on the development of the child's brain? Or is it better that the baby be breastfed with a tiny amount of medication in the milk that we do not know causes any problem? Not knowing does not mean there is no negative effect, but the alternative is to give the baby something with a *proven* negative effect.

There are good reasons why breastmilk has a positive effect on brain development. Formula contains no docosahexaenoic acid, a long-chained polyunsaturated fatty acid, important for brain development. But formula does contain higher amounts of potentially toxic heavy metals, which may have negative influences on the brain. These include lead, cadmium, manganese, and aluminum. Because artificially fed babies are more likely to get ear infections, they may be slower to develop language—the single most important factor associated with success in school. Though it is possible to be close to the baby when you are feeding with a bottle, most bottle-fed babies get much less skin-to-skin contact, which affects development. And if breastfed babies seem to wake more frequently to feed, they are getting more stimulation and contact while they are awake.

One other thing. Women have frequently phoned me in despair about having to stop breastfeeding. They know they are not well and need treatment, but they hate the idea of having to give up breastfeeding. As more than one mother has said to me, more or less, "The only thing that is going well in my life is the breastfeeding and the relationship I have with the baby. And they want to take that away as well."

So antidepressant medication does not usually contraindicate breastfeeding, if the above, and the risks of artificial feeding, are taken into account. Are some antidepressants better than others? Yes, some definitely are safer to try first.

Sertraline (Zoloft)

This drug is in the family of selective serotonin reuptake inhibitors, known usually as SSRIs. There are several available, but each is slightly different from the others, from the point of view of how much the baby will get when he is breastfeeding while his mother is on the drug. Sertraline is certainly the preferred antidepressant of this type in terms of the amount passed on to the baby. Studies on the babies show that their blood levels are usually too low to be measured. This would be a good medication to try first, and it is very effective for many women.

Paroxetine (Paxil)

Paroxetine is another SSRI antidepressant that should be safe. The information we have about it suggests it gets into the milk in only tiny amounts.

A recent article documented withdrawal symptoms in four babies whose mothers were on paroxetine during the pregnancy. This was interpreted by the popular press, incorrectly, that this information made taking paroxetine during breastfeeding a problem. This is not correct. In fact, breastfeeding did not prevent the withdrawal symptoms. This makes sense, since there is so little paroxetine in the milk. Perhaps pregnant women on paroxetine should, if they are able, stop the medication for the last month or so of their pregnancies, as suggested for fluoxetine (Prozac). But they should breastfeed their babies regardless.

Fluoxetine (Prozac)

Many mothers have nursed their babies just fine while taking fluoxetine. However, it does have disadvantages compared to the two previously mentioned antidepressants, and I would not consider it the drug of choice for the nursing mother. It has a long half-life, and it gets into the milk in more significant quantities than most other antidepressants of this type.

Nevertheless, if fluoxetine must be used (and I would suggest the alternatives be tried first), then it is worth continuing breastfeeding nonetheless. The baby can be watched and blood levels can be done, if necessary. Most babies whose mothers have been on fluoxetine have done well with no apparent side effects. However, it is true that because this drug is relatively new, we have no long-term follow-up on these babies.

A few babies have definitely had some side effects, such as severe irritability or lethargy. To prevent buildup in the baby's system, the mother who is taking the drug during pregnancy should stop the medication for the last four to eight weeks of pregnancy, if possible. (Fluoxetine is the only SSRI antidepressant presently approved for use during pregnancy.) If she cannot, she should switch antidepressants once the baby is born, to one that gets into the milk in smaller amounts and doesn't hang around in the baby's system for so long. If the mother can be off fluoxetine at the end of her pregnancy, and

for the first weeks or month after the baby is born, this is very helpful, as an older baby is better able to handle the drug than a newborn.

Tricyclic antidepressants

Most tricyclic antidepressants appear in the milk in very small quantities unlikely to be of significance to the babies. The main concern about these drugs is that they take a long time to start working (often three weeks or longer), but this is true for SSRI antidepressants as well. Also, a significant number of mothers taking them have side effects that they have trouble tolerating. However, if you have taken these medications before and have found they help, there is usually no reason to stop breastfeeding or to not consider breastfeeding, if you are going to start one of this family of drugs. Nortryptilene and dothiepin are two examples of tricyclic antidepressants that can be taken by nursing mothers.

Lithium

Lithium is a drug used for the "high" or "manic" phase of bipolar disorder, previously called manic depression. It is not effective against depression. This drug has always been considered to be contraindicated during breastfeeding. However, slowly, a change in attitude has taken place.

It has been found that lithium comes out in breastmilk in very variable quantities, from very low amounts to very high amounts. If you are one of those mothers who transfers only small amounts of lithium into your milk, it may be quite safe for you to take lithium and continue breastfeeding. Your baby will need to be watched and the amount of lithium in his blood measured, but you can continue to breastfeed.

If, however, the amount of lithium in the baby's blood causes concern, we now have alternatives to lithium for the treatment of the manic phase of bipolar disorder. Both valproic acid and carbamazepine have been used quite successfully for this problem. Both are compatible with breastfeeding, even in the large doses used for bipolar disorder, since only a small percentage gets into the milk.

Drugs to Treat High Blood Pressure

Many women are treated for high blood pressure around the time of delivery—before, during, or after. As with all medications given to mothers, the great majority of blood pressure lowering medications (antihypertensives) appear in the milk in only tiny amounts and are compatible with breastfeeding. Physicians should not prescribe medications that are a concern, and mothers should insist they get medications compatible with continued breastfeeding. No mother should accept the statement that she must take a particular medication, and that she must stop (or not even start) breastfeeding while on a particular medication. There are now so many medications available for the treatment of high blood pressure that the right drug can be used in the right circumstance.

There are several families of antihypertensives. They are grouped like this because if treatment with a particular drug from one family is not effective, it can be replaced by a drug from another family. It is unlikely that another drug from the same family will be effective, since it would work by the same mechanism. Or, if the drug is partially effective, but blood pressure is not controlled as well as is desired, the physician might add a member of another drug family to help control the blood pressure. Adding another from the same family would only increase the risks of side effects without necessarily increasing the control of the blood pressure.

Beta blockers

Propranalol is the original beta blocker. It is still an excellent drug for the treatment of high blood pressure, and is also used for the prevention of migraine headaches and the symptoms of an overactive thyroid. Being "older," it is not as often used as some of the newer beta blockers, which is unfortunate, since from the breastfeeding point of view, it is one of the best of this family. The amount that gets into the milk is extremely small and extremely unlikely to have any effect on the baby. Labetalol is another that gets into the milk in such small quantities that there should be little concern about the baby's intake. Metoprolol is perhaps better than both, from the point of view of safety during breastfeeding.

Atenolol, on the other hand, does get into the milk in larger quantities, and there is one case report of a baby getting into trouble while the mother was taking it. Many mothers have taken atenelol and breastfed fine and the babies were fine, but the one case report is worrisome. (It is interesting that many drugs have caused serious illnesses in children, yet we rarely see physicians hesitating to use them on children. The antibiotic cotrimoxazole [Septra, Bactrim] comes immediately to mind. Yet one single case report has resulted in widespread fear of using atenelol during breastfeeding.) I would agree that we should not prescribe atenelol to nursing mothers. Because we have so many alternatives, we don't have to. Atenolol is not better than propranalol, labetalol, or metoprolol, so why use it? Unfortunately, too many physicians prescribe the drug first, and then tell mothers they cannot breastfeed while taking the drug. The approach should be the opposite. Certain drugs should not be used while breastfeeding, so we shouldn't prescribe them—we should use something else that is acceptable during breastfeeding.

Calcium channel blockers

In general, members of this family are strongly bound to plasma protein (good, since only the unbound drug is available for excretion into the milk), and have relatively low oral bioavailability (also good). Levels in the mother's blood are usually low, and this is also positive from the point of view of breastfeeding.

Nifedipine, one of the more commonly used calcium channel blockers, fits this pattern and would be considered safe during breastfeeding. Verapamil is another that gets into the milk in only tiny amounts.

Angiotensin-converting enzyme (ACE) inhibitors

Again, in general, this family of drugs is characterized by strong binding to plasma proteins, and low oral bioavailability. Benazepril is a commonly used ACE inhibitor. It is estimated that the baby would get less than 0.1 percent of the total maternal dose, an amount extremely unlikely to cause problems for the baby. Captopril has long been used for children (including small infants) with cardiac problems. Because of its low excretion into the milk, the drug, in the baby, would only reach an estimated 0.002 percent of the maternal dose, an insignificant amount.

Magnesium sulphate

This drug, used for treating high blood pressure around the time of delivery, has frequently, in the past, been said to be incompatible with breastfeeding. It is difficult to understand why. Magnesium is normally found in the blood, incidentally, and is important for normal body functioning. The amount that gets into the milk is quite small, and the absorption of magnesium from the baby's intestines is quite low. There should be absolutely no concern about magnesium sulphate and breastfeeding.

Other medications used for high blood pressure

Some drugs are in a category of their own. Hydralazine is one such drug. It has been used for treating high blood pressure for years, even in infants. The baby would get very little through the milk.

Methyldopa shows up in the baby's blood only in tiny amounts and may have the beneficial side effect of increasing the mother's milk supply.

It is said that diuretics decrease the milk supply, but this has never been proved. Anything is possible, but since these drugs are rarely used these days, and are rarely necessary, they should not be prescribed for nursing mothers.

Birth Control Pills

It used to be said that mothers could not breastfeed if they went on the birth control pill. The concern was that the mothers would pass on hormones in their milk to the baby and thus influence the baby's hormone levels. This was an unnecessary concern because there are, already, hormones in the milk of a type similar to those found in the birth control pill, and the extra that would come into the milk while the mother is taking the birth control pill would make little difference in the quantity the baby receives. Physicians seem to have learned this very quickly, and many started to prescribe "the pill" to nursing mothers. Unfortunately, it was soon discovered that the estrogens in the pill, even in the small amounts found in the so-called mini pills, was enough, in at least some mothers, to decrease their milk significantly. This resulted, in many cases, in early and unnecessary weaning. Some physicians did pick up on this, and the word went out. Still, it is believed by some physicians that if the pill is started once the milk supply is well established—say, after six or eight weeks after birth—there is no concern about the milk supply decreasing. This is simply not true.

I have seen and spoken to nursing mothers who were started on birth control pills at five months after birth and later, who noticed a significant decrease in their milk supplies. Babies who had been content at the breast and were gaining well just breastfeeding, suddenly, within a week of the mother going on the pill, fussed, pulled at the breast, cried, and seemed insatiable, wanting always to return to the breast, but obviously frustrated when they were there. They were not getting the milk because of the decrease in supply, or flow (which may be more important).

In some cases, the mothers had taken the pill without problems while breastfeeding another baby, but then had problems with a subsequent baby. The decrease in the milk supply seems unpredictable. Even if the decrease is small, the reduced flow of milk may make the baby fussy and unhappy at the breast.

So what do I do?

Birth control is a very personal and intimate issue that needs to be handled with more than just a prescription for the pill. Physicians should discuss all options with the mother and her partner. The pill may not be for everyone, but it is the easiest thing for the physician to prescribe. It takes time to go over the other options that new parents have.

In the first place, the parents may not need birth control. The conception control that breastfeeding alone gives is significant, if certain guidelines are followed.

- The mother's menstrual periods have not resumed.

- The baby is younger than six months old.
- The baby is exclusively breastfed.

Second, not every couple is ready to resume sexual relations in the first few months after the baby is born. The fatigue and change of lifestyle that occur when a baby is born is not always conducive to a vigorous sexual relationship. Temporary celibacy is not a horror from which all new parents recoil. In addition, intimacy between two people does not always require "going all the way," as we used to say in the old days. A satisfying, close, physical relationship can continue without actual sexual intercourse.

Should the above approaches not be options for the family, other approaches are possible. Barrier methods (condoms, diaphragms) are available, and are extra reassurance for those who cannot believe that breastfeeding is a good method of child spacing. The IUD is a possibility. Remember though, that no method is 100 percent effective. A newspaper story a few years ago told of a woman who became pregnant even though she had had a tubal ligation, and the father had had a vasectomy.

So, what if the pill is the only option, the only acceptable way to go? Okay, there is now available a progesterone-only pill. Because it does not contain estrogens, its effect on milk production is said to be less or not at all. Some have even claimed that it increases the milk supply. None of the above has been proved, but certainly the effect is less with the progesterone-only pill than with the estrogen-containing pills.

When should one start the pill? It is better not to start too early. Six weeks after birth is early enough, and not too late. The chances of pregnancy occurring before this time are so low, even in mothers who do not breastfeed, that it is not worth the risk of the pill. The combination pill (with estrogens), if it must be used, should be delayed as long as possible, until the baby is taking other food, or after six months, so that any decrease in milk supply can at least be compensated for by increased food intake. However, remember that babies respond to flow, not to the amount of milk in the breast. A decreased supply may be an adequate supply, but if the flow to the baby is slow, he may not be content.

There is now available in Canada (and has been for several years in the United States) an injectable form of birth control (medroxyprogesterone, Depo-Provera) that requires an injection only every three months. Many physicians like it because it can be started anytime, and there is no "fuss or bother." In many areas of the United States, it has been frankly abused and misused, with minority and poor women being injected—sometimes without adequate information to make an informed consent—before they even leave the hospital. Indeed, considering that most women do not consider labor and birth a pleasant experience, especially with the lack of support and help that so many women experience in the hospital, one could argue that it is not possible for them to make an informed consent after living through such a terribly difficult and painful few days.

But there is an even greater problem. Research suggests that it is the drop in progesterone levels when the placenta is born that sensitizes the cells in the mother's breast that produce milk to the action of prolactin, the hormone that stimulates milk production. If there is no drop, there is no milk production. Thus, giving the injection of progesterone before the mother is discharged from hospital may, at least in theory, cut off her milk supply for at least three months. Which is the same as saying no breastfeeding for her baby. This has not been proven, but there are enough stories to suggest that it is quite possible.

New mothers should resist the temptation to accept the medroxyprogesterone injection (Depo-Provera) immediately after birth. Indeed, the manufacturer actually suggests that breastfeeding mothers not be given the injection before six weeks postpartum. Neither should it be given to mothers who do not plan to breastfeed until that time, because it is not necessary, and because many may change their minds about breastfeeding if they get a good milk supply.

Even six weeks after birth, I would urge mothers not to take the injection. They should first try the progesterone-only pill. If the milk supply remains abundant after one cycle of pills (28 days), then they can have the injection if they want. If the milk supply decreases with the progesterone-only pill, the mother can stop it, and the milk supply should start to return. On the other hand, if the milk supply decreases with the injection, there is no way to get rid of the injected progesterone.

I took the pill and my supply is down. What do I do?

Stop the pill. At this point, domperidone (a medication described in more detail in Chapter 5, Not Enough Milk) can bring back the supply very quickly—within a few days at most. Don't hesitate—it will work. And you should be able to stop it within 10 to 14 days.

Let your physician know that the medication you took decreased your milk supply. A conscientious physician will no longer prescribe the combined pill for breastfeeding mothers. He will not say, as many mothers have told me they have been advised, "You've breastfed long enough, anyway."

When Medication Is Recommended . . .

It is not possible to discuss every single drug in every single situation, and though there are occasionally situations when there is no option but to suspend breastfeeding while the mother is taking medication, this should only rarely be necessary. Remember the following:

- Breastfeeding is too important for the mother and the baby to stop just because the baby may get a small amount of medication. The risks of not breastfeeding need to be considered as well. Stopping breastfeeding for a ten-day course of metronidazole (Flagyl), for example, may result in permanent cessation of breastfeeding—and it is unnecessary to stop.
- It is rare for there ever to be one and only one medication available for the treatment of a particular problem. If a drug causes concern, a perfectly good substitute that is not a concern can usually be found.
- Sometimes drug therapy is not necessary. Unfortunately, medication is a quick fix. It is easy to give an antibiotic, when reassurance that the fever is caused by a virus is all that is needed. Even when treatment is necessary, medication is not always the only route. Postpartum depression, if serious, probably requires medication, and there are options available for the breastfeeding mother that do not require her to stop breastfeeding. But in milder cases counseling and support may be all that is necessary.

Drugs of Abuse and Recreation

These drugs are often looked upon in our society differently from drugs made by pharmaceutical companies because they are "not neces-sary," addictive, pleasurable or illegal, or all of the above. Some strong advocates of breastfeeding, who encourage mothers to breastfeed while taking antidepressants (quite rightly), balk at encouraging mothers to breastfeed after having ingested alcohol, or may suggest they should not breastfeed at all if they are smokers. This is very surprising to me, and seems to be a reflection of the new puritanism that has struck North America during the 1990s. A drug is a drug, and the breast does not know if it is illegal or recreational.

Alcohol

Many health professionals tell breastfeeding mothers that they must "pump and dump" their milk for two hours after each drink of alcohol (usually defined as one ounce, or 30 ml, of pure alcohol). I despise the expression "pump and dump," because it treats breastmilk as if it were some sort of disgusting fluid. In most cases "pump and dump" should be replaced by "sacrifice breastfeeding on the altar of our ignorance" or "sacrifice breastfeeding on the altar of our prudery."

Alcohol is a drug that passes freely from the mother's blood to her breastmilk. In this way, it appears in the milk in quantities greater than other drugs. But what sort of quantities? Do we really have to be concerned if the mother has a couple of drinks with dinner? No.

In many jurisdictions, you are considered too drunk to drive if you have 0.08 percent alcohol in your blood. In some others, the legal limit may be as high as 0.1 percent or as low as 0.05 percent. This is a blood level of alcohol that can cloud your judgment when you have to operate a vehicle, agreed. But if the mother has 0.08 percent alcohol in her blood, her milk will have 0.08 percent alcohol. Now this is a completely different situation. Wine is 10 to 12 percent alcohol, beer 3 to 5 percent, and hard liquor approximately 40 percent, occasionally more. So-called dealcoholized beer actually has 0.6 percent alcohol or more, that is seven times more than the mother's milk will contain if she has a blood level of 0.08 percent. You can drink a liquid that is 0.08 percent alcohol, day and night, and it won't affect you. So how is this likely to harm the baby?

The formula the baby would receive—while the mother is throwing away her milk because it has a tiny amount of alcohol in it—is known to put the baby at greater risk for a host of illnesses and problems.

One of the main reasons so many women in North America do not breastfeed or stop early is that they are given the impression that only saints should breastfeed. You can't have a drink; you have to be careful what you eat; you can't have a cigarette; you can't take an aspirin for your headache; you can't go out to a restaurant or to the movies because breastfeeding in public is not nice. There is a widespread belief that a woman who has a drink of alcohol has contaminated herself and her milk, and that her baby is better off without her milk and her breast.

A woman who is constantly drunk is a different case, but her baby is probably at greater risk of neglect or accidental injury than from the alcohol that might pass through in the milk.

Okay, you've heard or read that if a mother drinks more than a certain number of drinks a day when breastfeeding (the study said two drinks or more per day), the baby has not as good motor development at one year of age as babies of mothers who did not drink as much or did not drink at all. That's a fair amount of alcohol to be drinking on a daily basis—but is it the alcohol the baby gets while breastfeeding that is

to blame? One fault of this study is that the researchers depended on the mother's word regarding what she did or did not drink *during pregnancy*. The effects of alcohol during pregnancy are well known, and were well known at the time of the study. What heavy drinker will tell a researcher that she drank heavily during her pregnancy? Some, not all. We already know that alcohol during pregnancy affects the development of babies after they are born, and this may have been the real factor here—not the drinks consumed while breastfeeding.

Alcohol while breastfeeding? No problem, in moderation. No need to worry about "pumping and dumping." Just put the baby to the breast, even while you have your drink—why not?

Tobacco

On the other hand, smoking is not good for you or for your baby. There seems to be no doubt that babies exposed to cigarette smoke where they live are much more likely to have respiratory illnesses and to die of sudden infant death syndrome (SIDS, or crib death).

However, if you cannot stop smoking (nicotine is one of the most addictive drugs known), then you are better to smoke and breastfeed than smoke and not breastfeed. All the publicity about exposure to nicotine, about carcinogenic compounds that the baby receives, does not diminish the risks of *not* breastfeeding. Not breastfeeding also increases the risks of the baby for certain cancers. Respiratory illnesses are more common in breastfeeding babies whose mothers smoke than in breastfeeding babies whose mothers do not smoke, but they are less common and less severe than respiratory illnesses in artificially fed babies whose mothers smoke.

Any smoker, not just the mother, living in the same area where the baby lives, increases the baby's risk of sudden infant death syndrome. Breastfeeding decreases the risk of sudden infant death somewhat.

Stop smoking if you can. Cut down if you can't. If you or your partner must continue to smoke, do so outside, away from your baby. But breastfeed.

Marijuana

I am not advocating the use of marijuana, but some women will smoke marijuana whether I, or anyone else, advocate it or not. Does a mother who smokes a marijuana cigarette or two from time to time have to "pump and dump" her milk for a given time afterward, and feed formula instead?

No, she doesn't. Again assuming occasional use, there is no reason to stop breastfeeding after intake. There is no evidence that it is harmful to the baby to be exposed to small amounts that would be present in the milk.

However, chronic heavy use is a different story. It is possible that it decreases the milk supply by inhibiting prolactin secretion. More importantly, THC (the active ingredient) is concentrated in the milk, and chronic exposure could result in the drug accumulating in the baby. The long-term effects of this are unknown.

Breastfeed, and if you must light up from time to time, take it easy.

Narcotics

Occasional use of narcotics is not a contraindication to breastfeeding, though why are you doing this? Occasional use can easily become chronic use. Your baby needs you, and regular users are not usually in good enough shape to take care of their babies. A new life depends on you.

Use of meperidine (Demerol) or morphine for pain relief after surgery, for example, is not a reason to stop breastfeeding—again, because the amount that gets into the milk is tiny and not likely to harm the baby. This is understood by many (though not enough) health professionals. A mother who occasionally abuses narcotics does not pass on more in her milk than she would if the drug were given for legally accepted reasons. (Though street drugs may not be free of possibly dangerous contaminants.)

What of the mother who was a chronic user during pregnancy? Should health professionals be there to say that she can only breastfeed after she has made a solemn oath not to abuse narcotics? Put that way, no one will do it—the mother will formula-feed and her baby will be at risk for all sorts of problems. Indeed, formula-fed infants of chronic drug abusers, because of the lifestyle and health problems their mothers have, are at an even greater risk of serious illness than are formula-fed babies of mothers who do not abuse drugs.

Health professionals should not let this opportunity slip by. Giving birth and breastfeeding can be life-affirming events in a woman's life. Here is a chance to break with the past. Many drug abusers have low self-esteem. If we tell a new mother she can only breastfeed if she stops drugs first, we are telling her that she is no good, and we are setting her up for another failure. A better message is that we trust her with this baby, that we think she can make a go of it.

I realize that the above scenario does not always fit. Some drug users are too far gone. They will never be able to take care of their babies. But does this mean we should write off everybody? Let's give the mother and baby a chance.

When babies are born to mothers who were using narcotics regularly during pregnancy, the babies pass through several days to several weeks of withdrawal symptoms. These symptoms are often treated with narcotics—such as morphine—intravenously. At the same time, the babies' mothers are often told they cannot give their milk to the babies because of the narcotics that may be found in the milk. This is bizarre. The tiny amount of extra narcotic present in the milk will do no harm to a baby who is getting narcotics anyway in order to treat his symptoms of withdrawal. However, if we say to the mother that we cannot use her milk, we are sending out a very strong message: It's not the drug, it's you. And we are not giving the mother an opportunity to become involved with her baby in a way that is far more fundamental and more meaningful for her than merely touching the baby in the incubator.

The mother and baby will have to be followed carefully by their physician, and if drug abuse continues, the whole issue of breastfeeding or even her ability to care for her baby will have to be reevaluated. However, the mother just might make it work.

Methadone

A mother on methadone is usually trying to get off her dependency on street drugs. She should be encouraged to breastfeed. Again, discouraging breastfeeding only decreases the mother's feelings of self-worth, which may impair her abilities as a mother for this child.

At one point, the American Academy of Pediatrics recommended "allowing" breastfeeding only if the mother was taking 20 mg or less of methadone. Where this "20 mg" came from is not clear, but they have changed their stance and now do not specify that a certain quantity is too much. Most women are taking far more than 20 mg a day and breastfeeding and their babies are fine.

Cocaine

Cocaine appears in the milk, and since it is a very powerful stimulant and completely absorbed from the gut, a mother who uses cocaine should not breastfeed her baby for at least four or five hours after taking the drug. Occasional use, coupled with waiting after use, does not pose a danger to the baby from cocaine through the milk. But your baby needs you to care for him, unaffected by drugs.

Chronic, daily use of cocaine is too dangerous for the baby if the mother is breastfeeding. Do the best for your baby and yourself. Stop the cocaine.

If the baby has received cocaine through the milk, his urine will test positive for breakdown products of cocaine for several days to a week or even longer.

LSD

We do not know much about LSD and its transfer into the milk. Undoubtedly some gets into the milk, and it is a powerful hallucinogen even in tiny amounts. Do not take LSD while breastfeeding. If you have done so, wait 12 hours before breastfeeding the baby.

Medical Investigations (X-rays, CT Scans, MRI Scans)

All too often medical investigations are done for little reason. A breastfeeding mother should be absolutely sure that investigations she is to undergo are truly necessary, because she will frequently be told that she must stop breastfeeding for a certain number of days after the investigations are done. In fact, this is almost never necessary. Ordinary X-rays are not going to affect the milk, although mothers have often been told they cannot breastfeed after such procedures. There is no reason for a mother to wean, even temporarily, because of an X-ray.

On the other hand, most radiology department technicians or radiologists will tell the mother she must stop breastfeeding for a variable period of time after a kidney X-ray (intravenous pyelogram or IVP), lymphangiogram, or gallbladder X-ray (cholangiogram). These types of investigation are done with iodine-containing contrast materials (not radioactive), and the manufacturer of the dyes always advises interrupting breastfeeding for 24 to 48 hours after the procedure. Most radiologists will acknowledge that this is completely unnecessary, since the amount of iodine that gets into the milk will be negligible and will not affect the baby. Nevertheless, the prohibition on breastfeeding after these procedures continues because that is what the manufacturer suggests, and no medical professionals want to put themselves at medicolegal risk. The fact that many of these same investigations are done on babies with the same contrast materials seems not to stimulate inquiring minds to ask, "What are we worried about?" The answer, of course, is not that we are worried about the mothers or babies, but that we are worried about getting sued—even though nothing is likely to occur.

The same is true of CT scans, which use an iodine-based contrast material (not radioactive). And recently MRI scans have been a reason to tell mothers to suspend breastfeeding for 24 hours. The contrast material used for MRI scans is gadopentetate, a compound with a very short half-life (less than an hour), and thus one that will be completely eliminated from the mother's body within six hours (98 percent of a drug or material is eliminated after five half-lives). Furthermore, only a tiny amount of it is actually absorbed from the gut, estimated at 0.8 percent of the total eaten (the way the baby gets it). Thus there should be absolutely no reason to suspend breastfeeding after an MRI scan, yet the company recommends 24 hours. This is an astounding recommendation, given the behavior of this compound, and should be ignored.

Investigations using radioactive compounds present a different dilemma. We certainly want to expose babies to as little radioactivity as possible, but does that mean we must wait until the milk contains no radioactivity? Remember that radioactive studies are sometimes done on small infants as well as adults. They are conducted when we feel the value of the investigation outweighs the risk from the radiation the baby will receive.

The most commonly used radioactive compound for special studies is Technetium 99. It is used for lung scans, bone scans, brain scans, and several other types of scans. It has a half-life of six hours, which means that 98 percent of it will be out of the mother's body in 30 hours, more or less. Does this mean the mother should stop breastfeeding for 30 hours? Some would say that would be the best thing. However, I think this is unnecessarily long. The baby can get some radioactivity—we rarely hesitate to do a chest X-ray on a baby, for example. It's better not to give unnecessary radiation, but there also comes a point when the risk is infinitesimal. If the mother waits 12 hours (or two half-lives), 75 percent of the radioactivity will be out of her body.

Each mother and her physician will have to decide together when they feel the risk of breastfeeding outweighs the risk of the formula. Personally, I would not wait longer than six or 12 hours before resuming breastfeeding, but 30 hours would certainly be the maximum a mother should wait.

If the mother knows in advance that she will have this test, she can express and save her milk to cover the needs of the baby for the time required, without giving formula.

But in this day and age is it necessary to do as many of these scans as we do? After all, if the radioactivity is considered too hazardous for the baby, why is okay for the mother? Yes, of course, the baby is younger, but most nursing mothers probably have a good 30 to 60 years ahead of them. Certainly the brain scan should hardly be used anymore—the CT and MRI do a much better job. Remember, the CT and MRI scans do not require a mother to stop breastfeeding for even two minutes.

Radioactive Iodine Scans

One of the most common scans done on mothers who are breastfeeding is the thyroid scan. A significant percentage of women in the postpartum period develop an inflammation of the thyroid called postpartum thyroiditis, which may give the mother symptoms of an overactive thyroid—nervousness, fatigue, irritability, heart palpitations, weight loss. Typically, this occurs around three to six months after the birth of the baby, and the symptoms usually disappear after a couple of months. The mother actually may end up having an underactive thyroid after all the inflammation. Many physicians would like the mother to have a thyroid scan to differentiate between postpartum thyroiditis and Graves' disease, a much more chronic, and potentially more serious, problem. The scan can be done with I^{131} or with I^{123}. The first has a long half-life and shouldn't be used. With I^{123} we have new recommendations: the mother can resume breastfeeding after 12 to 24 hours, depending on the dose she is given. But another question to be asked is: Does this test need to be done?

The answer is almost never, at least to differentiate postpartum thyroiditis from Graves' disease. First of all, the chances are that a mother who has the symptoms of an overactive thyroid, say, five months after the baby is born, has postpartum thyroiditis. Furthermore, there are features of the blood tests that suggest one or the other, although these are not definitive. However, postpartum thyroiditis gets better spontaneously after six to eight weeks, whereas Graves' disease does not. Following the mother's blood levels of thyroid hormone will show, with postpartum thyroiditis, dropping levels by six to eight weeks after the initial diagnosis—earlier, if the diagnosis was delayed.

In the situation of a mother presenting with the symptoms of an overactive thyroid and compatible blood tests, the best approach would be not to do the thyroid scan. The mother can be treated for her symptoms, usually with propranolol, which is quite compatible with breastfeeding, and her symptoms and blood work should be followed. If it turns out that the blood tests continue showing evidence of hyperactivity of the thyroid without going down after six or eight weeks, then the diagnosis of Graves' disease becomes more likely. The mother can then be treated with propylthiouracil (PTU), which is one of the usual medications to treat Graves' disease, and one quite compatible with continued breastfeeding.

What if the mother has Graves' disease, though? Continued treatment with PTU is fine. But sometimes mothers are put into a situation where they are told the best treatment is destruction of the gland with radioactive iodine. The isotope (I^{131}) used is not the I^{123} that is the best choice for diagnostic scan, and is given in a dose to kill the cells of the thyroid gland. I^{131} has a much longer half-life than I^{123}—over eight days—which means that to avoid the baby getting any I^{131}, the mother would have to stop breastfeeding for 40 days (five half-lives). It is unlikely that even the most eager nursing baby would return to breastfeeding after being off the breast for 40 days. What a dilemma!

The problem is that women are not offered the range of choices. There are approaches to treating Graves' disease other than radioactive iodine. In the first place, PTU will work most of the time, along with propranalol, and can be used indefinitely as long as symptoms are kept under control. Second, surgery is an option. The mother can breastfeed immediately after the surgery (because the drugs used during surgery are not going to harm the baby, the amounts getting into the milk being tiny) as soon as she is awake and up to it. There are disadvantages to the surgery, too, but the mother should be offered this possibility. Perhaps in her situation radioactive iodine is the best choice, and the baby will have to stop breastfeeding. But maybe, just maybe, surgery is the best choice for her. The possibility should at least be explored.

MOTHERS' STORIES
DENISE

Denise was two months' pregnant when she found out she had cancer of the thyroid. Fortunately, the cancer was not an aggressive type, and she was offered surgery immediately, with a tiny risk for the baby, or surgery after she had had her baby. For various reasons, including the fact that she did not think she could face surgery with a new baby, she opted to have the surgery immediately. She was also aware that after the baby was born, she would have to have I^{131} treatment to kill off any cancer cells that might remain. This type of cancer is unlikely to spread, but it can. In order to make sure it did not spread, Denise was told that she should have a radioactive iodine (I^{131}) treatment by about six weeks after the baby's birth—and she would have to stop breastfeeding before her baby was six weeks old. The iodine would accumulate not only in the thyroid but also in her milk, since

iodine is concentrated in milk. It could also cause damage to the breast cells. Most authorities recommend that mothers stop breastfeeding a week before taking the radioactive iodine, to decrease the risk of trapping radioactive iodine in the milk.

I suggested Denise wait until the baby was six months old or more. At least the baby would get more breastfeeding, and Denise would benefit as well. What was the rush, exactly? The physicians were willing to wait eight or nine months to do the surgery for a cancer they *knew* Denise had. Why could they not wait six or seven months to do a procedure for a cancer they *didn't* know was there, especially since the risk was so low?

Pollutants in Breastmilk

Every so often, scare stories appear in the newspapers about pollutants (chemicals present in the environment) in breastmilk. Every time this happens, some mothers who otherwise would have breastfed decide not to, some mothers decide to stop earlier than they had planned, and many who do breastfeed are made anxious about their babies. Some environmental groups have a lot to answer for, since they have exploited the fact that breastmilk contains pollutants to further their own ends, laudable as those ends may be.

What in our world have we succeeded in *not* contaminating? Not much, and certainly I have never understood how infant formulas might have remained uncontaminated in this contaminated planet of ours. The toxins in breastmilk may be different from the toxins in infant formulas, but they are not worse just because they are different. It is true that our being at the top of the food chain results in some fat-soluble toxins being present in greater concentrations in humans than in cows or soy beans—dioxins are among these. But cows eat grass, hay, and grain sprayed with pesticides, and that makes their milk contaminated, too.

The processing of soy and cow's milk for infant formulas also results in their being polluted. Formulas contain heavy metals in concentrations far higher than those in breastmilk. Formulas contain much more aluminium (soy formulas up to 2,000 times the amounts in breastmilk), lead (there are no safe amounts of lead), cadmium, and manganese. These metals are all potential toxins to the brain and nervous system—and the latter three appear in formulas in concentrations about 100 times higher than those present in breastmilk. Why do we never hear about this in the newspapers? Why do the environmental groups never talk about contamination of infant formulas?

Breastfeeding is actually a very environmentally friendly thing to do. The infant formula companies are great polluters. The amount of land used to make milk for infant formulas is taken away from other land use. There is the environmental cost of growing soy beans and raising cattle. There is the environmental cost of transporting the milk or soy beans to the factory where formulas are made, the energy cost of transforming the base product into artificial baby milk, the transportation cost of moving the finished product to market. There are the tremendous energy and paper costs of marketing this often completely unnecessary product. Just think of the environmental costs of the advertising you alone received. Multiply that by the approximately five million mothers who give birth in Canada and the United States every year. And mothers are just part of the advertising blitzkrieg. Physicians, nurses, dietitians, hospital CEOs, and purchasing agents are bombarded with advertising. Waste? No waste with breastfeeding. But the number of tins of formula discarded every year amount to hundreds of millions in the United States alone. Where are we going to put them?

To suggest, as some have, that because of the toxins in breastmilk, women should breastfeed for only a short period of time, or not at all, makes as much sense as suggesting that the way to fight global warming is for everyone to buy an air conditioner.

One of the concerns over taking in dioxins and other environmental pollutants is that they may decrease the immune response. But studies consistently show that breastfed babies have a better immune response than do formula-fed babies. Another concern is that increased intake of these toxins will increase the risk of cancers. Yet studies show that babies who are breastfed have lower rates of cancer than babies who are not.

We should be very worried about what we are doing to the environment, if even mother's milk is polluted. But these findings should be a call to action, a call to a change in our way of doing things.

The best thing a mother can do for the environment, her baby, and herself is to breastfeed.

12

Maternal Illness and Breastfeeding

Myth: When a mother is sick, it is best she not breastfeed her baby.

Fact: Only rarely is there any illness that truly requires a mother not to breastfeed. Even when the explanations seem reasonable, they often are not. The risks of *not* breastfeeding almost always outweigh the risks to the baby of breastfeeding.

It may seem logical that if the mother has a cold or a rash or some other illness, the baby is more likely to pick up that infection if the mother continues breastfeeding. As it turns out, it is not more likely. The fact is, many, if not most, infectious diseases are most infectious before the mother even knows she is sick. By the time the mother has the symptoms of cough, runny nose, diarrhea, or rash, she has already passed on the infection to the baby. Most viruses, for example, are briefly circulating in the blood before the illness begins, and if they can pass into the milk, the baby will have been infected many hours, even days, before the mother is aware she is sick.

Is this bad? No, not at all. Indeed, it is good. The baby gets exposed to an infectious agent, while at the same time being protected by various anti-infectious agents in the milk. Though these anti-infectious agents in the milk are not a guarantee the baby will not get sick, their presence does usually result either in the baby not getting sick or just having a mild form of the illness. In fact, being exposed like this actually helps the baby develop immunity to that particular virus or bacterium—and this is what we want. Breastfeeding, by providing the baby with antiviral and antibacterial protection, allows him to be exposed to viruses and bacteria and other infectious agents in his surroundings, and to develop immunity to those viruses and bacteria without getting sick, or at least by getting only mildly ill. That's what immunizations do, essentially. The baby infected with the measles virus, for example, a weakened one, will develop immunity, usually without getting sick. Sometimes the baby does get sick after an immunization, with fever and irritability, or rash, but usually the illness is mild.

Protective Factors in Breastmilk

Health professionals frequently talk about the protective factors in breastmilk, and how important they are and why these are a good reason to breastfeed. Few act, however, as if these protective factors actually work. How else can we explain that so many health professionals tell a mother she must stop breastfeeding when she has a fever, or a cold sore or diarrhea?

Many people know that there are antibodies in breastmilk, but not as many realize that there are many different kinds of immune factors that help the baby resist and fight off infections. Here is a partial list of these immune factors and what they do for the baby.

Antibodies

Antibodies are the most widely known anti-infective factors in breastmilk, and when we hear people talking about the protection due to breastmilk, we almost always hear them talking about antibodies. In truth, antibodies are only part of a whole immune system in breastmilk—a system in which the various elements interact to give the baby the best protection possible during the first months and years when he is susceptible to many illnesses because he has not had much exposure to the world.

Although all the antibodies in the mother's blood are also found in the milk, most of the antibody in the milk is a particular type. The vast majority of the antibodies in breastmilk are secretory IgA antibodies (or SIgA). SIgA is present in particularly high concentrations in the colostrum, but even months and years after the baby is born—in fact, for the entire duration of breastfeeding—it is still present in significant amounts that help the baby fight off infection.

SIgA, like some of the other immune factors, provides the baby with "mucosal" immunity. It actually prevents viruses and bacteria from passing through the mucosal membranes—the "linings" of the body, such as the lining of the lungs or the intestines. Because the viruses and bacteria can't get through, they can't make the baby sick. This mucosal immunity prevents illness before it can begin.

The other antibodies found in the milk may be involved with mucosal immunity as well, but there is little known about what they do. It is unlikely that many antibodies are absorbed into the baby's blood from his gut. This is important when we discuss the woman who has auto-immune diseases, such as thyroid disease and idiopathic thrombocytopenic purpura. She *can* breastfeed.

The Enteromammary System

This is one of the most fascinating aspects of the protective effects of breastmilk. As a result of the mother being exposed to various bacteria and viruses, her milk will contain antibodies specifically directed at those very germs. For example, if a mother is exposed to *E. coli* bacteria, within hours of that exposure her milk will contain SIgA specifically made against *E. coli* bacteria. The baby is continually protected against those particular bacteria in his immediate environment, or at least the immediate environment of his mother, which is usually the same thing. Or if she is exposed to influenza virus, within hours of her being exposed, her milk will contain antibodies specifically directed against influenza virus. This is miraculous. Formula will never be able to replicate this— never.

White Cells

White cells of several sorts are normally found in breastmilk. The amounts are highest in colostrum, but even months after birth, the milk will contain many white cells in concentrations greater than those found in the blood. This concentration of white cells in the milk suggests that the breast is actively adding white cells to the milk.

It has been shown that the white cells in the milk retain their functions, which are similar to their functions in the blood. Antibodies and white cells often work together to more actively kill viruses and bacteria.

Lysozyme

Lysozyme kills bacteria by attacking them directly, breaking up the cell walls. It is sometimes present in the milk in greater quantities after the baby is one year old than when the baby is younger.

Lactoferrin

Lactoferrin attaches itself to iron molecules in the baby's digestive system, and this is one way in which it helps protect the baby against infection. Iron is necessary for some bacteria to multiply, and by binding iron in the baby's intestines, lactoferrin makes iron unavailable for these bacteria to multiply and grow.

It is thought that lactoferrin also directly inhibits the growth of bacteria, as well as decreasing the inflammation associated with immune responses.

B_{12} Binding Protein

In the same way as lactoferrin stops bacteria from using the iron in the baby's intestines, this protein interferes with bacterial use of B_{12}, a vitamin essential for bacterial growth.

Bifidus Factor

This factor encourages the growth in the baby's intestines of nonharmful bacteria, which will inhibit the growth of more dangerous bacteria that can cause disease.

Oligosaccharides

These sugars have special receptors on them that are similar to receptors on the cells of the intestines to which disease-causing bacteria may attach before they invade the bloodstream. The bacteria will attach to the oligosaccharides instead of the baby's cells, and the bacteria won't be able to cause illness—they will just leave the baby's body in a bowel movement.

Interferon

White cells (T lymphocytes) in breastmilk produce interferon. Interferon has many immune functions that may result in protection against viral infections.

Cytokines

Cytokines are small proteins that have a wide range of immune effects. They stimulate immune responses in white cells, but their main function may be to help the baby mature his own immune function.

These are just a few of the many immune factors in breastmilk. You can see how these work together to keep your baby healthy. Recently, formula companies have started to add a group of substances called nucleotides to their formulas, and are claiming that this addition protects the baby the way breastmilk does. This is clearly false advertising. Even recent studies have not shown an important effect of nucleotides on the baby's immune system. Nucleotides may have a role in immunity when the baby is under stress, such as after surgery, but none of this is proved.

It seems the main reason to add nucleotides is marketing. And as a result, far too many health professionals, as well as consumers, assume that the immune factors of breastmilk have now been added to formula. In this way, the companies perpetuate the notion that formula is always getting closer to breastmilk.

In summary, mother's milk contains many factors, antibodies, cells, and other elements that give the baby reasonable, though not guaranteed, protection against infection. When the mother develops some sort of infectious illness, it is almost always in the baby's best interests for her to keep breastfeeding. Babies who are breastfed when the mother gets fever, cough, rash, vomiting, diarrhea, or whatever, will likely be less sick than if they are prevented from breastfeeding.

In the presence of many illnesses, some health professionals will counsel mothers to not breastfeed "just to be safe." But this assumes that it is just as safe to feed artificially as it is to breastfeed, and this is simply not true (see Chapter 11, Breastfeeding While on Medication). Some specific situations are discussed below.

Infectious Diseases

Hepatitis

What is hepatitis?

There are many viruses that can cause the collection of symptoms we generally call *hepatitis* (jaundice, nausea, fatigue, abdominal pain). Seven of these viruses are named hepatitis A, hepatitis B, hepatitis C, down to G viruses. Expect in the next few years that there will be hepatitis H, I, J, and that eventually even all the letters of the alphabet will not suffice.

Other viruses, however, can also cause hepatitis-like illness, including infectious mononucleosis virus (Epstein-Barr virus), cytomegalovirus, and even some viruses that cause the common cold. It should also be mentioned that other illnesses, noninfectious ones, may cause hepatitis-like symptoms. Probably the most common example is hepatitis-like illness due to a drug reaction.

Hepatitis may be so mild that a person doesn't know they have it. Other cases are more severe, and in rare cases, fatal.

How is it transmitted?

Hepatitis is like most viruses: by the time a person is aware that they have an illness, they are less infectious than they were, and sometimes not infectious at all. Most viruses have a viremic phase (when the virus is in the blood), again, usually before the person is aware of any illness at all. When the virus is in the blood, small amounts of virus may also get into the milk. All this has happened before the mother notices any symptoms. By the time she realizes that she is ill, she has already passed the infection on.

Some hepatitis viruses (notably B and C) can cause both chronic-carrier states (that is, the person has the virus in their body, but has no evidence of actual infection) and chronic infection. These situations do raise the question as to whether breastfeeding is advisable.

Hepatitis A

Hepatitis A does not cause a chronic-carrier state or chronic infection. The acute illness is usually fairly mild, but can be severe, and symptoms usually last a fairly long time, often several weeks. Loss of appetite, nausea, and fatigue are typical symptoms—things nursing mothers could do without.

However, by the time the mother notices a yellow discoloration of her skin, the chances of infecting anyone else are pretty well nil. The viremic phase (when the virus is in the blood, and therefore potentially in the milk) has long passed, and even excretion of virus in the bowel movements has virtually stopped. So weaning at this point will do nothing to keep the baby from getting the virus.

How can this be treated or prevented?

Immune globulin can be given to the baby if the physician feels transmission should be avoided. Also, there is now an immunization for hepatitis A that will effectively prevent illnesses.

Hepatitis A infection in children tends to be particularly mild, but, as with adults, it can be severe.

The main concern, really, is continuing breastfeeding while the mother is feeling nauseated, extremely fatigued, and unable to eat. The adult with hepatitis will usually be in bed. The breastfeeding mother should go to bed with her baby and rest, sleep, and allow herself to be coddled. The baby can nurse in bed with her. The older child can be brought when he needs to nurse.

Hepatitis B

Hepatitis B, from the point of view of acute illness, is similar to hepatitis A, though often it is longer lasting. It can also cause additional symptoms, for example, arthritis.

Unlike hepatitis A, hepatitis B may cause a chronic-carrier state. In some parts of the world, 15 percent or more of all people are carriers for this virus. The chances of passing the virus on to the baby, either during pregnancy or birth, are significant.

How can this be treated or prevented?

In areas where many people are carriers of hepatitis B, the law may require screening of all pregnant women for the virus, and protecting of the newborn at birth with immune globulin and immunization. The success rate of preventing transmission to the baby is very high.

Even before the immunization was available, however, there was no proof that babies who were breastfed got the infection more frequently than those fed artificially. Indeed, at least a couple of good studies showed that the risk to the baby was the same, regardless of the method of feeding. Despite that, many physicians still counsel mothers who are hepatitis B–positive not to breastfeed. These doctors should, in fact, counsel these mothers to breastfeed, especially now that the risk of transmission with the immunizations is virtually zero.

Hepatitis C

Hepatitis C can cause acute illness similar to hepatitis A and B, but in most cases the disease is either unnoticed or very mild. The main issue with hepatitis C is the chronic-carrier state. A significant percentage of adults with chronic-carrier states do have chronic infections that will eventually develop into more serious illness (cirrhosis). What happens to babies infected with hepatitis C during pregnancy or delivery is not known, but it is suspected that they may be at considerable risk for developing chronic infection. We do not know for sure, however. Children are not adults, and they react differently to many infectious diseases—sometimes more severely, sometimes less, and babies infected during pregnancy or at birth might react quite differently from older children.

Current evidence suggests that there is no increased risk of the baby picking up hepatitis C through breastfeeding. There are some problems, however, with these studies. One is that they are based on only small numbers of mothers and babies. Everyone would feel more secure if larger numbers of women and their babies were studied. It is also possible that the situation could change over time—for example, as the baby gets older, the antibodies he received from his mother during pregnancy might decrease and he might then be more susceptible to infection with the virus.

Overall, given the risks of not breastfeeding, women should breastfeed when they are hepatitis C–positive.

Hepatitis D, E, F, G

Not much is known about these viruses or the risk of the baby acquiring the viruses through breastfeeding when the mother is infected. The chances seem negligible, and the mother should continue to breastfeed.

Human Immunodeficiency Virus (HIV)

What is HIV or AIDS?

HIV is thought to be a relatively new virus in the human population. There are various theories as to how the recent AIDS epidemic began, but we know that it is a serious, fatal illness that is transmitted through body fluids.

How is this disease transmitted?

We know that HIV is definitely passed from mother to baby. It is estimated that about a third of infections of the baby occur during pregnancy, and most of the rest occur around the time of birth. The question is: Can it be passed on through breastfeeding?

The answer: almost certainly. In a few cases, there appears to have been no other way the virus could have been passed to the baby except through breastmilk. Nevertheless, it is difficult to quantify how significant the increased risk to the baby is of getting infected through the milk. Various studies have shown everything from very minimal increased risk to double the risk, compared to that of a baby who is artificially fed. It should be pointed out that even the highest rates of transmission, with breastfeeding, are about 30 percent, which means that 70 percent of babies are not infected. However, because HIV infection, except in very rare cases, is fatal, the whole situation needs to be carefully thought out when a pregnant woman is known to be HIV-positive.

When the mother has been recently infected, she usually has a high load of virus in her body, and the risk to the baby is increased. When the mother is sick with AIDS, her viral load is high and the risks to the baby are higher. But what if the mother is HIV-positive, asymptomatic, and not showing signs of high viral load? There is no answer here, either, though the risks to the baby are certainly lower than in the first two situations.

To complicate the issue further, there is evidence that if the baby is actually infected at the time of birth, breastfeeding may give him immune factors that will delay the onset of his illness and maybe decrease its severity, though eventually, unless new treatment measures radically change the outlook, the baby will become sick.

How can transmission of this disease to the baby be prevented?

There have been some advances. It is now believed that treatment of the pregnant woman with medication during the last trimester, and treatment of the baby for six weeks after birth, decreases infection rates in the baby from about 15 percent to 6 or 7 percent. However, studies showing this did not include mothers and babies who were breastfed. All babies were fed artificially. This is unfortunate. It is possible that such treatment plus breastfeeding might protect the baby even more, though the risk may be increased. We just don't know.

The situation with HIV is always changing, and recent work has given new hope. There is now a drug that, when given to the mother during delivery and to the baby immediately after birth, seems to significantly decrease the chances of the baby picking up the infection at birth and from breastfeeding. And unlike most HIV treatments, it is extremely inexpensive. It has been tested in Africa and seems to work.

So what should mothers do?

As in all such situations, the risks of artificial feeding must be weighed against the risks of breastfeeding. In affluent situations, the risk of the baby getting HIV from breastfeeding, even if minimal, can outweigh even the significant risks of artificial feeding.

A study conducted in Durban, South Africa, in 2001 showed that *exclusively* breastfed babies have no increased risk of acquiring HIV from their mothers, when compared with babies who were exclusively fed formula. However, *partially* breastfed babies do have an increased risk. In previous studies, which have been used to show that HIV positive mothers should not breastfeed, the "breastfed" babies were almost all partially breastfed.

This is significant new information. It means that babies in those African countries where many mothers are HIV positive may not need to risk infection, disease, and death from formula feeding in order to protect them from acquiring the virus. I think it is also important to note that supplementing breastfed babies is not harmless, as so many people think.

We must not forget, however, that we have a Third World within our own First World. There are populations of people in Canada and the United States who are living in conditions that put babies at very high risk from not breastfeeding. Babies who are born to drug addicts are at significant risk of severe illness and death from diseases that can be prevented by breastfeeding, especially under the circumstances in which many chronic drug users live. Is it always the case that such babies should not be breastfed?

Tragically, until there is some way of preventing transmission through breastfeeding, under most circumstances, in an affluent situation it is probably better that the mother does not breastfeed.

But does that mean she can't give her baby breastmilk? Two possibilities aside from formula exist. Banked breastmilk has the advantage of providing breastmilk that still has some immune factors in it, though the method of processing the milk will definitely eliminate some immune factors, and significantly reduce others. Banked milk is expensive, which is its main drawback. But it is available.

It is also possible for the mother to use her own milk, have it heat treated, and then give it to the baby. The technology for doing this at home is not quite perfected, but could soon be. Heating milk to 60°C for 30 minutes apparently kills the virus. The local hospital, however, could do the heat treatment of the milk, if the mother or someone else took it to the hospital daily or every few days, depending on the quantities.

Herpes Simplex

What is herpes?

There are two herpes simplex viruses, which from the point of view of breastfeeding can be treated as one virus. Many of us have been infected with these viruses without actually knowing it. Type I virus causes mouth sores in children, and cold sores in adults, and can cause sores similar to chicken pox at any age. Often, though, people who have evidence of infection (antibodies against the virus in their blood) never have any symptoms.

Both can conceivably cause severe illness at any age, but are more dangerous for a baby less than a month old, especially when the infection is picked up at birth. However, the most severe disease occurs in the baby when he gets infected during the pregnancy, particularly during the first trimester. Infection then may cause the death of the fetus, or the baby may be born small, with severe neurologic deficits, liver disease, and skin lesions over his body.

How is this transmitted?

This virus is transmitted by contact with open sores that contain the virus. During pregnancy, the virus gets to the baby when the mother has the virus in the blood, and the virus passes over to the baby through the placenta.

How can herpes be prevented or reduced?

As long as the young baby is not in contact with an open sore, there is no reason to avoid breastfeeding. Obviously, if there is a sore right on the nipple, breastfeeding should be avoided on that side. Sores elsewhere on the mother's body can be covered (with a bandage) to protect the baby from infection.

Once the baby is older than about a month, there is much less risk of severe illness with this virus, though at any age it is possible to get severe illness.

Some babies or young children get ulcers in their mouths from herpes virus (herpetic stomatitis). This can be quite painful, and in some cases the child will refuse to eat or even drink, resulting in dehydration. Often the sores last a week or more. Breastfeeding babies will often be willing to continue taking the breast and getting milk from the breast and thus avoid dehydration. However, the mother may get inoculated with the virus on the nipple and areola, causing her to have painful sores. This does not necessarily occur. If at all possible, however, breastfeeding should continue.

Chicken Pox

What is chicken pox?

Chicken pox is caused by another kind of herpes virus, called varicella-zoster virus. Usually it is a mild disease, but an adult who gets this virus for the first time can be quite ill. It is particularly dangerous for the pregnant woman, for whom pneumonia due to this virus can be fatal. Occasionally even children can be quite sick with it, but this is uncommon. Generally, the older the child, the sicker he will be.

How is chicken pox transmitted?

Chicken pox can be transmitted to the baby if he has contact with any of the "pox." Like the viruses we discussed earlier, chicken pox has a "viremic" stage when the virus is present in the mother's blood and therefore potentially in her milk, but this would happen before she notices any symptoms.

There is one situation when the baby has to be watched quite carefully, and that is when the mother has not had chicken pox before and develops it just around the time of delivery, a few days before to a few days afterward. Because the mother has not previously developed any antibodies to chicken pox, she isn't able to pass any on to the baby. In that case, especially given the susceptibility of young babies to herpes viruses (the family of viruses to which chicken pox belongs) in the first month or so, the baby could develop very serious, even fatal chicken pox.

When would the baby be infected in such a manner? The mother who develops chicken pox around delivery has to have been infected several days, perhaps even weeks, before. When she is pregnant, the virus can cross the placenta and infect the baby. Or the baby can be infected when he is born, if he comes into contact with any pox that the mother has. Once the pox develop, the virus is no longer in the mother's blood and cannot appear in the milk. But the baby can be infected from virus originating in the pox, until they are crusted over.

Pregnant woman can prevent infection with chicken pox. Most women are immune by the time they are of reproductive age, but some are not. Women who are not should get the new chicken pox vaccine before conceiving, to prevent their getting ill during pregnancy or just after. It is a safe vaccine, and could prevent several deaths and complications in pregnant women and their babies every year. And the questions about breastfeeding when the mother has chicken pox would not even come up.

But what if the mother does get chicken pox? There are some complications of developing chicken pox early in the pregnancy, including death of the fetus. The baby may develop malformations and scarring of the arms or legs, and possibly nerve damage.

If the mother develops chicken pox more than about five days before the baby is born, the baby will probably have received antibodies from the mother across the placenta, and the chances of severe illness are much diminished. The baby may have been infected in the womb, and it is possible he will develop some illness, but he may not because of the transferred antibodies.

If the mother develops the rash within five days of the birth of the baby, the baby may be at risk of severe illness. In this situation, the baby should get varicella-zoster immune globulin, an injection of antibodies against chicken pox that gives relatively good protection against developing severe disease, though the injection is not a guarantee. The sooner it is given after exposure, the better the protection. Remember that if the mother has developed chicken pox, she was not immune, and

her milk may not contain antibodies against chicken pox virus, at least not immediately.

Many pediatricians and infectious disease experts suggest that if the mother comes down with chicken pox when her baby is very young, the mother and the baby should be separated until all the mother's pox are crusted and she is not developing any new pox, regardless of how the baby is fed. This occurs usually within about five days after the first chicken pox begin to appear, but the length of time the mother is infectious can vary a few days each way. Even if separation is decided to be the best approach, there is definitely no reason for the baby not to get the mother's milk. Indeed, the mother's milk can only be good for the baby, providing him with some protective factors against viruses in general and chicken pox in particular.

I believe, however, that this approach is overly and unnecessarily cautious. Especially once the baby is a little older—say, older than about a month—the severity of the illness seems to be much less. If the baby gets varicella-zoster immune globulin within 72 hours or so of contact, and continues breastfeeding, he is unlikely to become severely ill. I believe this is true also in the immediate postpartum period.

One complicating factor here is that the mother is often very ill with chicken pox if she develops it around the time of the birth of the baby, and it may not be practical to have the baby breastfeed. Again, however, it may be useful to have her expressed milk given to the baby, if this is possible.

Herpes Zoster (Shingles)

What is shingles?

Shingles is a painful rash that occurs in people who have previously been infected with chicken pox. The virus of chicken pox seems to live in the nerves that come out of the spinal cord—dormant for many years, perhaps for the lifetime of the person. For some reason, the virus suddenly becomes activated, the person develops a rash, usually on one side of the body, often in a very definite stripe. It may occur anywhere, but often on the face, chest, or abdomen. The sores look very much like the pox of chicken pox or herpes simplex virus infections, and can be extremely painful, or hardly painful at all. Sometimes the sores are not limited to one stripe from back to front on the body, but are all over the body, and thus may resemble chicken pox exactly.

How is this transmitted?

The sores are infectious to anyone who is not immune to chicken pox, but direct contact is necessary for infection.

Is breastfeeding when I have shingles dangerous for my baby?

This situation is quite different from that of the mother who develops a first infection with chicken pox. In the first place, the fact that the mother must have been previously infected with chicken pox means that she will have passed antibodies against chicken pox to her baby through the placenta. These antibodies stay in the baby's body for perhaps six months or longer after birth. Furthermore, the mother's milk, in addition to other immune factors, will contain antibodies to chicken pox virus. When the mother develops shingles, then, there is no need to separate her from her baby, and definitely no reason to suspend breastfeeding.

Cytomegalovirus (CMV)

What is cytomegalovirus?

In most children and adults, this virus (another member of the herpes family) causes a very mild illness. The most serious problem is when the mother contracts it during pregnancy, especially if she gets it during the first trimester. It may result in poor growth of the baby, neurologic abnormalities, liver disease, and death of the fetus. Babies who are born with this infection can be very sick, or may have no symptoms. It is thought that CMV infection is one of the most common causes of congenital deafness in North America. A baby may be born with only hearing loss, and not obviously have the worst symptoms of the infection. Babies and adults who have this infection often excrete virus, particularly in their urine, and thus are infectious for many months and even years.

Recently, it has been shown that young premature babies (younger than 28 weeks gestation) sometimes pick up cytomegalovirus from the milk and get ill from it. This does not appear to be true if the baby is older than about 28 weeks' gestation.

So is breastfeeding safe if I have this virus?

If you contracted the virus during pregnancy, so that your baby was born with this infection, he should definitely get your milk, even if the milk is shown to contain the virus. After all, the baby is already infected. There is a concern about adding more virus to the baby's system, but this is really more theoretical than real. The baby gets more from breastfeeding than just virus, though many health professionals do not take this into consideration.

Of course, sometimes these babies are born so sick that they do not feed well, and may require nasogastric feedings because they cannot suckle. Still, breastmilk feedings are the best for them.

What if your baby is a very small premature baby? Well, freezing kills CMV, so, perhaps, milk from a CMV-positive mother should be frozen before being given to the baby. Once the baby is no longer tiny—say, over 28 to 30 weeks' gestation—freezing the milk is unnecessary.

Cytomegalovirus picked up after birth, except in the case of the tiny premature baby, is almost always a mild disease, but as with all infections, there are exceptional cases that can be severe. Normally, however, the infection is asymptomatic, or causes a mild coldlike illness.

Except in the special situation of the tiny premature baby, breastmilk feedings and breastfeeding should be encouraged when the mother has CMV infection. Even in the case of the tiny premature baby, the milk need only be frozen before rethawing and giving it to the baby.

Infectious Mononucleosis Virus

What is mononucleosis?

Infectious mononucleosis is also caused by a herpes virus called Epstein-Barr virus. It is an infection of childhood, although it has the reputation of being an infection of young adults ("Kissing Disease"). By age three or four, possibly 75 percent of all children show antibodies in their blood against this virus, and by teenage years, almost everyone has been infected. In childhood, the illness is usually mild—no more than a cold or sore throat, but often without any symptoms at all. For this reason, infection with this virus during pregnancy or lactation is hardly ever an issue.

Is breastfeeding safe with mononucleosis?

If a mother develops infectious mononucleosis when she is breastfeeding, she should not stop breastfeeding. There is no evidence that there is a danger to the infant. In any case, once the mother has the illness, the virus has already passed into the milk several days or even weeks before.

German Measles (Rubella)

What is rubella?

German measles, or rubella, is usually a mild viral illness. It is a terrible problem, however, if a pregnant woman develops it during the first trimester of her pregnancy, because it can cause severe disabilities in the baby, including mental retardation, blindness, deafness, and liver disease.

However, German measles picked up after birth rarely causes any symptoms of illness. If anything, German measles in the mother, or her having had an immunization, infects the baby with either the wild or vaccine virus, and the baby becomes immune. There is absolutely no reason for a mother who develops German measles, or gets the vaccine while breastfeeding, to suspend breastfeeding.

Bacterial Infections

Bacterial infections almost never cause disease that would be transmitted through the milk. Bacteria, when they appear in the milk, have generally been circulating in the mother's blood—a situation usually associated with severe, even life-threatening illness.

Some bacteria live on us normally. One type of staphylococcus (*S. epidermidis*) does, and this is not only normal but expected. Some of us are carriers for certain bacteria that may be causes of illness, yet usually we do not become ill with these bacteria. Many health professionals who work in a hospital have *Staphylococcus aureus* growing in their throats or noses. Sometimes these bacteria change from being merely friendly neighbors in the same ecosystem to invaders. Of course, there are many theories about why this could happen, but the reasons are not clear.

Although bacteria can definitely be contagious, mothers and babies usually share the same bacteria (and fungi, for that matter). This is good because the mother develops resistance to bacteria, and she passes on this resistance to her baby through the milk.

So what happens if the mother becomes sick with a strep throat, for example? Should the baby be separated from her? Should the baby stop getting her milk? Of course not. Group A streptococcus, the cause of strep throat, is commonly carried by many of us. In winter, easily 20 percent of all schoolchildren have it in their throats, without necessarily being ill. Exposure to a bacterium does not mean illness, and a mother being sick does not mean her baby will get sick. On the contrary, if the mother continues to breastfeed, chances are that the baby will not get sick or, at worst, will get only mildly ill, though there is no guarantee. Nevertheless, the risks are less than those of taking the baby off the breast.

The majority of bacterial diseases require no separation of the mother and baby, and no restriction of breastfeeding.

Tuberculosis

What is tuberculosis?

Tuberculosis is primarily thought of as an infection of the lungs, but actually it can infect any part of the body. It is caused by *Mycobacterium tuberculosis* and it is coming back with a vengeance. When I was in training 30 years or so ago, the general opinion was that tuberculosis

was finished and about to disappear in the same way as polio had. Only a few older physicians warned against complacency, and they were not heeded.

How is tuberculosis transmitted?

Mycobacterium tuberculosis (the bacterium that causes the disease) is unlikely to get into the breastmilk, because it is unlikely to get into the mother's bloodstream. *M. tuberculosis* usually appears in the blood of young children only, often because of decreased immunity or malnutrition. Tuberculosis of the breast apparently can occur, but even in Africa where I worked, where tuberculosis was epidemic, I never saw a case of tuberculosis of the breast. It must be rare.

Two issues come up when the mother has tuberculosis. One is if she is coughing up sputum with *M. tuberculosis* in it (open tuberculosis, or sputum-positive tuberculosis). In that case, the mother is quite infectious. Luckily, with modern drugs for tuberculosis, even sputum-positive patients can be made sputum-negative within a few weeks.

But what do we do about the baby and breastfeeding?

The milk itself is not infectious, so the baby can get the milk. But can the mother and baby be in contact? There are those who say that if the mother is sputum-positive, she must be separated from her baby. I disagree. I believe the mother should be treated as soon as she is known to have tuberculosis. She can stay in contact with her baby as long as she wears a surgical mask. The baby should be given BCG (a vaccine against tuberculosis), and should be treated with anti-tuberculosis medication, at least isoniazid (INH).

As far as medication for the mother and continued breastfeeding goes, the drugs we use for treating maternal infection with tuberculosis are used for babies, as well (see Chapter 11, Breastfeeding While on Medication).

In summary, when the mother has tuberculosis, she can and should breastfeed her baby.

Syphilis

What is syphilis?

This is a sexually transmitted disease caused by a bacterium. Maternal syphilis is another bacterial disease that, like tuberculosis, in years past, has been given as a reason for mothers not to breastfeed. However, as with tuberculosis, this advice is essentially incorrect.

How is it transmitted?

Many babies whose mothers have syphilis are infected during the pregnancy. The risk is quite high; under some circumstances almost all babies whose mothers have syphilis during the pregnancy will be infected. There are protocols for treatment of these babies.

But the bacterium that causes syphilis does not appear in the milk. Occasionally, the mother will have active skin lesions and if these appear on the breast or nipple, or where the baby can touch them, especially with his mouth, there is a chance of infection in a previously uninfected baby.

How can I protect my baby while still breastfeeding?

Fortunately, appropriate treatment with penicillin will usually render the skin lesions noncontagious within about 24 to 48 hours of the first injection. The baby need be off the breast only a couple of days. If one breast has no sores, the baby can nurse from one side.

West Nile Virus

In the fall of 2002, a breastfeeding mother was diagnosed with West Nile virus. Material from the virus was discovered in the mother's milk, and antibodies in the baby's system. However, researchers were frustrated in trying to grow the virus from the mother's milk because something in the milk kept killing the virus. The (U.S.) Centers for Disease Control reported this and suggested that babies might possibly be at risk of catching West Nile disease from their breastfeeding mothers. Larry Gartner, a U.S. pediatrician who often speaks on breastfeeding topics, had this to say: "The West Nile Virus [WNV] report from the CDC [Centers for Disease Control] is of great importance, but we need to look at the facts. This is only one child. The child was entirely well and asymptomatic. The child is now apparently immune and presumably protected from future risk of infection. The mother continued to breastfeed the child throughout her illness. There is no evidence yet that any breastfeeding child has been ill from WNV infection. Finally, if a mother develops symptoms of WNV while breastfeeding, the greatest risk to the infant may come from interrupting the breastfeeding. Transmission of the virus almost certainly occurred during the period prior to the mother developing fever and headache, when the viremia was at its peak. Shortly thereafter, through her breastmilk she provided the infant with some immune protection as well as nonspecific antiviral agents. If the infant had not continued to receive breastmilk from the mother, the child might well have become clinically ill. Thus, the advice we need to give is to continue the breastfeeding even if the mother is symptomatic with what may be West Nile Virus infection—or any other infection—as

long as the mother is clinically able to do so."
(*Academy of Breastfeeding Medicine News and Views*,
Volume 8[4], 2002, p. 36.)

Noninfectious Maternal Illness

Thyroid Problems

One of the most common medical problems for the mother in the early months after the birth of her baby is thyroid dysfunction. This question has already been discussed in Chapter 11, Breastfeeding While on Medication. The issue is the use of radioactive iodine to diagnose and treat thyroid problems. Usually radioactive iodine need not be used, and thus it is not necessary to stop breastfeeding. If a nursing mother does get radioactive iodine, she will have to stop breastfeeding for a variable period of time, depending on the isotope and dose of radioactive iodine she will be getting. It's better not to take it.

Rheumatoid Arthritis

There is a general feeling among physicians that rheumatoid arthritis is worsened by breastfeeding. There is no good evidence that this is so, and the impression may be due to the fact that rheumatoid arthritis often seems to *improve during pregnancy*. Thus, the increased inflammation that occurs after the birth may be attributed to breastfeeding. Studies about the role of breastfeeding in the worsening of rheumatoid arthritis are definitely not conclusive.

More of an issue is the drugs the nursing mother might have to take for her rheumatoid arthritis (see Chapter 11, Breastfeeding While on Medication). There are several that the mother can safely take while continuing breastfeeding. Acetaminophen, steroids, and most nonsteroidal anti-inflammatory medications are

safe. With regard to others, there is divided opinion. One authority states that gold is not compatible with breastfeeding, while another says it is. One says that antimalarials are safe, while another says they are not. For various reasons, I would say that gold is okay, and so is hydrochloroquine. Of course, milk levels and levels in the baby of the various medications can be monitored, and changes made, if necessary.

Two new drugs now available for rheumatoid arthritis are Enbrel (etanercept) and Remicade (infliximab). Both of these are very large proteins that do not get into breastmilk, although mothers are frequently told they must wean to take these medications.

A mother who has pain in her joints and weakness of her muscles may not be able to handle the baby easily, but various pillows for support and splints for the mother's arms can help. The mother with arthritis can learn to nurse lying down, which will take most of the weight off her arms and allow the baby to be supported on a bed. Strategies can be found that will suit the mother and the baby in their own particular situation. For example, carrying a baby in a sling may take the weight of the baby completely off the mother's arms. A sling can also be used to hold the mother's breast, something that may be necessary, at least at first, since many young babies find it difficult to nurse on a breast that is not supported.

Multiple Sclerosis

As with rheumatoid arthritis, multiple sclerosis is a disease many physicians believe is made worse by breastfeeding, and probably for the same reasons—that there is often an improvement in the disease during pregnancy. In fact, there is no evidence that the disease worsens with breastfeeding.

Once again, the issue turns on the medications. Recently, various forms of interferon have been used to treat multiple sclerosis, and unfortunately mothers have been told they cannot breastfeed while taking this drug. There is simply no reason for mothers to stop when they are taking interferon. The molecule is too big to get into the milk. Even if it got into the milk, it would probably be destroyed in the baby's stomach.

Other issues do arise, as in the case of the mother with rheumatoid arthritis. Though pain is not a striking feature of multiple sclerosis, weakness is. Other neurological dysfunction, such as spasticity, may make it difficult for the mother to hold the baby and get him to latch on well. Again, with ingenuity, almost all problems can be overcome.

Postpartum Depression

Postpartum depression is a common problem and can range from just a mild feeling of being "down" to serious depression with a serious risk of the mother doing harm to herself and/or her baby. There are various treatments for depression, but the mainstay, especially in the more serious cases, is antidepressant medication.

Some physicians treat postpartum depression with hormones, but nursing mothers should avoid these, since the estrogens will often seriously decrease their milk supplies. Not always, but in many.

Several antidepressant medications are now available that are unlikely to get into the milk in any significant amounts, and can thus be used to treat nursing mothers with depression (see Chapter 11, Breastfeeding While on Medication).

Mothers who have bipolar disorder may be prescribed lithium. This drug can be used while breastfeeding, but the amount of medication in the baby's blood needs to be monitored. For most mothers, this is not a problem. Lithium can also be replaced by other drugs that are more compatible with breastfeeding, such as carbamazepine and valproic acid.

Surgery and Anesthesia

This question has already been addressed in Chapter 11, Breastfeeding While on Medication, but since it comes up over and over again, I will summarize here.

Most drugs used during general anesthesia are short-acting drugs that are not absorbed from the intestine. Most of the ones that can be absorbed will be present in the milk in only tiny amounts and will be there for only a short time, once the drug is no longer being given. The risk of the small amount of any of these anesthetic or tranquilizing drugs being found in the milk after anesthesia is virtually zero. The mother can breastfeed as soon as she is awake and up to it.

The same goes for drugs used for local anesthesia, such as in dental surgery. These drugs may appear in the milk, but they are not absorbed by the baby's digestive system, and so the baby will just get rid of them through bowel movements. No need for concern.

It is not possible to cover all the illnesses that a nursing mother might develop, but through an understanding of the importance of breastfeeding for the mother and her baby, and through persistence, a way to continue breastfeeding can be found in most situations.

13

Sick Babies,
Premature Babies, Special Babies

Myth: When a baby is sick, it is usually better that he is not breastfed or given breastmilk.

Fact: Not only is this untrue, but in the vast majority of cases, it is better that breastfeeding *continue* or that the baby *continue* to get breastmilk. Most of the prohibitions on breastfeeding arise from not understanding that breastfeeding is different from bottle-feeding, and that breastmilk is different from formula. Unfortunately, too many health professionals have been trained to believe that formula is better than breastfeeding when the baby is unwell.

There are rare instances when a baby's illness requires that the baby not be breastfed, but these are very rare instances, indeed. One such instance is a metabolic disease called galactosemia, in which the baby is unable to metabolize galactose, one of the two sugars that make up lactose, the milk sugar. (The other is glucose.) In the severe form, the inability of the baby to metabolize the galactose results in many problems, including severe liver disease, which can eventually lead to death if the intake of galactose is not halted. There are also partial enzyme deficiencies which allow the baby to metabolize some galactose. These babies may be able to breastfeed or at least partially breastfeed. There are other rare metabolic diseases that probably require the mother not to breastfeed, but we really don't know enough about breastfeeding, breastmilk, and these metabolic diseases. Often it is assumed that breastfeeding cannot be allowed, only because the physicians who are treating the baby need to control the intake of certain elements in the diet very strictly, and believe that this cannot be done when the baby is breastfeeding. Galactosemia is reported to occur in 1 in 60,000 live births, and it is one of the more common metabolic illnesses.

Another metabolic condition that is fairly common and is quite compatible at least with partial breastfeeding is phenylketonuria (PKU). It will be discussed later in this chapter.

In almost all other instances, it is possible for breastfeeding or breastmilk feedings to continue. Usually, when mothers are told it is not possible, it is because the physician is not aware of how breastfeeding works, or how to overcome the challenges involved with the mother's breastfeeding the baby.

What follows is a discussion of various infant or child illnesses that often result in mothers being told that they cannot breastfeed their babies. It is not possible to discuss every single illness a child might have, of course, but if certain principles are followed, a solution can almost always be found. What are these principles?

• Breastfeeding is important to the health and development of the baby.

- Breastfeeding is important to the health of the mother.
- Breastmilk is almost always better than any artificial feeding for the sick baby.
- Breastfeeding comforts the sick baby, and the fact that the baby breastfeeds comforts the mother.
- When mothers are told they must wean because their baby is ill, they should remember that many health care professionals do not understand much about breastfeeding, and that they may need to do further research on their own to determine if this recommendation is valid.

Acute Illness (Temporary Illness)

Gastroenteritis (diarrhea and/or vomiting due to a virus or bacterium)

An infection in the digestive system in an exclusively breastfed baby is very unusual and when it does occur, it is rarely severe. Once a child is taking other foods, especially if he is in contact with many other children, gastroenteritis becomes more common.

For many years, physicians had said that when a child has gastroenteritis, he needs to be taken off dairy products. This was an article of faith for many physicians even into the 1980s and persists to this day. On the other hand, early textbooks, at the beginning of the century, warned physicians not to encourage weaning of the baby from the breast during the summer months—the months when gastroenteritis was most common—because the protective effects of breastfeeding were known even then. The texts also stated that babies should not be taken off the breast during a "gastrointestinal emergency," as an acute infection was often called.

However, with a decline in breastfeeding after World War I, and the precipitous decline after World War II, most babies by the 1950s were not breastfed, or were breastfed for only a short period of time. Babies were getting severe vomiting and diarrhea, and often were not tolerating milk or formula. Disastrous instructions were sometimes given to boil skim milk and give it to babies with diarrhea and vomiting. This led to severe derangements in their blood sodium, which often led to convulsions and death. Dairy products became forbidden during gastroenteritis. As a pediatric resident in the 1970s and 1980s, I learned about taking the baby off his formula for a few days, then introducing half-strength formula and then full-strength formula. This approach of limiting milk intake has mostly been discredited, even for artificially fed babies.

It was never true for breastfed babies. First of all, breastmilk is not a dairy product, though this would seem to be a surprise to some. Dairy products (formula, cheese, ice cream, etc.) are those that include processed milk from other animals, such as cows or goats. But over the years, many babies with vomiting and diarrhea were taken off the breast because people thought that "what is true for formula must be true for breastmilk." It isn't. The best treatment for diarrhea and vomiting in the breastfed baby is breastfeeding. Breastmilk contains antibodies and other immune factors that will hasten the baby's recovery from the infection. Babies often tolerate breastmilk better than they do other fluids, since breastmilk leaves the stomach very quickly, often before the baby vomits it. The elements in breastmilk are much better absorbed so that the baby getting breastmilk is not starving. One of the causes of prolonged diarrhea in young children is starvation. The common approach of withholding food from the baby when he is ill is often done for too long, and the baby then gets "starvation diarrhea." Continued breastfeeding will prevent this. Finally, the child is comforted by breastfeeding when he is sick, and the mother is comforted by the child's breastfeeding. If this is repeated frequently in this chapter, it is because we tend to forget it too often.

It is important to understand that the main worry with an intestinal infection (gastroenteritis) is that it can lead to dehydration. The diarrhea and vomiting almost always will get better all by themselves without the need for specific treatment. As long as the baby keeps down more than he loses through vomiting and diarrhea, he will usually be okay. A child who is urinating six or seven times in a day, even if the urine is concentrated, is managing. He may not be as well hydrated as usual, but he will be okay.

One of the principles of feeding children with gastroenteritis is to give small amounts of fluid frequently. Large amounts are more likely to be vomited. Furthermore, due to a reflex called the gastrocolic reflex, a full stomach tends to stimulate a bowel movement. This is true for all of us, but babies have a much more sensitive gastrocolic reflex. Thus when a large amount of fluid gets into the stomach, the baby may then have a bowel movement. Had the reflex not been stimulated, the baby might have had time to absorb some more fluid from his gut. This makes sense, and has been a principle of feeding during gastroenteritis for many years. However, small frequent feedings do not mean the same thing when a child is breastfeeding.

Babies rarely spit up or vomit when they are suckling at the breast. This is due to the fact that while the baby is suckling, waves of muscle contraction continue along in his throat and move milk down, thus tending to prevent the vomiting. Vomiting while he is actually suckling is more likely to occur if the baby has gastroenteritis than if he doesn't, but still less likely than when he comes off the breast. Thus it is a good thing to let the baby drink from the breast, and then, even when he is no longer drinking, to allow him to suckle at the breast. Not only will this comfort him, but it may also decrease the vomiting, while giving him small amounts of breastmilk almost continuously.

What about electrolyte solutions?

Experience with electrolyte solutions was gained in developing countries where gastroenteritis is very common and often very serious, yet medical care is not always as well funded as in North America. Intravenous rehydration is a very expensive way to treat dehydration, and as we learned from the health care workers in developing countries, not even necessarily the best. The only advantage to intravenous rehydration is that we can control the amounts of fluids and electrolytes given. But just because we know what is given, that does not mean we are correcting the fluid and salt losses of the child correctly. Luckily, children usually have good hearts and good kidneys (unlike many adults), and even gross treatment errors can sometimes be tolerated by the child. However, the corrections we calculate are based on blood tests, and the blood tests do not always reflect accurately what is going on in the rest of the child's body, such as in the interior of the cells. Sometimes intravenous rehydration can be very tricky, and because of that, dangerous as well.

Oral rehydration was found to be effective much of the time, and for the majority of children, safer. Even if they vomited, they usually kept down enough liquid to become rehydrated. The solutions used for these acute gastrointestinal episodes was a rehydrating solution with a fairly high salt content, unlike the commonly sold oral solutions in North America, which can reasonably be called "maintenance solutions." They were not designed for "rehydration." They are also expensive—unreasonably so, considering that one of the main ideas of oral rehydration solutions was to reduce costs. In developing countries, these solutions cost only pennies. In North America, one brand (1999) cost about $12 Canadian per liter (quart).

In the majority of cases of diarrhea and vomiting seen in North America, especially in the breastfeeding child, the baby or child needs only breastfeeding. Only if breastmilk seems unable to keep up with the losses—an unusual situation—would some other fluid be necessary. Even if the mother's supply is down because the child is, say, 14 months old, and thus eating and drinking all sorts of other things as well as taking breastmilk, the mother's supply will usually increase with more frequent nursing. Indeed, I would say that if the child's losses are so great that breastfeeding cannot keep up, that would be an indication for the child to be evaluated by a physician, not just given extra oral rehydration fluids.

Older children will usually not drink these oral electrolyte solutions. They taste like sea water, and it is not surprising that a child, unless he is dehydrated, would refuse to drink it. Many of us grew up drinking flat ginger ale when we had the "stomach flu," and in the majority of cases, a variety of fluids in small amounts frequently will do the trick just as well as special, expensive oral electrolyte solutions.

The standard approach requires starting oral electrolyte solutions at the very first sign of "gastroenteritis." But what is the first sign in the breastfed baby? Breastfed babies can have many

bowel movements every day. On one day a breastfed baby could have five bowel movements, and on another 10 bowel movements. Does that mean he has an infection? Not necessarily. Breastfed babies can have yellow bowel movements one day, orange the next, and green the day after. Does green mean an infection? Not necessarily. Many breastfed babies spit up a lot. If they spit up and the bowel movements turn green as well, is that an infection? Not necessarily. What about if all the above happen? Still, not necessarily. We have to stop looking at the bowel movements and consider the baby. A happy, content, gaining baby with 12 green watery bowel movements a day, and lots of spitting up, is fine.

Breastfeeding, and breastfeeding alone, is all that the majority of babies with gastroenteritis need. Breastfeeding comforts the baby who is sick, and the fact that the baby will breastfeed comforts the mother.

What about lactose intolerance?

Lactose intolerance can sometimes be a cause of continued diarrhea, but it is not a reason to stop breastfeeding. Indeed, though it used to be said that the virus causing gastroenteritis injured the walls of the intestine, resulting in a depletion of the enzyme metabolizing the lactose in the milk, this may not be the only factor. It is also possible that the starvation we inflicted on babies and children with these infections was a partial cause of the child's developing lactose intolerance.

The best way to prevent lactose intolerance is to maintain feeding during gastroenteritis—and the best feeding is breastfeeding. If despite continued feeding, or if breastfeeding is interrupted, the child develops lactose intolerance, the gut will recover, and the lactase (enzyme that metabolizes the lactose) will recover as well. Continued breastfeeding will not somehow prevent the lactase from returning. On the contrary, because breastmilk contains factors that stimulate the growth of the cells in the intestines, it is probable the digestive system and the lactase will recover more quickly if the baby is kept on the breast.

My child got really sick!

Yes, it can happen, even if he is breastfeeding. But even if your child was admitted to the hospital and put on intravenous, it does not mean that he should not breastfeed. Breastfeeding keeps his nutrient intake up, and feeding allows more rapid recovery from his illness. Breastfeeding also comforts the child, and the fact that the child will breastfeed comforts the mother.

What medications
can the baby take for gastroenteritis?

Rarely do medications do any good, and they can do harm. For example, a commonly used drug to prevent vomiting not only does not work reliably, but can make your child excessively sleepy so that he does not take fluids adequately. Should you decide to take your child to the doctor, it may be difficult to evaluate why he is so sleepy. Is his illness worse, or is he being affected by the drug? Breastfeed your child and avoid medications unless their use really makes sense.

What Is Normal

Let us return to what is normal in the breastfed baby. This is important, because few health professionals have had any teaching about breastfeeding besides that it is good. They have very little in the way of practical experience about breastfeeding. Many have no idea that a baby who breastfeeds is different from a baby who is fed artificially. Below is information about

breastfed babies' normal bowel movements and spitting up.

Bowel Movements

During the first two or three days, babies pass meconium, a black sticky substance that accumulated in the intestines during pregnancy.

After the first two or three days, a baby who is breastfeeding well will start to have bowel movements that are lightening toward yellow or light green. A baby who has yellow bowel movements on day three or four of life (without any supplements) is getting a significant amount of milk. On the other hand, a baby who is still having meconium bowel movements on day four or five is definitely not getting much breastmilk and should be seen by a lactation specialist immediately.

Usually, during the first few weeks, exclusively breastfed babies can have many poops each day. But the amounts and color can be quite variable. One day, a baby can have three small yellow bowel movements, and the next day, 10 yellow or even green bowel movements. This is normal. Even if the bowel movements are always green (but not a dark green, which would mean that meconium is still present), as long as the baby is drinking well, gaining well and content, this is not a concern.

After the first few weeks, some babies may go from many bowel movements a day to none for many days. This may occur suddenly. The record I am aware of in a normal baby is 31 days without a bowel movement. As long as the baby is content and gaining, there is no problem.

Exclusively breastfed babies who are gaining well are never constipated, if we define constipated as having hard bowel movements. Even if they are not having bowel movements often because they are not getting enough milk, their bowel movements are not hard, only infrequent. If the bowel movements are hard, something is wrong; the baby should be seen by a doctor.

Spitting Up

Spitting up is common in babies. When mothers have a lot of milk, babies often spit up. The baby takes a lot of milk quickly, his stomach is full, and some will come up. Even if the milk comes through the baby's nose, this does not mean something is terribly wrong.

If the spitting up occurs an hour after the feeding is over, this also does not mean something is wrong or unusual.

Spitting up can be lessened by having the baby finish the first side before offering the second. Allowing the baby to nibble until he comes off the breast on his own can also often decrease spitting up significantly.

It is obvious that a baby whose mother has an abundance of milk can spit up a lot, can have frequent, watery, green poops, and can sometimes be miserable. All this does not necessarily translate into gastroenteritis. It may simply be a result of the mother's having a lot of milk and poor feeding information (for example, feeding the baby 10 minutes on each side). See also Chapter 9 on colic.

Other Causes of Vomiting and Diarrhea

Many babies have sensitive stomachs. Almost any illness can cause them to start vomiting or to have diarrhea. Something as medically benign as a cold or as serious as meningitis, or anywhere in between, may cause the baby to have vomiting or diarrhea. The infection or illness need not be in the digestive system.

If your baby has had a sudden change, if he does not look good or react normally, do not assume that all vomiting and diarrhea is gastroenteritis. Have your child examined by your physician. But remember, whatever is causing the problem, there is seldom a need to stop breastfeeding. One exception would be a blockage in the baby's intestines, but in that case he should not be getting *anything* by mouth.

What about prolonged diarrhea?

Vomiting during an acute infection usually lasts a day or two and then slows down and stops. Diarrhea usually does not last much more than a week or 10 days. But what if it should go on for weeks?

The most common cause of prolonged diarrhea (toddler diarrhea) is a too-slow return to a normal diet. Obviously, if your baby is under four or six months of age, his normal diet is breastmilk, and breastfeeding should continue throughout the course of the infection. If he has frequent or even watery bowel movements on breastfeeding alone, this is not really a big issue. This is normal.

However, the older child may continue having watery bowel movements if his diet includes a lot of sweet drinks—apple juice is a big offender—and not much food. Once the worst of the infection is over and the child wants to eat, he should be encouraged to eat, even if the diarrhea gets temporarily worse. Stopping food if the diarrhea gets worse only prolongs the diarrhea. A poor intake of fat will also prolong the diarrhea. So get the baby eating normal food (and that includes breastfeeding instead of sweet drinks), and his diarrhea will almost always improve.

Respiratory Infections

It used to be said that children should be taken off dairy products when they have respiratory infections. It was thought that dairy products would increase phlegm, or mucus production. It is not impossible, since some children do have allergic responses to dairy products and, possibly, increased mucus. However, once again, breastmilk is not a dairy product.

The main concern is that breastfeeding may be hard to do while the baby is having difficulty breathing. Fortunately, most colds, wheezing and even pneumonia are not so severe as to interfere with the baby's feeding. Indeed, if the child is having problems with nursing because of difficulty with breathing, you should have him evaluated by his physician or even at the emergency department, especially if simply unblocking his nose does not settle the problem. Unblocking the nose can be done with saltwater and an aspirator, just before feedings. The older child—say, over a few months of age—can also receive special medicated nose drops that are very effective, but you should be careful not to use them too often.

Stuffed Up

Is your baby's nose too stuffed up to nurse? Try these things:

• Use a rubber-bulb aspirator (available in drugstores) to gently suction some of the mucus out of the baby's nose.

• Take the baby to the bathroom, close the door, and run the shower while you both sit on the toilet. The moist air will often loosen up the mucus so your baby can breathe better.

• A drop of water—just a drop—in the baby's nostril will often make him sneeze and clear out his nose.

• If necessary, a medicated nasal spray may help.

In the unhappy circumstance that your child needs to be in the hospital, breastfeeding should not be interrupted. If you are being told he can take a bottle but not the breast, don't believe it. It is less stressful for the baby to breastfeed than to bottle-feed. There is absolutely no circumstance that I can think of in which some other milk would be preferable to breastmilk, so if your child is too ill to drink, he can still receive your breastmilk by tube into his stomach. If he can eat at all, it should be your milk. And if he can drink actively at all, it should be at your breast. The child is comforted by breastfeeding, and the child comforts the mother by breastfeeding.

Other Infectious Illnesses

Meningitis and Encephalitis

Children with meningitis (an infection of the lining of the brain) and encephalitis (an infection or inflammation of the brain itself) can be very sick. But not always. There are forms of meningitis caused by viruses that only give the child a minor illness. He may have fever and headache, but otherwise be well.

Usually children with these illnesses are admitted to the hospital until the course of the illness is clear, though often enough children with viral meningitis can be sent home.

A condition that may occur with these two illnesses is that the child's blood sodium can decrease to dangerous levels if the child gets too much fluid. This is due to more antidiuretic hormone (a hormone that acts on the kidney to reduce the amount of urine being produced—this hormone normally comes into action when the body needs to conserve water) being released from the child's pituitary than should be, probably because of the inflammation around the brain. It has been traditional for physicians to restrict the fluid intake of the child with meningitis or encephalitis to two-thirds of the normal intake for a child of his size.

This presents a dilemma for breastfeeding mothers. How do we know that the child is getting only two-thirds of his required intake if he is breastfeeding? The response has generally been to tell the mother not to breastfeed and to give the baby her expressed milk in a bottle so that the amount can be calculated. This is not the ideal solution. The child then does not get the comfort of the breast. Furthermore, some of the benefits of breastmilk, including immune factors, are always lost when we manipulate the milk in this way.

So what's the solution? The more serious the infection, the more likely it is that the problem of low sodium will arise. There is not a completely direct relationship, but it is there, nonetheless. It so happens that the sicker the child, the less likely he is to breastfeed—and vice versa, the less sick he is, the more likely he is to breastfeed. So in a way, nature provides. There is no reason not to allow breastfeeding during these illnesses, if the child is willing to breastfeed. His blood work will give an idea of what is happening, and restriction of fluid can be done at the intravenous, not at the breast. In any case, the chance of this happening decreases as treatment goes on, and after the first few days, no restriction is generally required.

Should there be a real need to restrict fluid, it can be done without taking the baby off the breast. The milk can be expressed, and, with a lactation aid, given to the baby on a "dry" breast that has just been "emptied" with the pump. The breast will still supply small amounts, but in any case, the two-thirds is just a number developed out of theoretic considerations—a guideline, not a magic wand. If physicians knew how to know that babies were actually drinking at the breast (and not just sucking), they would know that once the baby drank the amount allowed, he would probably just be nibbling, getting very little milk, but getting the comfort that is so valuable for him.

This approach to meningitis and encephalitis explains why so many pediatricians have had the attitude to breastfeeding they have. Breastfeeding, in my day as a resident, was often seen as an obstacle to "good medical care." The doctors needed to know how much milk the baby was getting, and we couldn't measure breastfeeding. In addition, breastfeeding mothers knew that their children would be unhappy if they couldn't nurse, and objected to not being allowed to breastfeed. This led many pediatricians and nurses to believe that these mothers were valuing the breastfeeding relationship over the best medical treatment for the children. What these health professionals sometimes missed is that there is more to "good medical treatment" than measuring precise amounts of fluids, and that there is real value in maintaining breastfeeding to help the ill baby.

Other Infections

There should not be a question of "allowing" breastfeeding in the case of any other infection that a child might have. If you are being told that your child with a bone infection, tonsillitis, ear infection, or whatever should not be breastfeeding, ignore this advice. It does not make sense.

> "How his mother nursed him, and dressed him and lived upon him . . . It was her life which the baby drank in from her bosom."
> William Makepeace Thackeray, *Vanity Fair*

Other Illnesses or Malformations

There are very few illnesses that require a mother to stop breastfeeding or providing her milk, though you would never guess it from the way mothers are advised. A sick baby does not need breastfeeding less, he needs it more.

Cardiac Problems

Cardiac problems can range from extremely mild to extremely serious. Some, probably the majority, of small holes in the heart close up by themselves without any need for treatment, surgical or otherwise. Some are life-threatening, though, luckily, this is only a small percentage.

Breastfeeding and feeding expressed milk (if the baby cannot nurse) are good for the baby because they provide him with immune factors that decrease his chances of getting infections. Any child in the hospital has increased chances of picking up infectious illnesses. For some babies or children with cardiac problems, even a mild case of gastroenteritis or viral chest infection can set them back seriously and possibly threaten their survival. Furthermore, breastfeeding comforts the child, and the fact that the child will breastfeed comforts the mother. Unfortunately, many pediatric cardiologists do not see the advantage of breastfeeding or even breast-milk, and may discourage the mother from breastfeeding for reasons that often are not valid, such as the following:

The baby needs to have his fluid intake and output calculated exactly.

In certain situations this may be necessary, but not usually. Even in circumstances where some pediatric cardiologists argue for measuring fluids exactly, others would not think it so necessary. No standard rule can be made, but what if the cardiologist insists on strict fluid intake measures? Of course, the baby cannot go to the breast. Or can he?

One stratagem that seems to work is to have the mother express milk from her breasts just before a feeding. The milk is put into a lactation aid, and fed to the baby while he suckles at the "empty" breast. Incidentally, scales are now available that are pretty good at measuring intake during a feeding. The baby is weighed before the feeding, and then after, and the scale gives an approximation of how much he got.

It is more work, of course, but the concerns about fluids can be addressed by careful physical examination and daily weighing. However, many doctors would rather just tell the mother that the baby has to be fed by bottle. On the other hand, if the baby really cannot suckle, bottles are more work than feeding the baby with a cup or using a nasogastric tube. The baby should be cuddled, skin to skin, next to the breast when being fed by alternative means.

It takes more work for the baby to breastfeed than to bottle feed.

This is not true, and there is research data, specifically for the baby with cardiac problems and also premature babies, to prove it. This is one of the oldest and most persistent myths of breastfeeding. And it could only be believed by someone who has never closely watched a baby breastfeed. The studies on cardiac babies show that the baby's oxygenation, for example, remains better when they are breastfed than when they are bottle-fed. Obviously, the argument that a baby has to learn how to bottle-feed, before he can be tried at the breast, is pure nonsense.

Babies with cardiac problems need extra calories.

Sometimes they do, and there are ways of giving the extra calories without taking the baby off the breast—such as using a lactation aid. However, babies metabolize breastmilk as if it had far more calories than the average formula. Unfortunately, since many physicians think of breastmilk and formula as equivalent, they do not seem to understand that breastmilk gives the baby more calories than the calculated amounts found printed in textbooks.

Babies with cardiac transplants can't breastfeed because the antibodies in the mother's milk will cause rejection of the heart.

I am surprised by this argument. It is used as well for mothers who have illnesses such as idiopathic thrombocytopenic purpura (ITP), or Graves' disease (see Chapter 11, Breastfeeding While on Medication). The fact is that the antibodies that appear in the milk are a very special type of antibody called SIgA, which is not specifically directed against the baby's heart, and, in any case, does not get absorbed from the baby's intestines. There are many nonspecific immune-enhancing factors in breastmilk, but it seems far-fetched that they would cause rejection of a transplanted heart, especially when the babies are taking powerful immune suppressants.

I believe that too many physicians still do not understand how much comfort a baby can receive from breastfeeding, and there are many other benefits to the baby from breastfeeding besides immune factors and calories.

Chylothorax

Some babies with cardiac problems develop chylothorax after surgery because the thoracic duct (which brings lymph back into the general circulation) is cut during the surgery. (With certain surgeries this is almost inevitable.) The baby's lung cavity fills up with this lymph. A drain is put in place, and the baby is given a formula containing special fats that decreases the lymph flow.

There is another approach. The mother can pump her milk, have it centrifuged and the fat skimmed off, and then the special fats can be added.

Robert, my son, had just undergone open-heart surgery for the correction of a congenital heart defect. He had sustained a complication that, according to Bobby's surgeon, 30 percent of pediatric open-heart patients will encounter, called a chylothorax.

Bobby was allowed no food by mouth for two weeks, but the drainage did not subside. The next strategy was to implement Portagen, a specialized formula that consisted of 15 percent long-chain fatty acids, as opposed to breastmilk which has 40 percent. For the next two days, Bobby was given Portagen via a tube placed in his nose, but instead of subsiding the draining increased. He was put back on intravenous feeding.

During that time I continued to pump and freeze my milk, praying for the day that he would be able to receive it. Pump, freeze, wait. After weeks of drainage and no food by mouth, Bobby's condition was deteriorating rapidly. I contacted a network of La Leche League Leaders and Lactation Consultants and we came up with a plan.

We needed a centrifuge, and didn't have one. My husband, John, decided we could spin the milk in our own Maytag washing machine. He drilled holes in pine boards and put them in the washer so the bottles could sit at the right angle as they spun. We also worked with researchers at Yale to find a way to aspirate the fat out of the milk, leaving the skim behind. I found an organic dairy farm that told me about the lab where they had their milk tested for fat content. The results showed that our "Maytag" sample had a lower fat content than the Portagen.

John then purchased a lab-quality centrifuge and set it up in our home. The tests showed that the centrifuged milk had .02 percent fat per 100 cc. of skim milk. We finally had fat-free milk! We took turns making the skim milk at night, and every day we brought in a fresh batch of milk for Bobby.

As Bobby began receiving my milk, the drainage started to subside. We slowly increased the amount of milk he was receiving and by the end of the week, Bobby was receiving one ounce (30 cc) per hour. When he could tolerate it, the milk was fortified with protein, carbohydrates, and special fats he needed.

Bobby began to thrive. The infections subsided, his skin began to heal, the bruises faded away and his vital signs improved. After three months in intensive care, Bobby finally came home. Initially we continued on the skim milk, but after a month, he had trouble gaining weight. We decided it was time to try full milk again, which we introduced very slowly. A month later, Bobby was receiving full-fat breastmilk. We are now doing the whole process backward and feeding the cream to Bobby at night to increase his calorie content. He is gaining weight beautifully and increasing his strength.

There was not a doctor at that hospital that would have denied that breastmilk saved Bobby's life, and several doctors bluntly told us just that.

The Premature Baby

I have always asked mothers who attend the breastfeeding clinic if they were breastfed themselves. One of the most common reasons new mothers say that they themselves were not breastfed (if they have a reason) is that they were born prematurely. The other common reason is that they were adopted. We now know that neither of these reasons is truly a reason not to breastfeed.

Indeed, the milk of the mother who delivers prematurely is, like the milk of all mothers, specially designed for her own baby. It has higher concentrations of protein, long-chained polyunsaturated fatty acids, and most immune factors. The colostrum of the mother who delivers prematurely has very highly concentrated amounts of immune factors. Unfortunately, at least in North America, very few premature babies get their mother's colostrum.

Why is breastmilk important for the premature baby?

The premature baby has all the same reasons to be breastfed as the full-term baby. In addition, there are some very specific reasons for the premature baby to get his mother's milk, even if he is not yet ready to take the breast.

• The premature baby's immunity is not as developed as the full-term baby's, so premature babies are more susceptible to certain infections. Furthermore, the premature baby is often living in an environment (the special care nursery) where infectious disease microbes are present in large numbers and are often quite resistant to many of the antibiotics commonly used. For this reason, breastmilk for the premature baby is not only important, but may be lifesaving.

• Premature babies, particularly very small ones, are at risk of some specific diseases. These include the following:

Necrotizing enterocolitis

This is a condition that damages the intestinal lining of the baby's gut and results sometimes in death of parts of the gut. It results in the deaths of many premature babies every year. Nobody knows exactly why it occurs, but infection is said to play a part. For this reason, breastmilk is the ideal food for the premature baby, and studies have supported the notion that breastmilk feeding helps protect babies against this illness. It may also be that extra concentrated feeding plays a role in causing the illness.

Premature retinopathy

Very small premature babies, in particular, are susceptible to eye conditions that may cause blindness. It is thought that oxygen at higher levels than the baby would have experienced while inside the mother are responsible for this. This results in a bit of a dilemma for the treating physicians, since, in order to save the baby's life, the physicians may need to treat him with oxygen. But if he gets oxygen, it may damage his eyes. Much of the work in neonatal intensive care units results from trying to keep the baby's oxygen at just the right level, not too low and not too high. Breastmilk has been shown to promote the development of the eye, especially the retina, because of the docosahexaenoic acid in it. There are studies that suggest, but do not prove, that premature babies who receive breastmilk have less severe oxygen damage to the eyes and more rapid recovery from any damage, than do premature babies who did not have any breastmilk.

• Premature babies are particularly susceptible to learning problems and neurological problems. Breastmilk contains long-chained polyunsaturated fatty acids, which help neurological development. A study on premature babies from England a few years ago showed that at eight years of age, premature babies who got their mother's milk had an eight- to nine-point IQ advantage over those who did not.

• Premature babies and their mothers have

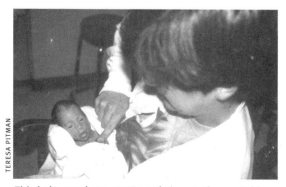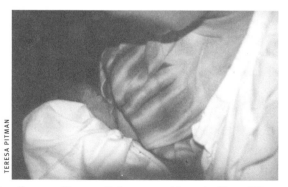

This baby was born at 28 weeks' gestation, weighing only 2 lbs 3 oz. She was fed expressed breastmilk until four weeks after birth; these photos show her first feeding at the breast.

greater problems bonding than do mothers of babies born at term. There are many possible explanations, including the fear of bonding on the part of the mother to a baby who might die, and long separations, with few opportunities to touch the baby, due to illness or hospital rules. Breastfeeding increases the amount of physical contact between mother and baby and can help them bond.

How will my premature baby be fed?

At first, many premature babies are not able to latch on and suckle effectively. It is a myth, however, that they need to be of a certain gestational age (say, 34 weeks) or a certain weight (say, 1500 grams) before they can be "allowed" to take the breast. It is also a myth that it is easier for a premature baby to take a bottle than to take the breast. Research has shown that premature babies are less stressed by breastfeeding than by bottle-feeding. This work has shown that a premature baby is likely to remain warmer, maintain his oxygen and carbon dioxide levels better, and is less likely to stop breathing or have his heart rate fall when he is on the breast than if he is taking a bottle. If a baby is ready for a bottle, in other words, he has been ready for the breast for a while already.

Smaller premature babies will usually be fed by nasogastric tube at first. This is a thin tube that passes through the nose or mouth into the stomach. Some prematures also need intravenous lines for various medical problems, but, of course, they can also receive some nutrients (glucose, calcium, vitamins, and others) through the intravenous. In fact, it is possible to nourish a baby totally through an intravenous, though it requires considerable skill and knowledge and a specialized pediatric department. It is not with-

out risk, especially in the very small premature baby, since his metabolic and nutrient requirements are not completely worked out. Most hospitals do not use this method of feeding for prolonged periods, except under extraordinary circumstances.

Larger premature babies may not need a nasogastric tube, but still not be able to suckle effectively. They can be fed by cup, spoon, or syringe.

Premature babies do not need to feed from a bottle. It is possible to argue for a long time about whether the bottle interferes with breastfeeding. I believe it does; others do not. But since it is not necessary to use it, why use it? If I am wrong, no harm has come from using a cup. If I am right, a lot of good may come from not using a bottle.

Putting the Premature Baby to the Breast

Whether or not the baby is capable of breastfeeding yet should not be the factor determining when he is first tried. Premature babies may take a long while to learn how to breastfeed. If the baby is born at 30 weeks (instead of the full-term 40 weeks), he may not take the breast for many weeks, but he still needs to learn how. If he is started on the breast only at four or five weeks of age, he has lost four or five weeks when he could be learning. After all, breastfeeding is a learning process, and it takes even some full-term babies a few weeks to get the hang of it. A premature baby needs even more time. Of course, if he is three days old and born at 30 weeks, he is likely just to nuzzle the breast, or to open up his mouth slightly when in contact with the breast. He won't latch on. So? He is learning. Every time the mother is with the baby, the baby and mother should be skin to skin, allowing the baby access to the breast. And if the baby seems hungry, she should make an effort to have him take the breast. Specialized help should be available to the mother and baby at these times.

Some special care nurseries use a nipple shield to help premature babies take the breast. Though I would not say that this approach is always wrong, I feel there is a rush to use it, when taking some time would be a better approach. There is work that seems to show that the baby will breastfeed better with a nipple shield, but I am skeptical. I believe the driving force should not be the idea of getting the baby out of hospital quickly. An early start at the breast, going slowly but surely, may be a better approach.

How early can a baby go to the breast? As soon as the baby is stable out of the incubator, which means he can be very young. There is a method of premature care, practiced at first in developing countries (first of all in Colombia), that is called "kangaroo mother care." It's named after the animal whose babies (joeys) are born very immature compared to other mammals, and who keeps its babies in a pouch for many weeks and months as the joey develops. This was adapted for human premature babies and seems to work very well. The premature baby is kept skin to skin with the mother, inside her clothing. He is kept warm by being in skin-to-skin contact with her, and being next to her allows for closer bonding between the mother and baby and much earlier and much more successful breastfeeding. In some units, even a baby who is still on a ventilator to help him breathe can be cared for in this way. Though many special care units in North America give lip service to kangaroo care, there are very few who follow it in any serious manner. Often kangaroo care in these hospitals means a few

minutes of skin-to-skin contact in a day, rather than the longer periods that would be better for the baby and the mother.

The baby can still have a nasogastric tube in his stomach and be fed through it, while at the same time being close to the breast and attempting to suckle. The mother can even express a little milk onto the breast or into his mouth to get him to understand what this is all about.

The principles of getting a premature baby onto the breast are essentially the same as those for getting a full-term baby latched on. The better the baby takes the breast, the better he will get milk and the less likely the mother will get sore.

There is no shame in leaving the hospital with a baby cup-feeding, however. As long as he is feeding adequately, why is the bottle somehow preferable or more natural than a cup or even finger-feeding? The baby can be discharged from the hospital feeding by these alternative methods, and he should get early follow-up from a specialist in lactation management.

"Inadequacies" of Breastmilk for the Premature Baby

There are very few pediatricians or neonatologists left who would deny that breastmilk is best for the premature baby, but despite everything, there are always a few holdouts. Nevertheless, at the beginning of the third millennium, very few neonatologists would agree that breastmilk *alone* is good enough for the premature baby.

A major reason for this is that many of the studies and much of the research on the nutrient needs of premature babies has been done in highly specialized units where the babies are very tiny, often below 1,000 grams (2 lb). These babies often have incredibly complicated and rocky beginnings. Yet, the majority of premature babies are not like that, and do not go to highly specialized units. What may be true for the baby weighing 900 grams (2 lb) may not be true for the baby weighing 1,500 grams (3 lb 5 oz) or 1,800 grams (4 lb), especially if he is not sick with respiratory problems.

Another problem is that it has been assumed babies born prematurely should be growing at the same rate as they would have had they not been born early (i.e., the rate that a baby grows inside its mother's womb). This is a logical assumption, but what is logical is not necessarily good, especially if we don't take all sides into consideration. There is no evidence that a baby who grows at "intrauterine growth rates" is better off when he is five years old or 20 years old than if he grew more slowly than that. The baby inside his mother is in a completely different physiologic situation than a baby who is outside his mother. Trying to force the same rate of growth in the baby outside may not be in his best interests. It *may* be best, but it has not been proven. What if the faster rate of growth just results in more fat cells being deposited, as some have postulated? In that case, matching the intrauterine growth rate may actually be less desirable.

It is also assumed that if the baby does not accumulate certain nutrients early in life, he will never do so. This is probably a false assumption, and has not been shown to be true for calcium, for example. The need for calcium was one of the major reasons used to justify adding nutrients to mother's milk. In one study, in Scandinavia, the more breastmilk (mother's own, plus banked breastmilk if necessary) a premature baby got, the denser (more calcium) his bones were at the age of two. This is in spite of the fact that babies get more calcium when they are given fortifiers in addition to breastmilk. But as we know from many situations with breastmilk and formula, what the baby is given to drink is not necessarily the same as what the baby absorbs.

Not Enough Calories

There is a problem getting a lot of calories into a premature baby using the traditional means of feeding. But there is an easy way to get around "not enough calories"—give more breastmilk. Amounts given to premature babies, based on the need to restrict fluids in some tiny, sick prematures, may not be enough to make them grow at a given rate. But a larger, well, premature baby could get a lot more fluids, on a kilogram for kilogram basis, than a sick, tiny one. And there are ways to increase the amount of fat the baby is getting as well, so that he gets more calories with smaller amounts of fluids.

Anything Else?

Aside from the question of calories sufficient for intrauterine growth, other matters come up. It is thought that there is not enough calcium, phosphorus, and vitamin D in breastmilk to allow the baby to mineralize adequately (with calcium) his rapidly growing bones. There have been problems, especially with very small premature babies, of their developing very soft bones with insufficient calcium deposited.

There is also a concern that there is not enough protein in breastmilk to allow for the very rapid growth of the premature baby.

Some very small babies are not able to metabolize lactose well. This results in loose, watery, green bowel movements in the baby, which in itself may not be of concern. However, because of the speed with which food travels through the gut in this situation, nutrient absorption may be diminished.

What About Insufficiencies in the Pre-term Formulas and Fortifiers?

This is not often discussed, because medical people seem much more willing to criticize breastfeeding and breastmilk than they do formulas. Yet there are real deficiencies in these products, which are, after all, made in factories by fallible humans based on inadequate data about the nutrient needs of the premature baby.

- In the first place, there are no immune factors in these products. Breastmilk contains dozens of factors, in addition to the well-known antibodies, which help protect the baby against infection. Not only do some of these factors protect the baby, but some stimulate the baby's own immune system to develop more rapidly and completely, so that the baby can protect himself.

  Something that has only recently been discovered is that there are factors in breastmilk that decrease inflammation. When the body fights off infection, there is usually an inflammatory reaction that occurs along with it. Many of the symptoms of infection are actually due to inflammation. Thus, the redness, pain, and swelling that occurs in an infected finger is actually due to inflammation. Inflammation is good in a certain sense, but it can also cause damage, and many of the bad effects of an infective process are actually due to the inflammation that occurs as part of the defense against the infection.

What is interesting about the immune factors in breastmilk is that they do not provoke an inflammatory reaction, at least not usually. This may be important in breastmilk's protective function against necrotizing enterocolitis, for example. A baby fed formula will not have these anti-inflammatory factors, and his chances of suffering damage from any infection are thus increased.

- There are no trophic factors in formulas, factors that encourage growth and development. Breastmilk contains many trophic factors, in addition to the epidermal growth factor mentioned earlier. There is nerve growth factor, for example, which may help in the development of the nervous system. A baby who gets formula but no breastmilk may not grow as well as a baby who gets breastmilk, because his digestive system may not be as developed and is thus less able to absorb nutrients.

- There is no docosahexaenoic acid (DHA) in infant formulas, even in formulas specially made for premature infants. The DHA would be there if it were easy, since formula companies quite rightly want their products to be as good as possible. But it is not just a question of adding some DHA. Long-chained polyunsaturated fatty acids need to be absorbed by the baby in certain proportions, or they can be toxic. Putting these fatty acids into the milk in those proportions doesn't work because they are not absorbed from formula in the same way as they are from breastmilk. Various long-chained polyunsaturated fatty acids are absorbed differently, and they are absorbed differently than from breastmilk. So, just as with iron and zinc, more DHA has to be put into formulas to get as reasonable absorption as from breastmilk, and this leads to possible toxicity.

DHA is important to the development of the baby's brain and retina. Even in full-term babies, there is good evidence that it makes a difference in the child's long-term cognitive development and school performance, and full-term babies are born with more DHA on board that has accumulated during the pregnancy for a longer period of time. The premature baby needs it more than the full-term baby does, because he lost several weeks of DHA transfer from the mother during the pregnancy, just as he did several weeks of iron transfer. DHA is actually an important component of every cell in the human body.

- In theory, there may be lots of this and lots of that in formula. Enough of everything, according to the bean counters. However, if the baby does not absorb it, then it may as well not be there. Just because it goes into the mouth does not mean that the baby benefits. Two good examples are iron and zinc, two minerals important to the body.

Iron is necessary for hemoglobin, which is responsible for carrying oxygen in red blood cells to the various tissues of the body. If hemoglobin in the red cells is deficient, the oxygen-carrying capacity of the blood is reduced, and there may be important consequences, including perhaps developmental problems in children. There is little iron in breastmilk, and there is a lot in infant formulas, yet the majority (probably over 90 percent) of the iron in formulas is pooped out by the baby, whereas close to 50 percent of the small amount of iron in breastmilk is absorbed by the baby. Essentially, the amount of iron the baby absorbs in each case is similar, but the breastfed baby gets less iron in his

intestines. However, large amounts of iron can cause problems, including constipation. Though some pediatricians deny that iron-enriched formula causes constipation, and, in fact, there are studies to suggest that it doesn't, many mothers find their babies are constipated on iron-enriched formulas.

Zinc deficiency causes slower growth rate. It can also cause a rare syndrome called acrodermatitis enteropathica, a mouthful if ever there was one. This syndrome causes an unusual facial rash associated with diarrhea and poor weight gain. This was not rare in artificially fed babies until it was realized what caused it. Though the formula companies in those days were touting their formulas, as they do today, as closest to breastmilk, there was not enough zinc in their formulas. In quantity, there was apparently enough, but because zinc is not as well absorbed from formulas as it is from breastmilk, it wasn't enough. Acrodermatitis enteropathica can occur also in breastfed babies if they are premature, but this is uncommon.

If these were the only two elements poorly absorbed from formula, it might not be such a big issue, but there are others, including DHA.

- Many elements in breastmilk interact with one another. Breastmilk is a living dynamic fluid, whereas formula is a chemical soup. As an example, lactoferrin is an important immune factor in breastmilk that attacks various microbes directly. It also works together with other immune factors, such as macrophages (specialized white cells), to further protect the baby. Lactoferrin is partially responsible for the high absorption of iron from breastmilk into the baby's blood, and it will bind iron to prevent its being used by bacteria, which require iron for growth.

But if we use breastmilk and fortifiers, don't we get the best of both worlds?

Possibly. What might be true, however, for the baby weighing 600 grams at birth, may not be true or necessary for the baby weighing 1,600 grams at birth. Unfortunately, many pediatricians and neonatologists have the one-size-fits-all approach. This approach results from so many of them not really believing that breastmilk is best. It also results from the dynamics of the neonatal intensive care unit, where there is so much to do, and so little time to do it. A factory approach seems the best approach. But it isn't, and it would be much better to individualize the feeding of premature babies.

There are risks to using formulas or fortifiers of breastmilk. There is the possibility of the baby becoming sensitized to cow milk protein. Some full-term babies do not tolerate formulas well. Why would premature babies tolerate them better? In fact, they don't. The whole point of using the fortifiers is to increase weight gain, yet if babies do not tolerate feedings, then feedings are cut back, and weight gain slows down.

It should be pointed out that there are no long-term studies on the safety of pre-term formulas or fortifiers. They were introduced into the market to respond to a need, but just because they contain more protein and more iron and more calcium that does not mean they are safe in the long term. No drug would be so cavalierly foisted on the market in the same way as so-called pre-term formulas and so-called fortifiers are. There is no reason to believe they are more unsafe than any other formula, but we have seen formulas sold that were lacking in basic elements or containing too much of certain elements and that have resulted in children becoming sick.

When should my premature baby start getting breastmilk?

As soon as possible. Though there are situations when this is not possible, either because of how ill the baby is, or associated abnormalities (say, a blockage in the intestines), most of the time the premature baby can be fed immediately after birth. By far the best food for him is breastmilk. In the first few days, the mother has colostrum that is rich in many of the elements the premature baby needs, including lots of white cells to protect him, lots of antibodies and lots of DHA. Small amounts of colostrum are better than large amounts of formula. Colostrum can be mixed in sugar water to be given to the baby, if necessary, to make up volume, though we do not really know what amount of fluid the premature baby needs in the first few days. Premature babies are at risk for hypoglycemia, especially if they have had a stressful delivery, so pediatricians are rightly careful about the blood sugars of these babies. Often premature babies, especially the smallest, will get an intravenous line. One advantage of the intravenous line is that it ensures the blood sugar is kept at a good level. If the baby has an intravenous, though, he does not need large amounts of food in his stomach. The small amount of colostrum, however, can be beneficial for preventing low blood sugar.

The early feeding of colostrum will also help develop his stomach and intestines so that he can tolerate feedings more quickly. Start expressing your milk, if your baby is unable to suckle yet, as soon as you can after the baby's birth. Many mothers find it easier to express colostrum by hand than with a pump.

Can my premature baby be fed only with breastmilk?

Yes, of course. The decision about adding something else should not be taken lightly. But because of perceived "deficiencies" of breastmilk, you may want to try some of the following.

Feed more. The feeding routines in neonatal intensive care units often result in holding back on the amount of fluids premature babies get. This is because babies on ventilators may go into heart failure if they get too much fluid, so it is a reasonable restriction. However, the healthy baby may have his fluids unnecessarily restricted as well, because "This is what we feed premature babies on day one, day eight, day 12, etc."

My experience in Africa was different. I was convinced at that time that babies needed to grow at intrauterine rates. But formulas were forbidden in our hospital. Mothers, at least partly because they were boarding with us as long as they had their babies in hospital, rarely had problems producing enough milk. And this was in spite of the fact, or maybe because of the fact, that they expressed by hand only. We had no pumps available. Most mothers, in fact, were expressing much more than we were calculating for their baby's requirements. When we fed the babies according to the rules, they grew, but not as quickly as they were "supposed" to. So we gave them more that they were supposed to get according to the rules. And they did grow faster. We gave them not 180 ml/kg/day, but 200, 250, 300 ml/kg/day, although I now realize that perhaps this was not necessary. But it did work. And many babies did gain at intrauterine rates.

Not only did the babies gain faster, but again, according to the rules, they were starting to approach "enough protein," and perhaps calcium and phosphorus as well. We did give them extra vitamin D, but that did not involve fortifiers.

We found that it was easiest to give a continuous flow of milk by nasogastric tube at the rate of 1 ml (for instance) every minute. This prevented distension of the stomach and diarrhea, at least most of the time.

I did not know at the time that the slow drip through a nasogastric tube might result in loss of fat in the tubing, but it worked anyway. There are now ways of decreasing the loss of fat in the tubing. One is ultrasonic homogenization of the milk. Though that sounds complicated, apparently it requires very little equipment and can be done anywhere. It results in much less fat sticking to the tubing.

One group of researchers found that premature babies could grow faster if they were fed "hindmilk" (milk from later in the feeding) rather than all the milk. Breastmilk increases in fat as the baby breastfeeds longer (or as the mother pumps or expresses milk for a longer period of time). The earliest milk is relatively low in fat (but still has some). If we put aside the first 30 milliliters (first ounce) or so, and the baby gets only the milk that is expressed after the first 30 or so milliliters, the baby will get more fat, and may grow faster. This is what these researchers found.

If the mother is producing more milk than the baby is getting, there are other options as well. Her extra milk can be set aside to settle, and the fat will rise to the top. The fat can then be skimmed off and added to the milk given to the baby. Every gram of fat gives nine calories to the baby, as well as those very important fats that develop the baby's brain and retina.

My baby needs more calcium and phosphorus.

It is possible, but is it really necessary to give the extra as fortifiers made from cow's milk? Calcium can be added to the breastmilk straight from vials of calcium chloride or gluconate added to intravenous solutions. Why not? Phosphorus is manufactured as a pill and can be dissolved into breastmilk. Vitamin D is given as a liquid and can be added to breastmilk as well.

My baby is not digesting the lactose in the milk.

This is usually the problem of the very small, premature baby. The younger and the smaller the baby, the less lactase he has in his intestines to metabolize the lactose. But the fact that your baby is not metabolizing the lactose is not a reason for him not to get your breastmilk. Commercial lactase is available, which can be added to your milk and then the mixture set aside for a few hours. The lactose is thus broken down before the milk is fed to the baby.

So would you say that no baby needs "fortified" breastmilk?

That is a very general statement, and there are always exceptions. The babies I worked with in Africa were "special" in a way. They were the hardiest and the largest. We had very little equipment in our nursery. If a baby couldn't make it with only a little oxygen, he didn't survive. This is different from neonatal intensive care units in affluent countries where, truly, miracles are being wrought.

Before modern medicine, it is unlikely that a 600-gram (1.5 lb) baby would have survived. Mother's milk was not designed for such an eventuality, and it is quite possible that something would need to be added to breastmilk to make sure the baby did not become seriously deficient in certain nutrients. On the other hand 1,500-gram (3 lb) babies often survived even without special care nurseries. Breastmilk may be enough for one, but not the other. It seems too often the baby "needs" fortifiers added to his milk, not because of his needs, but simply because he is in a special care nursery.

But if we are going to add fortifiers, why do these fortifiers have to be made from cow's milk? Why not human milk? This has been done in the past and can still be done. Milk banking gives us the option of human milk fortifiers. Not only can milk banks provide "premature" breastmilk, but breastmilk can be fractionated (divided up) so that a bank can provide fat, or protein, or even antibodies. This is not commonly being done, or perhaps at all, right now, but consumer pressure will eventually make it happen.

In the final analysis, the decision over fortification of human milk should be made on an individual basis. Each baby is an individual. Each baby has different needs depending on his size, how long he was in the womb, whatever illnesses he may have in addition to prematurity, and many other factors. Parental desires are often not taken into account here, and parents are often told there is only one way to do this. This is almost never true.

I was producing plenty of milk at first, but now the amount has gone down.

This is a common complaint of mothers expressing milk for a sick or premature baby. Around three or four weeks after the baby is born, many mothers feel their supply is down. This occurs despite their maintaining pumping or expressing, or even increasing it. Why this should happen is not clear, but it may be due to fatigue. Of course, taking estrogens may play a part, so if you are taking estrogens for some reason three or four weeks after the baby is born, perhaps it is better you stop them. If there is no obvious reason for a decrease, and the amount of milk is definitely decreasing, this is a good time to use domperidone. Domperidone quickly returns the milk supply to where it was, and the mother is usually able to stop taking the drug within a few weeks.

Cytomegalovirus (CMV)

Cytomegalovirus is a virus that can cause severe damage to the baby during the first trimester of pregnancy. The effects vary widely—it can cause miscarriage or stillbirth, or there may be no obvious problems at all. It frequently causes neurologic damage or liver damage, and may result in the baby being born underweight. It is said to be the most common cause of congenital (that is, the baby is born with it) deafness in North America.

Infection with cytomegalovirus after birth does not usually cause serious illness. Occasionally, it may cause a generalized swelling of the lymph glands, which can result in an illness similar to infectious mononucleosis, but usually infection causes no symptoms or a mild coldlike illness. Therefore, there is no reason for a mother who is infected with cytomegalovirus (people infected with it may be shedding the virus, and are thus infectious for many weeks or months) not to breastfeed or to provide her milk for her baby, even if her baby is premature.

Recently, however, fairly severe illness has occurred in very premature babies who were fed their mother's milk containing cytomegalovirus. Note that these babies were very small, under 28 weeks' gestation, and that older babies were not seriously affected.

If there is a chance that the mother has CMV infection and is passing the virus in the milk, should she still give her milk to her baby? Of course. If the baby is very young, however, under 28 weeks' gestation, it is better that her milk be frozen and then thawed before it is given to the baby, as freezing kills the virus.

Hypoglycemia (Low Blood Sugar)

There is a certain amount of hysteria in North America about hypoglycemia or low blood sugar. In some hospitals, every baby is being tested for hypoglycemia and many are being given formula to raise their blood sugar.

The "normal" blood sugar level of newborn babies has never really been determined with precision. As with many tests, what is normal for an adult or an older child is not necessarily normal for a newborn baby. Part of the issue is that many of the studies to determine "normal blood sugar" were done in the days when immediate feeding was not the rule, when feedings were scheduled, and when many, if not most, babies were being formula-fed. Furthermore, at such times, separation of mothers and babies was the rule.

The risk of a low blood sugar for the full-term, healthy baby who is demonstrating no symptoms is also difficult to determine, and there is probably no risk at all. Studies have not shown that low blood sugar without symptoms caused the full-term baby without any risk factors (being the baby of a diabetic mother, for example, would be a risk factor) any problems at all. This is undoubtedly due to the presence of other "fuels" or foods being available for nourishing the baby's brain. These include free fatty acids, lactic acid, and ketone bodies.

The usual method of measuring the blood sugars of babies, with a heel stick and putting a drop of blood on a glucose stick, is not accurate, even when the measurement is done with a special machine. This method of testing, which was designed initially for diabetics to test for high blood sugars, is just not a precise enough method on which to base decisions. It tends, in newborn babies, to underestimate the blood sugar. The only reliable method is to take blood from the baby from the vein and send it to the laboratory for a proper blood sugar test.

So, not only do we not know the normal blood sugar for a newborn, but we are not certain that low blood sugar without symptoms actually causes any problems, and the test we normally use is not reliable.

Risk Factors

Certain babies are at risk of becoming hypoglycemic, and there is no doubt that a low blood sugar level can be dangerous for the baby. Severe drops in blood sugar may cause convulsions, brain damage and even death, so this is not a problem to be toyed with. The infant of a diabetic mother, particularly if the mother is a juvenile onset diabetic who needs insulin injections, is most at risk. If the mother's blood sugars are under control during the pregnancy, this lessens the risk but does not completely eliminate it. Others who are at risk of low blood sugar are babies who were born prematurely. The more premature they were, the greater the risk, since these babies do not have a lot of glycogen (a complex sugar broken down when the body needs glucose) stored in their livers, and the mechanisms they have for increasing their blood sugar once it begins to fall are not well developed. For the same reasons, infants who have been malnourished during the pregnancy and are small for the length of the pregnancy are at risk because of a lack of storage of glycogen, but they have better-developed mechanisms for raising their blood sugars because, although they are small, they are more mature, physiologically speaking, than premature babies.

Finally, any "stressed" baby may have a drop in blood sugar. Cold is a stressor for the newborn baby, and one of the best ways of making a baby cold is to separate him from his mother. True, the heat lamps under which newborns are often put do keep babies warm, but the mother is also quite capable of keeping the baby warm. There is good evidence that skin-to-skin contact with the mother, after the baby has been dried off, keeps him as warm as any heat lamp or incubator. Furthermore, if the baby is kept skin to skin with the mother, he may start to suckle at the breast, which he cannot do while under a heat lamp, stressed by separation from his mother and getting tubes stuck down his nose and throat. If he suckles at the breast, he will get some colostrum, and colostrum is the best food a baby can get to help prevent low blood sugar. Formula is not, because various nutrients in formula stimulate production of insulin—the hormone that lowers blood sugar. Not only does insulin lower blood sugar, but it also decreases other nutrients newborns can use when they cannot get glucose. These other nutrients include free fatty acids and ketone bodies, and have been shown to protect the babies from the effects of low blood sugar, since the brain can use these biochemical products to nourish itself. On the other hand, colostrum does not stimulate insulin production. It has not been proved, but it has been observed by some that babies' blood sugar levels seem to respond more rapidly and stay up better if they get colostrum rather than formula. One reason may be that insulin is not released in response to colostrum.

Normal, Full-Term Babies and Low Blood Sugar

There is absolutely no reason to test healthy, full-term babies at birth or in the hours that follow birth, unless there are symptoms suggestive of low blood sugar. We would expect that a healthy, full-term, unstressed baby would maintain his blood sugar quite nicely, thank you very much.

The healthy, full-term baby should be skin to skin with the mother within minutes of birth. If he latches on, great, and if he drinks, better yet. He will be warm, he will have gotten colostrum, and his chances of having a low blood sugar level are virtually nil. The baby and mother should be left alone.

Infants of Diabetic Mothers

The infant of the diabetic mother is in a different situation. Such an infant is at risk for low blood sugar because he has been exposed to the mother's high sugars during the pregnancy. His pancreas secretes insulin in order to decrease the sugar, because his pancreas is working fine, unlike his mother's. When he is born, the mother's glucose is no longer available to him, but his insulin secretion may not respond immediately to his lower blood sugar level, and this over-production of insulin may result in the baby's blood sugar dropping dramatically. In addition, because insulin decreases ketone bodies and free fatty acid levels in the baby's blood, the brain cannot get nourishment from these alternative sources, as it can in the normal baby.

The mother can reduce the risk of her baby's getting low blood sugar by keeping her diabetes under control during the pregnancy. If the baby is not exposed to prolonged periods of high sugar, his pancreas does not have to produce more insulin. This is particularly true for the mother who has gestational diabetes (diabetes only during pregnancy). There is some evidence that infants of mothers who have type I diabetes (insulin-dependent) are still at a higher risk than babies of other mothers, even if the mother's sugars are very well controlled during the pregnancy—for reasons that are not clear. Nevertheless, even for these babies, good control decreases the risk of lower blood sugars.

So what is to be done? In many hospitals, infants of diabetic mothers are removed from the mother, taken to special care and given formula immediately. They are fed formula frequently, and if the blood sugar drops despite the formula (it takes time to absorb formula), the babies are often given glucose by intra-venous. They are often kept separated from the mothers, and the mothers are rarely encouraged to express or give their milk to the baby, as if formula were somehow better. But it isn't.

There is another consideration. Although it has not been proved conclusively by any means, there is real concern that early introduction of cow milk protein (as found in most formulas), may predispose the genetically susceptible baby to developing insulin-dependent diabetes later in life. (There is now some evidence that there may be a preventive effect of breastfeeding on adult onset diabetes as well.) Of course, we must prevent or treat hypoglycemia, but isn't it ironic that by treating the consequences of the mother's diabetes, we may be setting the stage for the development of diabetes in the baby later on? If there were no option, it might be necessary to take that risk. But is there truly no option to giving the baby formula in the first day or two? There are, in fact, a few.

Some mothers are producing quite a bit of colostrum even before the baby is born. Even small amounts of colostrum could be expressed in the few weeks before the baby is born. Though in theory expressing this colostrum might start labor, this is unlikely. But it wouldn't be necessary to start expressing until the baby was at about 38 weeks' gestation. A few milliliters of colostrum every day, collected and put together, could equal a fairly substantial amount of milk after a couple of weeks. The baby could be fed this colostrum at birth, if it becomes necessary to give him something immediately. Of course, it would be best if this colostrum were given to the baby via a lactation aid at the breast (see Chapter 5, Not Enough Milk). But it could also be given by finger-feeding, cup-feeding, or, if it were truly urgent, by bottle or nasogastric tube. However, if it is that urgent to raise the blood sugar, we should not be depending on oral feedings anyway. An intravenous needs to be started.

When it is urgent to treat a baby's dropping blood sugar, we cannot depend on the colostrum, sugar water, or formula being absorbed rapidly enough from the stomach to prevent the dropping sugar. Only an intravenous will ensure the blood glucose does not fall to dangerous levels, and sometimes, in severe cases, not even then, though such a situation is quite rare. If the baby is having symptoms associated with low blood sugar, starting an intravenous is absolutely essential.

But what if there is only a risk of low blood sugar—no symptoms, but just a risk—and no colostrum is available yet. Wouldn't formula be better then? I don't think so. Here is my take, and what I would want for my baby. I would much prefer he get an intravenous of glucose than formula. Actually, in my own experience of treating babies in special care with a risk of hypoglycemia, sugar water alone, by mouth, prevents the blood sugar from dropping. Again, it could be used at the breast with a lactation aid, but it could also be given by finger-feeding or cup, as with the colostrum. It is true that something containing protein, such as colostrum, is preferable to sugar water alone, but if sugar water does the trick, why not?

Furthermore, there is an option to formula which altogether too many health professionals do not even consider. And that is banked milk. Many will not agree with my approach as outlined above. They feel strongly that protein-containing food must be given to the baby, and sugar water, in the absence of colostrum, is just not good enough to prevent later drops in the baby's blood sugar. This is not a false argument, though I think that very often sugar water works. However, if you are diabetic and are being told that your baby will need formula after delivery, look into getting banked breastmilk ahead of time, so that it can be given to the baby instead of formula.

It goes without saying that the baby's being on an intravenous does not prevent him from going to the breast and learning to breastfeed. It does not mean he shouldn't get the mother's colostrum if he is not interested in breastfeeding. On the contrary, every effort should be made to get the baby breastfeeding, or at least getting the mother's expressed colostrum.

Thus, after all is said and done, it is almost never necessary to feed a baby formula, even if the mother is diabetic.

Large Babies

Large babies (over 4 kg or 8 lb 12 oz, or over 4.5 kg or 10 lb, depending on the hospital routines) are frequently tested for hypoglycemia. This routine began because infants of diabetic mothers are often very large. (Insulin is the major fetal growth hormone.) But, in fact, most large babies are not infants of diabetic mothers and have no more increased risk of hypoglycemia than babies who are smaller. The practice is continued, often, because the pediatrician will argue that the mother's high blood sugars may not have been picked up, and this is an infant of an "unrecognized" diabetic mother. Or that because the baby is so big, the stress of labor and birth is greater. Or that the reason the baby is being tested is that "This is what we've always done."

The problems of the testing do not change just because the baby is large. And the approach to preventing low blood sugars is no different in the large baby. Keep the baby warm, skin to skin with the mother. And get him feeding early, at the breast, of course. If the baby does not feed well, use compression to express colostrum into his mouth. If he seems to need to feed, extra sugar water at the breast with a lactation aid is the best way to get extra fluid and calories into him, because he will be getting some colostrum as well.

Premature Babies

Premature babies that are very small are often at serious risk of low blood sugar, especially if they are stressed by cold or respiratory difficulties. They should be fed early for many reasons, including to prevent hypoglycemia, but even if they are fed formula they cannot often be fed enough to assure maintenance of their sugars. So very small premature babies are often on intravenous. If that is the case, the sugar can be maintained with intravenous glucose, while the mother is expressing her colostrum to be given to the baby by mouth. Even drops may help to keep the sugar up, help develop the gut, and provide the baby with antibodies and other immune factors.

The larger, well, premature baby may not actually be at greater risk of hypoglycemia, but it is important to start feeding early. Separating the larger, healthy, premature baby from the mother just because he is premature is not always or even frequently necessary. Just as a full-term baby can be at the breast within minutes of birth, so can a baby born at 36 weeks and weighing 2 kg (4 lb 6 oz). It may take him longer, but it may not. If he feeds, terrific. If he latches but does not get milk, he can get some sugar water through a lactation aid. If that's difficult, then use cup- or finger-feeding. The procedure is always the same. The breast is best. If not breast alone, supplements can best be given at the breast. If that's not possible, other feeding methods are available, the bottle being the last resort.

Small-for-Gestational-Age Babies

These babies are born with a small weight for the amount of time they spent in the mother's uterus. A baby born at 39 weeks' gestation, and weighing 3.5 kg (7 lb 11 oz), is appropriate for gestational age. But if he was born at 39 weeks and weighed 2 kg (4 lb 6 oz), he is small for gestational age. A premature baby born at 1.5 kg (3 lb 4 oz) at 32 weeks' gestational age is appropriate weight. A premature baby born at 32 weeks' gestation but weighing 1.0 kg (2 lb 3 oz) is small for gestational age.

There are several known factors that may cause a baby to be small for gestational age. These include defects of the placenta that do not allow nutrients to get to the baby, maternal high blood pressure (though only when quite severe), uncontrolled maternal diabetes (mildly elevated blood sugars usually result in a bigger-than-average baby), and maternal smoking. Most of the time, the cause is unknown.

These babies are essentially malnourished during the pregnancy. Thus, they have low reserves of fat and glycogen, and, if stressed, may not be able to maintain their blood sugar in the normal range. These babies do have alternative energy sources (ketone bodies and lactic acid) available to nourish the brain. If they start getting breastmilk early and frequently, they are not likely to get low blood sugar.

The Baby with Trisomy 21 (Down Syndrome)

It can be devastating to learn that your baby has Down Syndrome. But one of the best things you can do for your child is to breastfeed. Babies with Trisomy 21 often have difficulty at first with breastfeeding. But once they get going, they do well.

They have problems for several reasons. Most are hypotonic, at first. This means that they don't have much tone in their muscles and they tend to be "floppy." This makes it difficult for them to latch on well, especially because some also have large tongues. They are often not demanding, and thus go into a phase early on where they don't demand, therefore don't get fed, therefore don't demand—a cycle that can occur with normal babies as well.

Some babies with Trisomy 21 have cardiac problems, ranging all the way from very mild to very severe. The approach to the baby with cardiac problems is the same as with other babies with similar conditions. The combination of Trisomy 21 and severe heart problems makes things quite complicated, but only because of the difficulty so many pediatric cardiologists have with breastfeeding.

Some babies with Trisomy 21 have intestinal problems, notably a problem called duodenal atresia, which is a block in the area of the intestine just past the stomach. If the baby is born with this, he cannot take anything by mouth until this problem is repaired surgically. The mother during this time should be expressing her milk and saving it to be fed to the baby once he can take oral feedings. Unfortunately, some surgeons are sold on the notion of predigested formulas being better for babies who have just had their intestines operated on. Breastmilk is not only easy to digest, but also includes enzymes that digest the breastmilk protein, fat, and carbohydrate. Because breastmilk also contains anti-inflammatory properties, the healing of the gut is likely to be less traumatic and more rapid for the baby.

Time and patience are necessary to breastfeed a baby with Trisomy 21, and almost always pay off. Alternative feeding methods should be used until the baby is ready to latch on. The mother and baby need experienced help for this. The most important step in getting any reluctant baby to latch on is for the mother to develop a good milk supply.

Most babies with Trisomy 21 will, with good help, be able to latch on by the age of three or four weeks, sometimes later—but again, this depends on the mother's developing a good milk supply.

Cystic Fibrosis

Cystic fibrosis is an inherited disease most common in people of northern European origin, although it may occur in other groups also.

Children with cystic fibrosis have difficulty digesting their food because they have very low amounts of the enzymes that come from the pancreas and break down the fats and proteins to be absorbed into the body. Thus, though they may take in a lot of food, they may not gain weight well.

In addition to these problems with digestion, they also have frequent lung infections. Their lungs become filled with thick secretions that are hard to cough up.

Twenty-five years ago, most children with cystic fibrosis were expected to die quite young. Now many are growing into adulthood. Except for those with the mildest symptoms, though, children and adults with cystic fibrosis need constant medical supervision and care.

Some women with cystic fibrosis are now having their own children. Early on, there was some concern about the quality of the milk these women could produce, but there is now sufficient evidence that the milk is fine and that their babies thrive on breastfeeding. Any baby of a mother with cystic fibrosis will always be a carrier for the disease, but he won't actually have it unless he also inherits a gene for cystic fibrosis from his father.

Babies with cystic fibrosis are occasionally identified at birth as having this disease, and sometimes it is diagnosed prenatally. Their meconium is sometimes so sticky that they develop a blockage of the intestines called meconium ileus. This is seen almost exclusively in cystic fibrosis babies. In some places, the meconium is tested, after the baby is born, for various pancreatic enzymes to determine if he has cystic fibrosis. Usually, though, cystic fibrosis is diagnosed a bit later because of the baby's poor weight gain or recurrent lung infections, or both.

Very few babies with cystic fibrosis are breastfed, unfortunately, at least in North America. Yet for the same reasons that all babies should be breastfed, babies with cystic fibrosis should most certainly be breastfed. The immune factors in breastmilk would help the baby fight off the recurrent infections that are such a problem with cystic fibrosis. Furthermore, breastmilk contains the enzymes lipase and protease, which help digest the food the baby gets and which he himself cannot provide. There are not enough of these enzymes, but there are some, and in the mildest cases there may be enough to prevent malnutrition simply by breastfeeding. In more severe cases, the malnutrition can be diminished.

Why are babies with cystic fibrosis so rarely breastfed? In part, because some medical professionals feel that if the baby is not perfect, the baby needs formula, while in truth the opposite approach should prevail. In addition, as soon as the disease is suspected or diagnosed, the baby is often put on bottle feedings for at least three days so that the amount of fat that is lost in his bowel movements can be measured. This helps the medical people to decide the appropriate quantity of replacement enzymes to give—but it interferes with breastfeeding.

Most babies with cystic fibrosis will need replacement enzymes. In bottle-fed babies, these are generally added to the bottle. This is more of a problem with breastfeeding, however, so often mothers of babies with cystic fibrosis are told they must stop nursing and give bottles instead. The mother may be urged to give "special" formulas that do not require as much digestion.

This approach does not take into account the special relationship of breastfeeding, something that could provide significant benefits to a child facing a chronic, lifelong illness. The infant or toddler who is frequently in the hospital, undergoing painful or frightening procedures, will surely benefit from the comfort of the breast, but few health professionals seem to see this.

How can you continue breastfeeding and still give the necessary enzymes? It's not that difficult. The mother simply expresses some milk, mixes it with the enzymes, and gives it to the baby with a lactation aid at the breast. On occasion, these enzymes may cause irritation of the nipples, but with care, and by giving the enzymes early in the feeding so that the baby's saliva will wash the residue off the nipples, this is not usually a problem.

I also think that taking the baby off the breast in order to measure the amount of fat in the baby's bowel movements compared to the baby's fat intake is not necessary. The amount of enzymes given could be on a trial-and-error basis, as they are anyway. The measurement of fat lost in bowel movements only provides a starting point.

Cleft Lip, Cleft Palate

One of the most common abnormalities that prevents babies from breastfeeding is cleft palate. A cleft may be partial or complete. It may be one-sided or occur on both sides. Usually, a cleft palate is an obvious deformity and is noticed immediately at birth, or, with prenatal ultrasound, sometimes even before birth. However, it is possible to have a partial cleft palate that involves only the soft palate (the back part of the roof of the mouth), and sometimes this cleft is so small that all that is noticeable is that the baby does not seem to have a uvula (the fleshy thing hanging at the back of your throat).

A cleft palate makes it difficult for the baby to breastfeed well, because he cannot form a good seal and cannot hold on to the breast well. Neither can he draw milk out of the breast well. However, it seems some babies can latch on if given the opportunity—perhaps not the majority, but some. Unfortunately, many cleft palate programs deny the possibility of a baby ever breastfeeding with a cleft palate, and encourage mothers not to try. This results in a self-fulfilling prophecy. Since most mothers don't even try, no such babies actually get breastfeeding. Mothers who try are often discouraged because the baby won't take the breast, and because everyone is telling them it doesn't work. But the fact is that some babies without cleft palates also don't take the breast at first and then do later on. I cannot say that I have had tremendous success with babies with cleft palates, but I have often seen them very late, once they have been bottle-feeding for some time.

In some centers, babies with cleft palates are fitted with obturators, mouthpieces that fit into the cleft and seal it, and allow better and easier feeding, including breastfeeding. This is the way babies in Switzerland are treated, and the Swiss are reported to get a lot more babies breastfeeding. In North America, it is obvious that most cleft palate teams do not understand or care that there is a difference between breastmilk feeding (via bottle) and breastfeeding. But there is a difference.

In centers where obturators are used, they must be replaced every few weeks—an expensive proposition, but it is believed that this expense is justified, not only because more babies get breastfeeding, but also because repair of the cleft is easier and speech is ultimately better.

When a baby is born with a cleft palate, the mother should start expressing her milk as soon as practical, usually within a couple of hours of birth. It is important she develop a good milk supply, because even if the baby latches on poorly, in the presence of an abundant milk supply he only has to swallow the milk as it pours into his mouth. A good latch is not always necessary. Furthermore, the mother can use breast compression to keep the flow going. This is the same principle as the squeeze bottle, which is frequently used to feed babies with cleft palates.

The mother should also try the baby at the breast within minutes of delivery, just as any other mother would who wanted to get started in the best way. In the first few days, babies only need small amounts of milk, and the baby might learn in those first days how to adapt to the mother's breast. Any milk he needs can be given by cup, which is better than a bottle. The best milk is breastmilk, of course.

If, even with good help, it does not appear possible to get the baby with a cleft palate to breastfeed, he can still be fed breastmilk. However, with the use of obturators, perhaps more babies will, in fact, get breastfeeding, even with cleft palates.

Babies with cleft lip alone should not have real difficulty with breastfeeding. The mother can position the baby in such a way that her breast seals over the cleft in the lip. Thus, if the cleft is on the right side (it is rarely midline), the mother can feed the baby on the left side using a cross-cradle hold, with the baby leaning slightly upward (best position anyway), and on the right side using the football hold. Or the mother can use her finger to seal the cleft. Nonallergenic tape can also be used. However, once the alveolar ridge (where the teeth will eventually be) is involved, the situation becomes more difficult, but not impossible.

Surgery

The age at which surgery is done for cleft lip and palate varies from center to center. Usually, it is too late to get a baby breastfeeding who has been fed by bottle. But it is still worth a try to put the baby to the breast after surgery.

The baby with the cleft lip should usually get breastfeeding. It used to be the rule of many surgeons to tell the mothers that they could not resume breastfeeding until 10 to 14 days after the cleft was repaired. The babies would have to be fed by spoon or eyedropper, an extremely difficult procedure in a four-month-old who is used to rapid flow and who needs the comfort of the breast after surgery. The surgeons felt that breastfeeding would result in poorer wound healing, perhaps even in the stitches pulling out and destroying the repair. There was no evidence at all that this would occur with breastfeeding, and no reason to believe it. Most surgeons no longer instruct mothers to stop breastfeeding after surgery, or if they do, only for a day or so (though even this is probably not necessary).

Whether or not a baby will eventually breastfeed with a cleft palate, however, it is still worthwhile for him to get breastmilk for all the reasons discussed elsewhere. In addition, babies with cleft palates are prone to ear infections, and it has been clearly demonstrated that babies with cleft palates who get breastmilk by bottle have fewer ear problems than those who get formula by bottle. If for no other reason, breastmilk feedings should be encouraged for the baby with cleft palate.

Phenylketonuria

It is not possible to discuss every possible illness a baby or child might have or how to encourage breastfeeding in that particular situation. For this reason, I will discuss this quite rare illness, and show how, with an approach that emphasizes the mother's and baby's right to breastfeed and the importance of breastfeeding to both mother and baby, a solution can often be found even for some complicated situations.

Phenylketonuria (PKU) is what is called an "inborn error of metabolism." There are dozens, if not hundreds, of these illnesses, which are usually quite rare. Some have been described in only a handful of children in the world. The cause is often a single enzyme that is absent or not functioning. In the case of PKU, it is an enzyme that changes phenylalanine (an amino acid) into tyrosine (another amino acid). Because the enzyme is absent, phenylalanine builds up in the baby's blood. High levels of phenylalanine eventually cause mental retardation, seizures and other problems.

Most North American jurisdictions screen the baby's blood for this abnormality within a few days of birth. If a low phenylalanine diet can be instituted within the first few weeks, most of the problems associated with PKU can be prevented, or at least decreased significantly.

For a long time, it was thought that breastmilk could not be given to babies with PKU, because it was assumed that since standard formulas had too much phenylalanine, and formulas were just like breastmilk (hmm!), breastmilk would have too much. Several years ago, however, it was discovered that breastmilk had a lot less phenylalanine than most standard formulas. Since babies need some phenylalanine, workers in this field began to believe that the baby with PKU could get at least some breastmilk.

At the Hospital for Sick Children in Toronto, a new plan was instituted for mothers who wanted to breastfeed. The dietetic department would calculate how much low-phenylalanine formula the baby needed. This was based on his initial blood levels, and also on the levels in his blood with treatment. Adjustments were made on a weekly basis. However, the amount of phenylalanine in breastmilk was now taken into account. An estimate of the amount of breastmilk and special formula the baby needed was made, and the mothers were instructed as follows:

1. The baby would be weighed before each feeding (a scale was provided).
2. The baby would be breastfed on each side for 10 minutes and then reweighed.
3. The rest of the feeding (weight gain as determined by the scale subtracted from the total calculated amount the baby needed) would be given by bottle as low-phenylalanine formula.
4. By following the baby's phenylalanine levels weekly, adjustments to the calculated amounts would be made.

Anyone who has read Chapter 5, Not Enough Milk, should immediately understand why this approach would not work. Aside from the inconvenience of weighing babies before and after each breastfeed, and of carrying the scale everywhere the mother and baby went, the baby eventually got used to the bottle and stopped breastfeeding. Mothers were nervous about feeding the baby 10 minutes on each side, and worrying about whether the baby would get too much breastmilk, and their letdown reflex was inhibited.

However, taking some basic principles of breastfeeding into account, it was possible to change the situation completely. Instead of the above regime, the dietetic department calculated the amount of special formula the baby needed. This was given early in the feeding with a lactation aid, so that the baby got the entire amount of calculated formula during the feeding, and then nursed until he did not want any more. There was no problem with the baby preferring the bottle, and the baby was able to suck on the breast as long as he wanted rather than being pulled off at a given time. At least one baby breastfed 18 months in this way. No need for scales or bottles. No need for timing. The babies' phenylalanine levels were well controlled.

In some atypical cases of PKU, the baby can do fine with breastfeeding alone, but these are uncommon variants of an uncommon illness—most babies with this illness cannot breastfeed exclusively. But unfortunately, many workers in the field believe the babies cannot breastfeed at all.

Breastfeeding Before Surgery, and After Surgery

Up until recently, many babies were forced to fast, beginning at midnight, if they were going for surgery in the morning. We can be thankful that this approach is disappearing, though some anesthetists still insist on it. Parents whose babies need surgery should find a hospital with more enlightened policies.

However, it is still the rule in many hospitals that babies need to be off milk, including breastmilk, for six hours before the planned surgery. This is often a terrible hardship for the breastfeeding mother and baby. Many breastfeeding babies and toddlers continue to wake up during the night to nurse. Trying to prevent nursing can be a torture for the mother, and her baby. Those who insist on it just do not appreciate how traumatic it can be for all involved.

Some children's hospitals, such as Boston Children's and Philadelphia Children's, now have protocols that allow breastfeeding up to three hours before surgery, a much more reasonable approach. Unfortunately, most Canadian hospitals, including the Hospital for Sick Children in Toronto, are miles behind such progressive hospitals.

After surgery, if there is no reason to restrict oral feedings (as there may be with some abdominal surgeries, though not hernia operations), the breastfed baby can go to the breast as soon as he is awake from the surgery. It is a great comfort for the baby to be able to breastfeed. Surgery is a frightening business for the adult who has some comprehension of the need for the procedure, the pain they may feel afterward, and the absence of friends or family at their side when they wake up. A child cannot understand all these things. Many hospital protocols require the baby or child to drink a clear fluid and not vomit before being permitted to go to the breast or drink milk. This is yet another example of the thinking that formula=breastmilk and breastfeeding=bottle-feeding. Breastmilk is not

formula, and the inflammatory reaction that would occur with the baby aspirating formula would not occur with the baby aspirating breastmilk. Breastfeeding is an active and complex process. A baby who is awake enough to breastfeed has the gag reflex necessary to avoid aspiration. Bottle-feeding is more passive, and a baby can get milk from a bottle with little active participation.

When Your Baby Is Hospitalized

One of the challenges for mothers who want to establish or continue breastfeeding when a baby must be hospitalized is that some hospitals do not encourage or even permit parents to stay with their children. Even if the hospital policy says that parents can stay, staff may do all they can to discourage it. Mothers are often told they need to go home and rest, that they will do their baby more good if they get a good night's sleep, that their presence is making the baby "unsettled." This can be really hard for the mother to deal with, since she's already feeling emotional about her baby's illness and is probably exhausted from worry as much as from the sleepless nights in the hospital.

The hospital may permit parents to stay with their children, but not provide any sleeping facilities, so that the mother spends the night sitting beside her baby in a hard chair.

Usually when these mothers go home, as they have been told to, they don't sleep anyway. They are too concerned about the baby they've left behind, and probably need to get up at least once in the night to pump milk.

It is even more difficult for the mother who has other children at home. She finds herself torn between her baby, who needs her comfort and her milk, and her family, who also need her.

Support from your partner, family, and

friends is critical in making this situation work. Be firm with hospital personnel about how important breastfeeding is for you and your baby. Your baby needs breastmilk and breastfeeding more when he is ill, not less. You may be able to get your partner or someone else to stay with the baby while you take a nap, and have that person come and wake you if the baby wakes up and wants to nurse. If you have other children at home, you may be able to arrange to have them brought to you at the hospital, or (if you live close by) you might be able to go home for short visits. Some hospitals have "family rooms" near the pediatrics or neonatal unit, where the entire family can come and spend most of the day near the mother and the sick child.

If you simply can't stay in the hospital, be sure to express or pump your milk during the times you are separated from your baby. This can then be fed to your baby while you are away. Keeping up a good milk supply will make it easier when your baby is with you full-time again.

Most reasons for not breastfeeding sick children are based on nothing more than a lack of understanding of how breastfeeding works, and of the nature of breastmilk. If there is a will to keep breastfeeding, ways can most often be found to manage this. But it takes commitment.

14

Special Situations: Adoption, Breast Surgeries, Relactation

Myth 1: A mother who is adopting a baby will not be able to breastfeed.

Myth 2: A mother who has had breast reduction surgery will not be able to breastfeed.

Facts: Neither of the above is correct. The mothers in both situations may not be able to breastfeed exclusively, but they should be able to breastfeed, given good support. And some can, in fact, breastfeed exclusively.

Myth 3: Once a mother stops breastfeeding, she cannot restart.

Fact: It may be difficult to restart, but it is not usually impossible. It may even be possible to return to exclusive breastfeeding.

Situation 1:
Breastfeeding the Adopted Baby

Breastfeed an adopted baby? Most people are astonished to find out that this is even possible. Can a mother breastfeed a baby she hasn't given birth to? Can she breastfeed even if she's never been pregnant?

Yes, frequently she can. She may not be able to produce enough milk to completely feed her baby—she may need to supplement—but her baby will still get significant benefits from even a small amount of breastmilk.

It is obvious that there is more to breastfeeding than just the nutritional value of the breastmilk. Breastfeeding gives confidence to the mother and helps her establish a special, physical relationship with her baby that cannot be duplicated. This occurs whether or not the baby is getting milk from her breasts. The baby also gets security and warmth and a physical relationship with the mother, which cannot be duplicated by a rubber and plastic bottle.

I am not saying that a mother cannot love her baby if she bottle-feeds. I am not saying that the baby cannot develop security and independence and love for his mother if he is not fed at the breast. Of course, all this is possible. However, the act of breastfeeding is special.

I would encourage any mother who is adopting a baby to seriously consider breastfeeding. Here's how.

Getting the Baby to Take the Breast

In my opinion, getting the baby to take the breast is far more important than making milk. Even if the mother eventually produces only drops of milk for her adopted baby, she can still breastfeed if the baby takes the breast. Thus, this is the first priority.

Will a baby take the breast if there is no milk? Well, babies suck on pacifiers all the time, and a baby who is not getting much milk from the breast may still be happy to suckle when he is sleepy or simply wants some comfort. Using a lactation aid with banked breast milk, or formula, if necessary, can encourage the baby to keep suckling.

More and more, adopting mothers are able to nurse the baby as soon as the baby is born. This is good. It is much better this way than in the old days, when the adopting mothers could not even hold the baby for 10 days after birth or longer. Several of the adopting mothers that I have followed in the clinic were able to put the baby to the breast in the delivery room. The increase in open adoptions means that often the adoptive mother and the birth mother have met and gotten to know each other before the birth, and frequently the birth mother has encouraged the adopting mother to breastfeed.

However, this situation must be handled with some sensitivity. The sooner the baby starts breastfeeding, the better, but not at the expense of making the birth mother's experience more painful. In some situations, it is also worthwhile to consider having the biological mother nurse the baby during the first few days, especially if it is impossible for the adopting mother to put the baby to the breast.

When this possibility is brought up, reactions can be strong. Many urge the adopting mother not to allow the biological mother to breastfeed, because she might change her mind about giving up the baby. This has not happened in any of the few cases I am aware of, in which the biological mother did, in fact, breastfeed for a day or a few days. But it is a possibility. After all, one cannot push the "bonding" that breastfeeding promotes and then turn around to say it does not occur when the mother is about to give up the baby for adoption. Personally, I believe the "bonding" of breastfeeding is a slow, gradual process, not a

lightning flash—at least, not usually. Still, I understand the fear of the adopting mothers who do not want the biological mother to breastfeed.

There are advantages for the biological mother to breastfeeding during the first days. She should have fewer problems with engorgement when the milk increases on day three or four, if the baby has been nursing well. In some cases, the biological mother has even donated her milk to the adopting mother to use for the baby. This allows the biological mother to develop an emotional tie with the baby, even when she does give him up. This may not be such a bad thing. On the contrary, it may be a good thing. And, of course, the baby will get the colostrum so important for his health.

If the biological mother does not breastfeed, and if the adopting mother cannot yet, for whatever reason, put the baby to the breast, it is far better that the baby not get bottles or pacifiers during this time. Alternative methods, preferably cup- or, perhaps, finger-feeding, should be used to feed him. Cup-feeding, when the mother is not present to feed the baby, would be preferable, since the main use of finger-feeding is to help a reluctant baby get to the breast. The longer the mother and baby are separated, the more difficult it may be to get the baby to take the breast once they are together. All efforts should be made to get the adopting mother and baby together as soon as possible after the birth.

If you will not be able to have the baby you are adopting right away, and the biological mother will not be breastfeeding, this would be an indication to use domperidone, because you want to have as plentiful a milk supply as possible to encourage the baby to take the breast. When you bring the baby home, if supplementation is necessary, I think this is a case where it is imperative that the baby be supplemented with a lactation aid at the breast. The issue here is to get the baby breastfeeding.

If the baby is reluctant to take the breast, do not despair. It can be done (see Chapter 10, When the Baby Refuses the Breast). As mentioned there, the better the milk supply, the more likely the baby is to take the breast eventually. Interestingly, however, out of many dozens of adopted babies we have followed in the clinic, only two refused the breast initially, and of the two, one eventually took the breast well (by about two weeks of age) and breastfed exclusively for about five months. In the other case, the mother did not produce much milk and the baby refused the breast, but the mother did not persist in trying to get the baby to breastfeed.

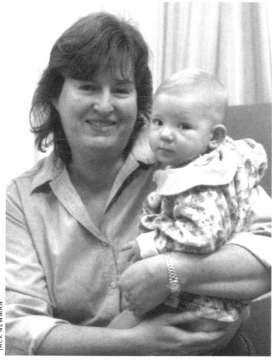

JACK NEWMAN

This adopted baby was breastfed exclusively for about five months, and is still breastfeeding at one year of age.

Making Milk

The adopting mother should start inducing milk production as far ahead of the birth of the baby as possible. Sometimes, as in the case of a surrogate mother, the adopting mother will know within weeks of conception that she will get a baby and will have almost nine months to prepare for breastfeeding. In other cases, the adopting mother may have only a week or less advance knowledge.

I will describe the "ideal" situation, at least from the point of view of producing milk. A little background might be helpful.

During pregnancy, among other hormones (chorionic gonadotropin, for example), the placenta is producing increasing amounts of progesterone and estrogen. At the same time, the pituitary is producing increasing amounts of prolactin. These three hormones cause the growth and development of the breast tissue during pregnancy, but the production of milk is inhibited by the progesterone and estrogen in the mother's blood. Once the placenta is delivered, after the birth of the baby, the placental hormones obviously are no longer available, and prolactin now can exert its effects on the breast without the inhibiting effects of other hormones. It is probably for this reason that it takes a few days for the milk production to increase after the birth of the baby. Research suggests that it is the fall in progesterone after the delivery of the placenta that sensitizes the milk-producing cells of the breast to the effects of prolactin. If this fall in progesterone does not occur, then milk is not produced. Such a situation may arise, for example, if pieces of the placenta remain in the uterus (retained placental fragments) or if a too-early injection of medroxyprogesterone (Depo-Provera), for contraceptive purposes, is given.

Unfortunately, and quite possibly to the detriment of breastfeeding success, too many physicians, particularly in the United States, are giving new mothers injections of medroxyprogesterone within a day of the baby's birth.

Given six or more months to prepare, and assuming there are no contraindications to the use of any of these drugs, I would suggest the following to the adopting mother, which would, I would hope, "simulate" the situation that occurs during pregnancy—high progesterone and estrogen levels with high prolactin levels. However, it is difficult to know how closely any of these hormonal regimens would come to the situation during a normal pregnancy. I have now used this protocol with several mothers, and it works quite well. The first mother who was on this protocol has become so interested in adoptive nursing that she has become a lactation consultant and has a website about adoptive nursing (http://www.asklenore.info/breastfeeding/abindex.html). She has helped some 400 women from around the world breastfeed their adopted babies. This is the protocol—and two variations—that she has developed with my help. All mothers going on any of these protocols need to be followed by a physician with the support of an experienced lactation specialist. Though domperidone is relatively safe, there are side effects associated with the use of birth control pills, and your doctor needs at least to know you are on these protocols and what medications you are taking.

The Regular Protocol

This protocol requires a long lead time, so it will be most successful for a mother expecting a baby through surrogacy (meaning you have the whole pregnancy to prepare) or another kind of adoption that is planned well before the baby's birth. Most of the women who have followed this protocol were able to meet most if not all of their baby's breastmilk needs and sustain until weaning.

1. At least six months before the baby is due (the longer the better, if the mother can start as soon as she knows a baby is on the way it would be great), take an "active" birth control pill each day (that is, do not take any sugar or placebo pills that may be included in the birth control pack. Skip on to the next cycle's supply without a 7-day break). Also begin taking 10 mg domperidone four times per day for 1 week. Then increase the dosage to 20 mg four times per day. The breasts may swell. This is normal. The birth control pill actually suppresses milk supply mimicking what happens during pregnancy. *No pumping or herbs until six weeks before the baby is due.* Pumping before the breasts are ready is unnecessary and will not ultimately make a difference to your milk supply. We have found that Diane 35 and Ortho 1/35 have worked well as the birth control pills for this process, though there is no reason to believe other pills might not work as well.

2. About six weeks before the baby is due, the mother should stop the birth control pill and continue the domperidone dosage of 20 mg four times a day. The mother should experience vaginal bleeding. This is normal withdrawal bleeding. If the mother does not experience withdrawal bleeding and is fertile, it is recommended that she be examined for potential pregnancy.

At this point, the mother should begin pumping about every three hours. Note: Stopping the birth control pill while maintaining the domperidone and then pumping, should cause a rapid decrease in the mother's serum progesterone level while causing an increase in the mother's serum prolactin level. This process attempts to mimic what happens after a normal pregnancy and birth. This should cause the mother's milk supply to increase substantially.

Once the mother has started pumping she can add the herbs blessed thistle (390 mg per capsule) and fenugreek seed (610 mg per

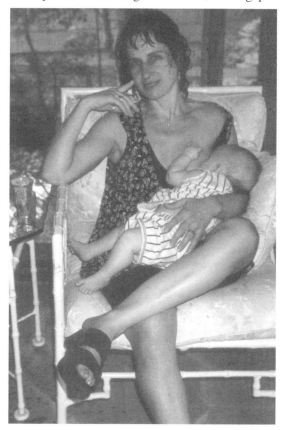

A mother and her exclusively breastfed adopted baby, who never had a drop of formula. He was breastfed for more than a year.

capsule). The recommended herb dosage is three capsules of each, three times a day with meals. The domperidone should be taken half an hour before meals for best absorption. Many mothers on the protocols have noticed a significant increase in their milk supplies when they began to add oatmeal to their diets regularly.

3. It's helpful to pump at least once during the night. A mother's serum prolactin levels naturally rise between 1 a.m. and 5 a.m. Pumping during the night takes advantage of this natural occurrence. Additionally, research has shown that frequency of breast emptying is more influential on milk supply than duration of breast emptying. The more often the mother pumps, the more milk she can store, and the better her supply will be.

The arrival of the milk supply while pumping follows a particular pattern. It begins with clear drops, which become more opaque and whiter in color. Drops will appear, followed by milk spray, and then a steady stream of breastmilk. It may take a few days, a week, or two, or more for the mother's milk supply to come in. Everyone responds differently.

4. Once the baby arrives, the mother should continue the domperidone dosage of 20 mg four times a day and continue until either she achieves a full milk supply or is ready to wean her baby off the breast. The mother should put her baby to her breast as soon as possible, in the delivery room if she can. She should feed her baby "on demand" and as often as possible.

While the mother's milk supply is still building, it is helpful to pump after each feeding at the breast, if that is practical. This will help to increase her milk supply, until it is well established. The mother should maintain the herbs fenugreek and blessed thistle and continue until her milk supply is well established and throughout the entire time she is breastfeeding if necessary. Once the mother's milk supply is well established it might be possible for her to slowly decrease the domperidone and even eliminate it completely. See the section on "stopping the domperidone."

The Accelerated Protocol

Not all adopting mothers are lucky enough to have several months to prepare for breastfeeding. This accelerated protocol will help you develop a milk supply as quickly as possible. It's also been successful for mothers wanting to relactate. Milk production may be lower with this protocol than that achieved with the regular protocol, but remember—there is more to breastfeeding than breastmilk.

Diane 35 is taken for 30–60 days non-stop, only active pills, no sugar pills, together with the domperidone 20 mg four times per day. If significant breast changes occur within 30 days, the birth control pill is stopped while maintaining the domperidone, and the pumping schedule begins.

Significant breast changes include an increase in breast size (one cup) and breasts that feel full, heavy, and painful.

Milk production may not be as great on the accelerated protocol, but one can never predict and the supply is usually sufficient to provide a significant amount of the baby's needs. The mother should use the feeding tube device (lactation aid, see Chapter 5) filled with either breastmilk or artificial infant milk to breastfeed her baby while she is going through the protocol. Many adoptive mothers and intended mothers have asked the birth mother to provide breastmilk for a limited amount of time ranging from two weeks to one month or more. Many birth mothers are happy and willing to provide the child with a healthy start in life. At least one birth mother has reported that providing breastmilk helped her to cope with the adoption process. Many surrogate mothers have provided expressed colostrum and breastmilk for their couples to give their children.

If the mother has four weeks or less or even if the baby has arrived, the Diane 35 (once a day) is started immediately, together with 20 mg of domperidone four times a day. If the mother can take the Diane 35 together with the domperidone for at least 30 days, she may produce significant amounts of milk.

Once the mother has completed at least 30 days on the combination of Diane 35 and domperidone and has experienced significant breast changes she can stop the Diane 35, maintain the domperidone and begin pumping with a double electric breast pump. A hand pump is just not up to the job. Of course, if she already has the baby she should be putting the baby to the breast. Significant breast changes include an increase in breast size (at least one cup) and breasts that feel full, heavy, and painful.

Refer to the regular protocol, earlier in this chapter, for details on the pumping regimen and the use of herbs.

Remember that if the mother is fertile, and does not wish to get pregnant, she should use a nonhormonal method of birth control at this point.

The mother should store as much breastmilk as she can. Once her baby arrives, or if her baby is already here, the baby should be fed on demand. The baby should be supplemented if necessary using a feeding tube device filled with either the stored breastmilk, or artificial infant milk until the mother's milk supply is well established. Remember, not all the milk has to come from the mother. Whatever amount of breastmilk she can provide to her baby is a precious gift. There is more to breastfeeding than breastmilk.

Note that the birth control pill and domperidone are both approved by the American Academy of Pediatrics for use in breastfeeding mothers.

The Menopause Protocol

If the mother is menopausal due to surgical removal of her reproductive organs or naturally occurring menopause, she can still breastfeed and bring in her milk supply. A woman does not need a uterus or ovaries in order to breastfeed. All she needs are breasts and a functioning pituitary.

The first step is to stop the mother's hormone replacement therapy and replace it with Diane 35 (once per day). Diane 35 contains enough estrogen and progesterone to keep the mother's menopausal symptoms at bay while at the same time developing the milk-making apparatus of her breasts. The mother also needs to take domperidone (10 mg four times a day for the first week and then increase to 20 mg four times a day). It is a good idea for the mother to stay on the combination of Diane 35 and domperidone until she experiences significant breast changes. At least 60 days, on the combination of Diane 35 and domperidone is recommended for menopausal women. Significant breast changes include an increase in breast size (at least one cup) and breasts that feel full, heavy, and painful.

Once the mother has completed at least 60 days on the combination of Diane 35 and domperidone and has experienced significant breast changes she can stop the Diane, maintain the domperidone and begin pumping with a double electric breast pump.

Refer to the regular protocol, earlier in this chapter, for details on pumping regimen and the use of herbs.

If the mother experiences menopausal symptoms, it is best she not resume hormone replacement therapy but rather try taking soya products to control her symptoms. Soya milk and/or soya butter are good choices because they contain phytoestrogens, but the mother should eat only enough to stop hot flashes because too much will decrease her milk supply.

What to Do If the Mother Does Not Experience "Significant" Breast Changes:

Significant breast changes include:

- Breasts increasing in size by at least one cup size.
- Breasts full, heavy, and painful.

These symptoms are indications of adequate growth of the milk-making apparatus of the breasts. If the mother does not experience significant breast changes within 15 days of beginning either of the protocols, she may want to consider increasing her progesterone intake. There are two reliable ways to do this:

1. Replace her current birth control pill with Diane 35. This medication has twice the amount of progesterone that is in the 1/35–type birth control pills.

2. Continue on the current 1/35 birth control pill and add 1 mg of progesterone another way, such as by adding half a pill of Provera 2.5.

Adding progesterone usually solves the problem but the first option works better than the second option because of the anti-androgynous nature of the progesterone contained in the Diane 35.

A word of caution about creams—they do not provide the needed level of progesterone in a reliable manner. An oral form of progesterone is a better choice.

More on Domperidone

Domperidone has been discussed in Chapter 5, Not Enough Milk. In the case of the adopting mother, however, will the mother be able to stop the domperidone while she is breastfeeding? It is impossible to say. We have now had about 10 mothers altogether who have been able to produce all the milk the baby required (this does not include mothers using the protocols previously, but only those taking domperidone and pumping). Most have required taking domperidone through the entire nursing period, though some were able to reduce the dose. It is worth trying to at least decrease the dose. Many mothers who do well with the maximum dose (20 mg four times a day) will be able to continue to produce all the milk the baby needs with, say, 20 mg three times a day, or 10 mg four times a day. If no effort is made to decrease the dose, then we will never find out if there are mothers who continue to produce plenty of milk even if they no longer take domperidone at all.

Dropping the dose can be done slowly, say by 10 mg (one tablet) per day every week or so. If there is no obvious change in milk supply and the baby remains happy and growing, then drop another pill, and so on.

The fact remains, however, that most adopting mothers will need to stay on the domperidone for the entire time that the baby is nursing, if they want to maintain a full milk supply.

If the mother does not produce all the milk the baby needs, then a different situation comes up. Is it worth taking a drug, which, though it seems quite safe and is distinguished by a lack of side effects, is still a drug—in order to keep the amount of supplement at, say, 300 ml/day (10 oz/day) rather than 420 ml/day (14 oz/day)? I would say not. What about keeping it at 300 ml/day (10 oz/day) rather than 600 ml/day (20 oz/day)? Hard to say. Again, in my opinion, the breastfeeding is primary, not the amount of supplement.

How long should I breastfeed my adopted baby?

See Chapter 19, Breastfeeding the Toddler. It seems to me there is absolutely no reason to stop earlier just because the baby is adopted. On the contrary, given that adopted babies are at greater risk of having behavior problems in their teen years, a longer nursing period—not a shorter one—would be reasonable. The mother should not try to force the baby to stay at the breast if he is not interested at 18 months, say, but she should not stop nursing earlier just because he is adopted. Even if the mother is producing only small amounts of breastmilk, as the baby gets older, the act of breastfeeding becomes more and more important than the breastmilk itself.

Once the Baby Is Taking Solids

Many mothers who have an insufficient milk supply believe that once the baby is taking solids, they will be able to stop the supplement and/or the domperidone, if they are taking it. And often enough that works, though the transition from breast and supplement to solids or from domperidone to no domperidone should be gradual, rather than hurried. Remember that a baby tends to like good rapid flow at the breast, and if the mother stops the supplement at the breast, or decreases the domperidone too quickly, the baby may fuss at the breast. He may pull away and cry, go back to the breast and suck a while, then cry some more. This may happen even if there is a fair or even reasonably good milk supply. In such a situation, the mother may find that she needs to continue using the lactation aid to supplement. One trick that often works is to feed the baby solids first, so he is not too hungry. In this situation, the baby might be far more patient at the breast and not need the rapid flow.

> "Who fed me from her gentle breast,
> And hushed me in her arms to rest,
> And on my cheek sweet kisses prest?
> My Mother."
>
> —Anne Taylor, "My Mother"

Relactation

Relactation refers to restarting breastfeeding with the same baby after it has been stopped for some reason.

As with breastfeeding the adopted baby, it is best that the mother get help from someone experienced in relactation. This is probably not your family doctor or pediatrician, and not all lactation consultants have much experience with helping mothers relactate. Also, as in the case of breastfeeding the adopted baby, there are at least

two issues to address: getting the baby to take the breast and increasing the milk supply. The degree of success of the mother who wishes to relactate depends very much on the following factors.

Milk supply before weaning

If the mother had a good milk supply, even an abundant milk supply, it may be possible to rebuild that supply. Even if the milk supply was not abundant before weaning, it may still be possible to build up the milk supply, because often "not enough milk" is not that at all. Rather, it is poor breastfeeding technique resulting in the baby not getting the milk available. Of course, even if the mother is incapable of producing enough milk (an unusual situation), this does not mean she should not try to relactate. *Some breastmilk is better than none. And breastfeeding is more than breastmilk.* A low milk supply, however, may make it difficult to get the baby to take the breast again.

How long it has been since the baby was taken off the breast

The longer the baby has been off the breast, the more difficult it will be to get him back to it. But I have seen some babies who have returned to the breast after an amazingly long time. In one situation, the mother had never put her four-month-old to the breast because she had been told that she could not breastfeed when she was taking the medication she was on. This was incorrect information, and when she found this out, she came to our clinic with her four-month-old to start nursing. The mother had never pumped her breasts or expressed her milk. I had strong doubts that the baby would take the breast, but he did. Eventually, the mother produced a fair bit of milk, and she was still nursing the baby when he was six months old. (I did not follow up longer than that.) In another case, a mother decided she wanted to breastfeed after she left an abusive partner who had forbidden her to breastfeed. Her baby was three months old when she came to us to start breastfeeding. This baby did not take the breast easily, but eventually he did, and I have heard the mother and baby went on to breastfeed very well.

In general, however, the shorter the time period after weaning, the easier it will be to get the baby to take the breast.

How long the baby breastfed before weaning

Generally, the longer the baby breastfed before weaning, the easier it is to get him back to the breast. This is a general rule only, and many exceptions occur. However, if the baby was breastfeeding well and exclusively for 16 weeks and was off the breast only two weeks, it is much more likely that he would take the breast than if he had never really breastfed well or had breastfed only eight weeks and was off the breast for two weeks.

The baby who is younger than a month or two, however, is in a somewhat different position. As you may have read in Chapter 10, When the Baby Refuses the Breast, if the mother's supply is abundant, many babies who would completely refuse the breast suddenly, for no obvious reason, take the breast between four and eight weeks of age, though on occasion this may occur even later. I have seen one such baby who finally decided to take the breast at four months of age. I have no explanation for this, except, perhaps, that if the milk supply is abundant, most babies eventually will take the breast.

However, many mothers probably stop trying before the baby decides to do the right thing.

The mother's determination

In many cases of relactation, the mother has to be very determined to get the baby breastfeeding again. In some cases, it is actually quite easy. In other cases, we expect that it will be easy, and yet it may not work. Or we think it impossible, and it works beautifully.

The mother who wants to relactate will have to put some work into it. Determination and the refusal to give up easily are the keys.

Relactation When the Baby Willingly Takes the Breast

If the baby takes the breast, this makes things a lot easier, in general. If he'll take the breast, start offering it, more and more. Especially at night, when some babies will be happy to suck even if they get little or no milk. Take the baby into bed with you, and let him suck on the breast as much as he wants.

There may be two patterns of acceptance actually. One is that the baby will take the breast and nurse as long as there is some reasonable flow of milk, but once that slows down, the baby will start to pull off. Or he may take the breast to soothe only, much as he would take a pacifier. He may not really care about milk flow. Or the baby may be content to pacify sometimes and drink others, combining the two patterns. It is important to recognize these patterns, I believe, because it will help in the process of relactation.

If the baby does, indeed, take the breast, it would be best to stop all artificial nipples as soon as possible. This may not be possible immediately, but it should be possible some of the time, at least. The best way is to provide any supplement with a lactation aid. The supplement should be given before the baby gets too upset at the breast, as soon as the milk flow slows down. The mother will know when the flow slows, because the baby no longer sucks with that open mouth wide–pause–close mouth type of sucking. The pause tells the mother the baby is getting plenty of milk still, but once that pause disappears, the baby is getting little milk, and will probably soon start to fuss. The flow should now be increased with the lactation aid.

If the baby pulls off and screams despite the lactation aid, perhaps cup-feeding or finger-feeding is possible. You are unlikely to get a four-month-old to finger-feed (though it's worth trying), and some mothers are not comfortable with cup-feeding a baby under six months of age (though it is easy for many young babies to cup-feed), so a bottle may be necessary sometimes. The mother should not become frustrated because the baby is not always willing to stay at the breast, and sometimes giving a bottle helps to make the baby less frustrated. There is a fine line between determination to keep at it, and knowing when not to push too hard.

On the other hand, the baby who is sucking at the breast mostly for comfort may not be too keen to get extra milk, especially if he has just fed. This baby may pull off as milk starts to come from the lactation aid. Go a little more slowly. Use compression to get him used to receiving milk from the breast. Keep him at the breast as much as he will stay there, even if he doesn't get much milk. As the milk supply increases, he will grow accustomed to getting more milk at the breast. You can use the lactation aid [with the bottle fairly low] so that only small amounts of supplement will get to him. Or if you are using a manufactured lactation aid,

use the smallest tube available. If you wait until the baby gets quite sleepy before starting the lactation aid, you may find he will accept it more readily.

As the baby accepts the breast more, and gets more milk from the breast, you will find that he may stay at the breast for whole feedings and that he will always accept the breast. Remember how to know the baby is getting milk at the breast. Perhaps if he drinks several minutes with the open mouth wide–pause–close mouth type of suck, he won't need any supplement. This should all come naturally. Don't hold back the supplement if the baby obviously needs it. Don't give it if the baby breastfed well. If you are not sure, offer it, and if he does not want it, he will pull off the breast.

During all this time, keep working to increase your milk supply. Even if the milk supply is good, if you cannot manage to keep the baby at the breast for all feedings, it is worth increasing the supply.

Increasing the Milk Supply

The milk supply may be increased in several ways. (Refer also to the accelerated protocol described earlier in this chapter.)

Expressing milk

Getting milk out of the breast stimulates the hormones of lactation to start working again. Whether you do this with your hand, or a pump, or directly into the baby (breast compression), getting milk out of the breast will increase your supply. Of course, the best way is to use compression to get more milk into the baby. Since the baby gets the milk directly, it eliminates some extra work for the mother.

If you are going to use a pump, get a good one

(renting is often less expensive), especially one that can pump both breasts at the same time. It is also worth learning to express by hand, since once you are used to it, it is often more convenient than having to hook up to a pump. Many mothers prefer it to the "industrial" approach of the machine.

You should express *after* feedings at the breast, not before, since you want your baby to take as much of your milk as possible directly. Always use breast compression once the baby does not nurse on his own. Express manually or with a pump as often as is reasonable in your circumstances. See also Chapter 5 for more information on compression.

Herbs

Herbs have been discussed in Chapter 5, Not Enough Milk. Fenugreek (*Trigonella foenum-graecum*) and blessed thistle (*Cnicus benedictus*) are two that I have found useful. It should be said that very little scientific study has been done on these herbs, but nevertheless, they do seem to work for some mothers. They tend to work better early in lactation (before the baby is six or so weeks old), but can work at any time. The mother has to take a lot (teas probably don't do the trick, as the mother would have to drink so much that she would be in the bathroom most of the day), and I generally suggest three capsules three times a day of each.

Other herbs used to increase the milk supply are fennel *(Foeniculum vulgare)*, goat's rue *(Galega officinalis)*, and garlic *(Allium sativum)*. As I have not used them or had any experience with them, I cannot comment. At least it can be said that they will probably do no harm.

Domperidone

Domperidone has already been discussed. It should be started as soon as the mother has decided to relactate. This drug gets into the milk in only tiny amounts, but in the case of relactation, when the mother's supply is not yet full, the baby will get even less. Though there has never been a drug that has no side effects, domperidone is generally safe for the mother and also for the baby, since only very small quantities pass through the milk. This is the medication of choice for helping with relactation.

Metoclopramide (Maxeran or Reglan) works well, but is associated with many side effects in the mother, including depression after long-term use. Unfortunately, in the United States, domperidone is not available.

Relactation When the Baby Will Not Take the Breast

If the baby will not take the breast, the best hope is to increase the milk supply. Again, babies will go where they get milk. It is sometimes possible to trick a sleepy baby to take the breast, but it is better not to fight him. In the first two months, babies will often take the breast on their own, between four and six weeks of age, if the mother's supply is abundant.

If all the best efforts with the help of a good lactation consultant do not seem to get the baby to the breast, a nipple shield might be worthwhile trying. I believe it is a last resort only.

It is worth increasing the milk supply regardless, since, even if the baby never takes the breast, at least he will get breastmilk. A good supply is important, too, if you are going to use a nipple shield.

When my first child, Ruthie, was born, I looked forward to breastfeeding her as the natural and obvious way to nurture her. Two of my sisters had wonderful experiences breastfeeding their babies, and they provided me with plenty of support, encouragement, and information even before Ruthie was born.

My labor with Ruthie was relatively short and easy. She was born a healthy 3.1 kg [6 lb 13 oz], and nursed immediately following her birth. During our 48-hour hospital stay, she roomed in with me, was fed on demand, and I thought that everything was fine, despite the fact that I developed sore, cracked, bleeding nipples from the second day on. [*Of course, everything was not fine, and Ruthie was not latched on well, as shown by the sore, cracked, and bleeding nipples!*]

After we got home, on the fifth day of her life, Ruthie began to refuse the breast. At that time, we had many visitors arriving from near and far to see the new baby, and our home was full of commotion. When I tried to put Ruthie to the breast, she fussed and cried, and I could not get her to calm down and take the breast. I was not willing to simply give her a bottle. In despair, I called up my midwife, who referred me to a lactation consultant.

With the help of the lactation consultant, we succeeded in getting Ruthie to the breast, with improved positioning, and she had what I believe was her very first good feed.

Unfortunately, when we got home, she continued to refuse the breast. The lactation consultant then advised me to begin to express milk, and she attempted, over the phone, to describe how to finger-feed Ruthie. At that time good breast pumps were unavailable where we lived, but I did manage to get hold of a poor quality electric pump. We did not manage with the finger-feeding, which seemed cumbersome and complicated. Both my husband and I were exhausted and stressed out, so we proceeded to bottle-feed Ruthie, with whatever milk I could express, in addition to supplementing with formula.

During the following days, we got into a routine of pumping my milk as often as possible, while feeding Ruthie whatever milk I expressed, by bottle. I offered her the breast now and then, but to no avail. She continued to fuss and cry and push away. I was exhausted, worn out, and discouraged.

When Ruthie was 11 days old, I woke up one morning with a high fever. One of my breasts was warm and tender. I called my doctor, who had me come in for an "after hours" private visit, at a very high price. The price was high in more than one sense, as she told me that I had mastitis, and I must immediately start taking antibiotics, and immediately stop breastfeeding. She told me to bind my breasts in a tight wrap, and to absolutely forget about breastfeeding. [*Very poor advice, but unfortunately advice that is still given out by some health care professionals.*]

As determined as I had been initially about breastfeeding, I must say that after all I had been through with Ruthie, this brought a certain element of relief. I was sick, exhausted, and worn out physically and emotionally. In a way it was just what I needed: "permission" to give up, and resort to the predictable and simple alternative of bottle-feeding. I rationalized that a baby can do "just fine" on formula, and can be loved and nurtured just the same as a breastfed baby.

Ruthie did seem to do fine on formula. But as

I recovered from the mastitis, started getting more sleep, and began to adapt to life with a new baby, my sadness about not breastfeeding her grew stronger. It was almost a feeling of grief. Whenever I saw another baby breastfeeding, such as in the pediatrician's office, tears would come to my eyes, and I would go home and cry over the loss of breastfeeding Ruthie.

One day, I read in one of my baby care books that it is possible to switch from bottle-feeding to breastfeeding. I was excited at the idea that maybe, just maybe, it could be possible in my situation with Ruthie. At the time she was about six weeks old. I tried to put her to the breast, just out of curiosity, to see what she would do. I had no expectations whatsoever. To my amazement, Ruthie latched on to the breast, and remained calm. It had been over four weeks since I had last tried to express milk. Ruthie was completely bottle- and formula-fed, and yet, she sucked at my breast. She stayed there for about five minutes.

I was very worried that if I tried again too soon, she would begin to fuss and refuse the breast, as she had that first week. I tried again a few hours later, and again she latched on and sucked, this time for about 10 minutes. I decided that I would keep trying, every few hours, and gradually try to increase the time that she was at the breast, as long as she was calm and willing.

On the second or third day of this, I called the lactation consultant to get some guidance and advice on how to proceed. Ruthie was still getting all of her feedings as bottles of formula, but she was at the breast for 15 or 20 minutes, five or six times a day. The LC told me to keep her at the breast for as long as she wanted, as often as she wanted. She advised me to decrease the amount of formula she was getting by about a third to half the amount, and to take Ruthie to be weighed twice a week. She said that the weight gain could slow down during this time that I was rebuilding the milk supply, yet it was important to know that she was not losing weight. I could not tell at that point how much milk Ruthie was getting at the breast. I was keeping her at the breast for long periods of time, sometimes for hours, while she would doze off and sleep intermittently. I kept a log of the bottle-feeds, and the amount of formula and number of bottles gradually decreased. I think I didn't believe that she would ever get back to exclusive breastfeeding, but compared to what I had been through, I was thrilled at the idea that she would be even partially breastfed, and I'd be able to nurture her at the breast.

I remember that breastfeeding her during this time became my absolute one and only priority. Ruthie was my first child, so I was able to devote all of my time to her. I rented movies to watch while she was at the breast for long periods of time, I read, talked on the phone and even slept while feeding her. I was on the phone with the LC almost daily to report our progress, and get her advice and encouragement.

After about two weeks, the bottle-feeds decreased to about twice a day, once in the afternoon, and once right before bedtime. I think there was a period of four or five days where we always kept an emergency bottle "just in case," which she sometimes needed, and sometimes did not, until she eventually did not need any supplement. About three weeks after beginning relactation, Ruthie was exclusively breastfed.

This was a triumph for me. I had been extremely motivated and determined, and I also could not have done it without the help and support of my husband, who took upon himself all the chores, in addition to long hours at work, to enable me to completely devote myself to breastfeeding Ruthie.

Ruthie continued to nurse until she was 16 months old.

This mother and baby were able to restart breastfeeding because the mother was determined and had plenty of support from her family and a lactation consultant. However, if she had used a lactation aid instead of bottles to supplement the baby, it is probable that the whole process could have been easier and faster. In addition, the use of fenugreek and blessed thistle, plus domperidone if needed, to increase what she felt was a low milk supply, might also have helped to bring about exclusive breast-feeding more rapidly.

As is obvious from this nursing couple's story, things can work even when the situation is not ideal. We have learned a lot over the years, though, and I think more mothers would succeed with relactation—and succeed more quickly—using these new techniques.

Of course, the real goal is to have all new mothers starting breastfeeding with good help and support, so that relactation isn't necessary.

Last Word on Relactation

If you stopped breastfeeding because you were given poor information (for example, you were told you must stop because of medication, or X-ray), do not forget to give feedback to the people who gave you this wrong information. These professionals will not change their ways if they do not hear that they gave poor information. Let them know nicely, but let them know. Most

health care professionals are not maliciously trying to stop you from breastfeeding (though some are). They would be pleased to know that your baby did not have to stop breastfeeding, and they may take that into account the next time a similar situation arises.

Breastfeeding After Breast Surgery

Breasts, Women, Surgeons, Society

The phenomenon of women getting cosmetic surgery on their breasts is something that has always intrigued me. I do not want to judge other people, and I hope I have not done so too often in this book (except with regard to health professionals, many of whom really do need to shape up with regard to their knowledge of breastfeeding). But I cannot understand how women would subject themselves to such major surgery in order to change their breasts so that the breasts are "more attractive" to men. Frankly, it seems to me that it is best to run, not walk, from a man who is attracted only to the size or shape of a woman's breasts, or for whom the size or shape of the woman's breasts is a major factor in whether he would be interested in her.

I realize that this is a function of our society, as well. Just as we live in a bottle-feeding society, we live in a society where breasts are for sexual attraction, for selling beer and automobiles, not for nurturing babies. When fashion dictates that a certain breast size or shape is fashionable, many women feel they have no choice but to conform.

I also realize that not all breast surgery is cosmetic, and that breast reduction surgery is sometimes done for medical reasons. Nevertheless, much surgery done on women's breasts is unnecessary, and even when necessary, is done without consideration of future breastfeeding.

This becomes obvious when one considers that many surgeons will operate on a woman's breast through an incision that follows the border of the areola (a periareolar incision). This incision, in many cases, decreases the present or future milk supply considerably. Not in all women, and not always enough to make a difference, but this incision probably interrupts nerves that send impulses to the brain to release the lactation hormones. This incision also is done where the ducts converge into a smaller area and are thus more susceptible to damage. The extent of the damage would depend on whether the incision completes the circle of the margin of the areola or is only partial, and whether, as in breast reduction, the areola and nipple are actually moved.

Why is the incision made in this area? Surely pain after surgery is greater in this area than it would be on the part of the breast closer to the woman's chest. Perhaps technically it is easier, but I doubt it. The incision is placed here because it looks better. Ah, yes, that's it, isn't it? Breasts are to attract men, not to make milk. Surgeons assume the woman would be more concerned about having attractive breasts than about breastfeeding. Of course, this may be true at the time the surgery is being done. But often women regret not being able to breastfeed because of surgery done many years before.

I try to be objective about this, but I do not find the periareolar incision more attractive. On the contrary, I find it less attractive. It is jarring to see that scar surround the areola—and you can see it, that's for sure.

To emphasize the point yet more—I have seen a few women who had breast surgery because one breast was much different in size from the other. The women wanted to have the breasts look the same. They went to a surgeon and were told there were two options: to reduce the larger breast, or augment the smaller one. The surgeon, in all cases, encouraged the women to reduce the larger breast! I am not sure why the surgeon would push this option— perhaps because of concerns about breast implants, or because the woman herself said she would prefer smaller breasts. However, by reducing the larger breast, in all cases, the surgeon's choice resulted in serious compromise of those women's ability to breastfeed. What was obvious on even casual examination was that the smaller breast was not fully developed, that it did not have a lot of milk-producing tissue. It would have been more logical to me to augment that side and leave the other alone, significantly improving the mother's chances of breastfeeding success.

Finally, even when surgeons do operate on the breast and make the incision in the "body" of the breast, they often make circumferential incisions (following around the curve of the breast). Circumferential incisions are likely to cut many more ducts than are radial incisions (where the incision goes in the direction of chest to nipple). There are really no surgical advantages to making circumferential incisions, and they should be avoided.

Breast Reduction, Breast Augmentation

One of the major problems is that breast reduction or breast augmentation surgery is often done on teenagers, before they have ever thought of having children, and, in our society, of using their breasts for what they were really designed to do, nurture those children. As well, even if the question of breastfeeding comes up, the answers are often incomplete or just plain wrong.

The women undergoing the surgery will often be told either that it will not interfere with breastfeeding at all, or that they will not be able to breastfeed at all.

In fact, breast augmentation, if done by placing the sac that enlarges the breast through an incision under the breast near the chest wall, should not interfere with breastfeeding. If however, the surgery is done through the areola, then even augmentation surgery can have a devastating effect on the mother's milk supply.

If the surgery is done through the areola, the milk supply is compromised. For some women who might otherwise have been able to nurse triplets exclusively, this may not be of much consequence. But some new mothers have just enough milk for their single baby. These women, if they had had breast augmentation or reduction done this way, would now be pushed into the "not enough milk" group.

The question of breastfeeding after breast reduction or any surgery through the areola is not "Will I be able to breastfeed?" but rather

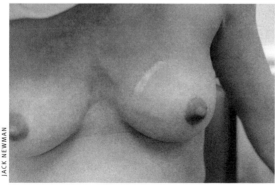

Scar from operation to drain a breast abscess. This circumferential incision is more likely to interfere with future breastfeeding than if the incision had been made at right angles to this incision.

"Will I be able to breastfeed exclusively?" And the answer to that will not be known unless the mother gets the best possible start with breastfeeding and gets good help and support. Even then, it may not be possible to say definitively, because many women inexplicably produce a lot more milk for one baby than for another.

The approach to breastfeeding should be to get that good start, to get that good help, and if the baby really does not appear to be getting enough from the breast, then to supplement (if possible, with banked breastmilk) through a lactation aid. Again, there is more to breastfeeding than breastmilk. And with a lactation aid, a baby and a mother can breastfeed for as long as they want. Years, if they want.

If a woman has had breast surgery, especially the type that involves a periareolar incision, and especially where the nipple and areola have been moved, then it might be worth starting fenugreek and blessed thistle as soon as the baby is born, as soon as the mother is up to it. This may allow for a better start (babies breastfeed better when they get more milk, and if they breastfeed better, they stimulate the breasts to produce more milk) and more successful breastfeeding.

If it turns out that the baby does, in fact, need to be supplemented, a lactation aid should be used. Once the baby is a little older, it might be worth trying domperidone.

Again, the idea here is to breastfeed, not necessarily to produce all the milk the baby needs—though obviously this would be best. But best is not always possible, and sometimes it is better to settle for a good breastfeeding relationship with some supplementation (again, donated breastmilk through a milk bank would be the best supplement, rather than formula).

What about blocked ducts?

Many women who have had surgery on the breast worry about having blocked ducts, but in my experience this is *not* more common than in women who have not had the surgery. The treatment of blocked ducts in the woman who has had surgery is the same as in the woman who has not. (See Chapter 7, Sore Breasts.)

If you have had breast surgery, or are adopting a baby, you can breastfeed. You may not produce all the milk the baby needs, maybe not even more than a small percentage of what the baby needs. But even this small amount of milk will benefit your baby, and you will both benefit from the nursing relationship.

If you have stopped breastfeeding and wish to relactate, in most cases you will be able to produce milk. With luck and determination, you should be able to get the baby back to the breast.

Unhelpful Medical Professionals

One of the hardest situations for new parents is when their baby is in the hospital, needing medical care, and they find themselves dealing with medical professionals who are not supportive of breastfeeding. Unfortunately, this happens quite frequently because most doctors and nurses have almost no training in breastfeeding, do not understand why it is important, and have no clue about how to help mothers breastfeed successfully, especially in situations where the baby may be ill or unable to go to the breast.

Remember that physicians give medical *advice*, not commandments. This is still your baby, and you have the right to make the decisions. Ask lots of questions about why your doctor is recommending weaning, or formula supplementation, and ask to see the research supporting those recommendations. You do not have to produce research supporting breastfeeding; it is the normal, optimal way to feed a baby.

Sometimes it turns out that your doctor is recommending weaning because he believes it will be easier for you, the mother—you'll be able to go home and get some rest while the nurses feed the baby formula. The nurses have been discouraging you from pumping because they think you'd prefer to get more sleep. Let them know that breastfeeding is important to you and your baby.

It might help to put things in writing. When Teresa's son and daughter-in-law had a premature baby and were told he might need supplementation with formula to prevent low blood sugar, they wrote out a list of the supplementation approaches that would be acceptable to them: the mother's expressed colostrum; adding sugar water to the mother's expressed colostrum; or, if needed, donated breast milk, which they would arrange to collect from mothers they knew personally. All supplements were to be given by gavage tube and not by bottle. If it were absolutely necessary, an intravenous system could have been started. The hospital said they would have to sign a waiver to give their baby the donated breast milk, which they were happy to do. Fortunately, the baby's mother produced plenty of colostrum and other supplements were never needed. Parents have also made little cards saying "No formula" or "No bottles or pacifiers" or "I'm an EXCLUSIVELY breastfed baby" to put in their baby's isolette.

But it can be a difficult struggle. You are already worried about your baby's health, and you don't have the energy to get into a battle over breastfeeding. It may help you to know that if you keep up your milk supply, almost all babies can be brought back to the breast. So if the medical staff insists on giving your baby bottles and/or formula, continue pumping and perhaps take the herbal supplements recommended elsewhere to keep or develop a good milk supply.

Ask that they use the milk you pump as much as possible to feed your baby, and when you bring your baby home you can start the process of transitioning him back to the breast.

IV

You and Your Breastfed Baby

15

Breastfeeding and Other Foods

Myth: Breastmilk is missing some things that are important to the baby's health.

Fact: Breastmilk is the perfect food for human babies, and is all the vast majority of babies need until the middle of the first year of life (around six months). Other animals produce milk that is quite suitable for their own babies and which is missing nothing. Why would humans not make milk appropriate for their babies?

While this seems obvious, many people—including some professional medical associations—think that human milk is missing lots of things. They calculate that breastmilk may not provide enough vitamin D or iron. But their thinking uses the artificially fed baby as the model of normal. Breastfed babies do just fine on breastmilk alone, without anything added, for about six months, despite these calculations.

Vitamin D

Vitamin D is a fat-soluble vitamin, which means it can be stored in the body to be used in periods of scarcity. It can be obtained from the diet, although not easily (liver is a good source, but . . .). For that reason, in most North American jurisdictions, vitamin D has been added to milk. But the easiest way to get vitamin D is through exposure to the ultraviolet rays of the sun. Ultraviolet radiation reacts with chemicals (previtamins) in the skin to produce vitamin D. Note that it is not necessary for it to be sunny for you to get vitamin D this way, since ultraviolet rays pass through cloud cover. It is true that clouds and pollution decrease the amount of ultraviolet radiation, but most people get enough from outside exposure. Rickets, the disease caused by a lack of vitamin D, is now rare in North America. Incidentally, exposure to the sun through glass (as through a window) does not expose you or the baby to ultraviolet rays, and will not give you vitamin D.

During pregnancy, the mother passes on vitamin D to the baby, and if the mother herself has adequate supplies of vitamin D, the baby will have enough on board at birth to keep him going for at least a few months. Breastmilk has small amounts of vitamin D, but these alone would not be sufficient to prevent vitamin D deficiency.

One reason vitamin D deficiency has not disappeared is that people go outside less and less, and have less ultraviolet exposure. The recent concern about getting "too much sun" is valid, but as with so many things, it has resulted in an overreaction. A study in Wisconsin a few years ago showed that exclusively breastfed babies did not develop low vitamin D levels during the first six months of life, even though their ultraviolet exposure during the winter months was effectively nil. If the baby gets some ultraviolet exposure, especially during the warmer months, and has stored up plenty of vitamin D during pregnancy, there is no need for extra vitamin D.

Research suggests that if the baby is wearing only a diaper, he needs about five minutes a day of sun exposure to get plenty of vitamin D. In cooler weather, with just his face and hands exposed, 10 to 20 minutes a day is enough. If you live in the far north, or if your baby is dark-skinned, you may need up to 30 minutes of exposure to the sun three or four days a week. Remember that vitamin D is stored in the baby's liver, so it isn't essential to get those five minutes every single day, and that your milk does contain some vitamin D as well.

It is true that some mothers do not have adequate stores of vitamin D when they become pregnant, and thus the baby may not get enough vitamin D stored up during pregnancy. Some reasons: the mother is dark-skinned, doesn't get vitamin D from her diet, or does not get much sun exposure. Why is dark skin a concern? Darker skins developed in people who were living in areas where there was a lot of sunlight, to protect the skin from sun damage and perhaps even an overdose of vitamin D. Actually, it might be more accurate to say that light skin developed as an adaptation for people who live

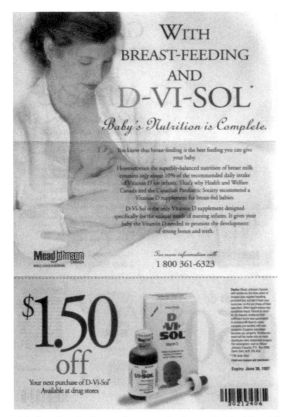

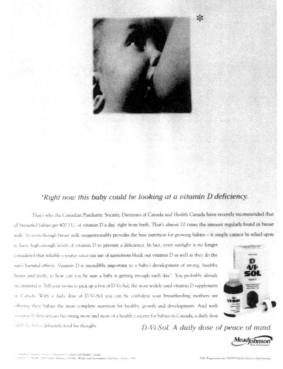

Ads for vitamin D supplements for breastfed babies. The one on the left is directed to mothers, the one on the right to pediatricians. By implying that breastmilk is incomplete, the ads make people doubt that breastmilk is, in fact, better than formula, since the formula-fed baby does not seem to need extra vitamin D.

in climates where there is *not* very much sunlight. But nature didn't anticipate African mothers living in Norway. People who have dark skin but live in areas where there is less available sunlight (or where the weather is too cold to expose their skin to the sun much of the time) may not be getting enough vitamin D.

In North America, there are many women now who are veiled and who have gotten almost no sun exposure for many years. In such a situation, it is not certain that extra vitamins, at least in the doses usually given during pregnancy, will provide enough vitamin D for the baby to store up adequate amounts. When there is a risk of vitamin D deficiency, the baby should get extra vitamin D.

However, this situation applies only to a small percentage of mothers and babies. The majority of exclusively breastfed babies do not need extra vitamin D.

Why is this an issue? First of all, if we say that all breastfeeding babies need vitamin D, we are saying that breastmilk is incomplete. One formula company, which also makes vitamin D, has come up with pamphlets and advertising for parents that trumpet, "With breastfeeding and (our brand of vitamin D), baby's nutrition is complete." Message received, loud and clear. Of course, formula-fed babies do not need the supplement of vitamin D, because formulas are complete. Well, they aren't, but we pretend they are. In addition, vitamin D is not given away, at least in the drugstore. It is free from the sun, but in the drugstore it is pretty pricey. So another reason to breastfeed—that breastmilk is free—is gone.

Iron

Exclusively breastfed babies get all the iron they need during the pregnancy, and from the small amount of iron that is in the breastmilk. There are good reasons for there to be small amounts of iron in breastmilk. Mother Nature knows best. One is that iron is needed by many bacteria in order to multiply, so having only a little iron around decreases the growth of these bacteria. There is even a protein in breastmilk, lactoferrin, which binds to available iron and prevents its use by bacteria. Lactoferrin also makes it possible for about 50 percent of the iron in breastmilk to be absorbed by the baby, and thus be available for use in the making of red blood cells.

Iron from formulas or cereals is poorly absorbed. Probably less than 5 percent of the iron from cereal, for example, is actually absorbed into the body. Thus, a lot has to be added, and this results, frequently, in the baby getting constipated. Though studies have been done that do *not* show an increase in constipation in formula-fed babies getting high iron formulas, this is not what seems to be happening in the real world. The only exclusively milk-fed babies I have seen with bowel movements that looked like rabbit droppings were being fed iron-enriched formula.

In general, a baby who is exclusively breastfeeding needs no extra iron until after six months of life, more or less. There are exceptions. Babies born quite premature probably do need to get extra iron because they did not get the stores of iron from the mother that are usually transferred during the final 12 weeks. If the baby has lost a lot of blood around delivery or for other reasons, he may need extra iron, but this would be an unusual situation.

The best way for a six-month-old or so baby to get iron is through his food. Iron-enriched cereals are not necessary, and, as mentioned earlier, may be constipating. The easiest way for a baby to increase his iron intake is through meat. There are others, but this one is easiest. More on starting solids below.

Water

Breastmilk is about 90 percent water. There is no need to give the baby extra water, even in hot weather. Several studies on exclusively breastfed babies in hot climates showed that extra water does the baby no good. If your baby seems thirsty, put him to your breast.

Does the baby need extra fluids or calories in the first few days?

Hardly ever. Often it seems like it because so many babies are so poorly latched on that they cannot get the milk that is available. There is milk (colostrum) present, but many babies don't get much of it. There is nothing wrong with keeping the baby at the breast for long periods during the first few days, if the baby is truly latched on and if your nipples do not hurt. If your nipples do hurt, or if you are not sure the baby is getting on well, get help with the latch from someone who knows what she or he is doing. If the baby is well latched on, and your nipples are not sore, lie down with your baby and let him nurse. Compression works particularly well in the first few days to help the baby get more milk. Once the milk becomes abundant, after the first three or four days, the baby will get milk much faster.

Hypoglycemia (Low Blood Sugar)

The premature baby, the stressed baby (who has had a difficult birth, for example, or who has gotten cold), or the infant of a diabetic mother are at risk of developing low blood sugar soon after birth. Not all of them do, but the risks from low blood sugar are too great to be ignored in high-risk babies.

However, the healthy, full-term baby should not be tested routinely for blood sugar. Why not?

- Nobody really knows what a normal blood sugar is in a healthy newborn.

- The sticks used for the test are not made for testing low blood sugars. They were made for testing *high* blood sugars. Many factors particular to the newborn make them quite inaccurate.

- Even if the blood sugar is somewhat low, no one knows what this means. There is no evidence that a slightly, or even somewhat, low blood sugar in a baby with no symptoms causes any problems. This is because the healthy, full-term newborn has other sources of energy for his brain that protect him.

Thus, the asymptomatic baby should be at the breast from birth, since the best way to prevent cold stress and to prevent low blood sugar is early breastfeeding, with the baby and mother in skin-to-skin contact. Colostrum is better for preventing low blood sugar than the formula that is all too often suggested by health professionals as the first choice. Colostrum stimulates the production of ketones, which is one of the alternative fuels a newborn baby can use to nourish his brain. Colostrum does not stimulate insulin production the way formula does, so it is better for preventing low blood sugar, but, of course, the baby has to *get* the colostrum, and that means early feeding and a good latch.

What if my baby is at high risk? (I have insulin-dependent diabetes.)

This does not mean that he needs to be fed formula. Since the heel stick and paper measure of blood sugar is not a good way of knowing the baby's blood sugar (although it can be used as a rough screen), and since the only way to get a good measure is to take blood from a vein and send it to the lab, why not start an intravenous with glucose to protect the baby's sugar? This is what I would do, and this is what I would request if I were a diabetic woman who had just given birth. I would not want my baby exposed to nonhuman milk protein—even if the evidence that formula can cause diabetes were not as strong as it is.

Yes, it's more difficult, but if blood is being taken anyway, it's not that much more difficult. True, in some hospitals, the baby of a diabetic mother is given formula without tests being done. But this is not a good policy.

Yes, it's more expensive to run an intravenous in a baby. But this will prevent low blood sugar without interfering with the establishment of breastfeeding. A baby can be at the breast when an intravenous is running. If it seems to be unnecessary, and the baby is nursing well, the intravenous can be taken out. It will only be needed for a short time, until the baby is getting plenty of breastmilk.

If I were a diabetic mother, I would also start expressing and freezing colostrum during the last two or three weeks of the pregnancy, and let the hospital staff know that if they want to supplement the baby, they should use this colostrum. The colostrum can be given to the baby while he is breastfeeding through a lactation aid, perhaps with some sugar water added, if the mother has not been able to save very much.

These steps will help to prevent low blood sugar and at the same time not interfere with breastfeeding. Another option is to use banked milk for the infant of the diabetic mother.

Jaundice

Jaundice has been dealt with in a separate chapter. If the baby is breastfeeding well, there is no need to stop breastfeeding or to supplement breastfeeding. If the baby is not breastfeeding well, we should not stop breastfeeding, we should fix it.

Other "Reasons" to Supplement

A mother may be told that her baby needs to be supplemented because he hasn't passed urine, because his urine is red, because the baby is fussy, or because the baby is not settling.

Again, the approach should be to keep the baby at the breast. If the baby is not breastfeeding well, the mother should be helped to latch the baby on properly so that the baby *does* breastfeed well. If the baby is getting enough milk, but the mother is sore because the baby is feeding for long periods, fix the latch, do not give the baby a supplement. The mother can also use breast compression, as described in Chapter 5, Not Enough Milk, to increase the flow of milk. When supplements are truly required, expressed breastmilk is the best choice, and it should be given by one of the alternative methods discussed in Chapter 5. If expressed milk isn't available, a little sugar water given with a lactation aid will also work just fine.

Solid Foods

A generation or two ago, many physicians were recommending that babies be started on special infant cereals as early as three or four weeks of life. Six weeks was about as long as anyone would wait. Why so early?

Infant cereals were invented as a supplement to *formula feeding*. It was known that formulas were incomplete (most formulas at that time were made at home) and cereals were developed to overcome these nutritional inadequacies. (Actually, formula is still nutritionally incomplete. See Chapter 11, Breastfeeding While on Medication.) One of the biggest problems was the lack of iron in homemade formulas. So cereals with added iron were started early to prevent anemia. It is interesting to note that the problem of anemia was actually the problem of the *artificially* fed baby.

Since the 1930s, cereal has become a sort of magical food, something so special that many parents do not consider it a solid food, as if it were in a class by itself. Many mothers have said to me, "He hasn't started solids, but he's been on cereal for the past four weeks." Interesting concept. Of course, sometimes bottlefeeding mothers are adding the cereal to the bottle of formula, so I guess it doesn't seem like a solid food to them.

My personal experience with my own children has given me some perspective on this. My wife and I started cereal with our first two children when they were about six months old. Both spat it out immediately. We tried it a couple of times and they kept spitting it out. So we gave them the food they really wanted, which is what was sitting on our plates. With the third, we didn't even bother with the cereals.

The current mantra is to start solids at four to six months. Many breastfeeding mothers are told by their physicians to start solids at four months—just to be sure, I guess. Hidden in there is the suggestion that her breastmilk probably isn't good enough on its own.

I once sat beside a mother on the subway who was obviously just returning from the doctor's office. She had a sheet in her hand (which I read over her shoulder—couldn't help myself), that stated something like this:

Your Baby is Four Months Old
Start rice cereal, one or two tablespoons once or twice daily for a week.
At four months and one week, start oat cereal.
At four months and two weeks, start mixed cereal.

It went on until five months, when, presumably, the mother and baby would be seen again, and given careful instructions as to what to do for the next month about solids, including the stern warning about not starting fruits before vegetables. The mother would leave with another instruction sheet outlining the teaching she got so that she wouldn't make any mistakes.

What on earth is this all about? Preventing allergies? Sounds reasonable. One food only per week, so that if the baby has an allergic reaction, the parents will know what food caused it. And how will they know it's an allergic reaction? Because the baby gags on the cereal? Well, that could mean he doesn't like it, or it could mean he just isn't used to eating solids and he's learning. The same with vomiting food. If the baby gets diarrhea after eating, does this mean it's an allergic reaction? Not at all. Babies develop loose stools for any old reason, including that they are developing a cold, which would cause them to have a stuffy nose. Ah, a stuffy nose—so diarrhea with a stuffy nose is an allergic reaction? No, it might just be a cold. A lot of sugar in the solid food might cause loose bowel movements, too. What about a rash? Babies get rashes all the time, including hives, and even hives do not necessarily mean they have had an allergic reaction. Even if they are allergy-related hives, the reaction may be to a viral infection or some other cause, rather than the food. What about a rash around the mouth? Any six-month-old child who eats a strawberry will have a red rash around his mouth afterward. The strawberry (or tomato) has an acid juice that irritates the baby's skin. It's irritation, not allergy. There is such a thing as allergy, and allergies can be serious, but this is not the way to prevent them or detect them. It's an exercise in futility.

When mothers were being urged to start solids at three or six weeks, it was necessary to be very careful, but it was also inappropriate advice to be giving the baby solid foods at that age. When babies are starting solids around the middle of the first year, there is no need for such vigilance, except, perhaps, if the family history is a very allergic one. If you do have a strong family history of allergies, waiting until your baby is at least six months old and showing a definite interest in other foods is important. For your baby, introducing foods one at a time and avoiding those that frequently lead to allergic reactions might be a good strategy. Common allergens include cow's milk, peanuts or other nuts, seafood, eggs, wheat, and citrus fruits—but, of course, it is possible for an individual baby to have an allergic reaction to any food.

But even when you need to be somewhat cautious because of allergies, I'd encourage you to be as relaxed as possible about feeding your baby solid foods.

Philosophically, I am concerned that we are taking a normal process (eating) and thinking of it as something risky. There are, of course, concerns about our food and what goes into it, what is good food, and what might cause allergies and all that, but I think focusing on these risks can take all the pleasure out of eating for our children.

An Easier Approach

This is the way I would suggest babies start solids. This is an approach that depends on the baby's demonstrating that he is *ready* to eat solids.

One thing that is quite extraordinary about babies, especially breastfed babies, is that it doesn't matter how long they sleep—they always seem to wake up when the mother herself sits down to eat. I don't know how they know, but they know. In the first few weeks, especially, mothers and fathers are not always eating at the same time, but the baby does not

wake up when the father sits down to eat. Only when Mom does. It's miraculous, actually.

In any case, this means that the baby is often breastfeeding, or on the mother's lap, or at least at the table, when the mother is eating. Around four months of age, sometimes earlier and sometimes later, the baby will become very interested in this eating process. He will watch the food on the fork, from your plate to your mouth, and there is no doubt that this is fascinating for him. By six months of age, many babies will try to grab that food, and try to put it into their mouths. They're ready to eat, aren't they? Why make it a particular day? How is the baby so different at four months of age than when he was three months and 30 days, or at six months of age than when he was five months and 30 days?

Yes, I hear that some parents like schedules; they feel more secure with schedules. True. But having a baby is an opportunity to get away from that structured, scheduled approach to life. It's not bad. Life with children will be a lot easier if you learn early on to go with the flow rather than try to make them conform to schedules.

So what should the first foods be? If a baby is starting to eat at five to seven months of age (as most will, if left to do what they want), it really does not matter. There are some foods that are not a good idea, such as round slippery ones that can go down the wrong way into the lungs. If this happens, it is quite serious, so such foods must be avoided. Peanuts come immediately to mind. Highly spiced foods might be reasonable to avoid, since burning the baby's mouth with hot chilis might not be the best approach to getting him eating. But some babies will surprise you with their enjoyment of garlicky foods and other strong flavors.

Some foods are considered "highly allergenic." Egg white is one of them, but I would guess that it is less so if the baby is starting solids at six months rather than three months or three weeks. If allergies are a concern for your family, you might want to wait until your baby is over one year old to try him with egg whites. But generally, you can be very easygoing. If the baby grabs for your steak, cut off a piece and let him have it. He'll chew on it, he'll turn it into mush, he may not eat much at all. That's not the point. On this day when he is five months and three days, it is not important that he eat a lot of steak, or potato, or avocado or whatever.

What is important is that he start eating solid foods. He is ready. He wants to. Physiologically he is ready or almost ready. Soon he'll have teeth (the first two usually come out around six months of age, but babies actually can eat fine without teeth), and soon he'll be sitting up all by himself. He's shown you that he has the hand-and-eye coordination to pick up food and put it into his mouth. And he can chew.

So, let the baby eat what he wants, off your plate. Of course, you can mash it up for him, and if you can mash it up with a fork, that's good enough. It will be easier for him to pick up if it's not pureed. He may gag occasionally, and throw up the food. It looks dramatic, it's scary, but rarely does anything serious happen. Gagging or choking is a protective reflex to prevent the food going down the wrong way, and this reflex is very strong in babies of this age. Just don't give him a plateful of food and then leave the room.

But wouldn't it be better to have vegetables before fruit? No, not at all. Why? The usual answer is that if the baby eats fruit first, he'll get used to the sweetness and won't take vegetables. This is not true. In the first place, he has been getting sweetness all along, both figuratively and literally. No fruit tastes as sweet as breastmilk. Actually, if you think about it, the sweetness of breastmilk is a mystery. Why do formulas, which have, we are told, the same amount of sugar as breastmilk, not taste sweet (actually, they taste pretty awful). Just goes to show that measurement isn't everything.

Here are my suggested guidelines:

- No need for one food a week.
- No need for fixed amounts (e.g., 1 tablespoon, twice a day). Let him eat as little or as much as he wants.
- No need for special or commercially prepared baby foods, including baby cereals. No need for baby foods at all.
- No need to avoid particular foods (with a few exceptions).
- No need for a particular order for introduction of foods.

Easy Finger Foods

Your baby wants to feed himself? Try these to start:

—small chunks of ripe banana
—small chunks of peeled ripe peaches or plums
—pieces of cooled, baked sweet potato
—tender cooked meat (such as beef stew meat)
—pieces of cooked carrots
—grated apple or pear

Waiting Longer than Six Months

Some parents, for various reasons, want to wait longer before introducing solid foods—some as long as a year. It is not clear to me why they want to do this, especially since most babies are showing clear indications by six months that they want to eat. However, a baby who starts solids well at seven months of age is at no disadvantage compared to a child who starts at six months or four months of age.

Although there is evidence that a baby who is exclusively breastfed for six months has fewer allergies than a baby who is not breastfed exclusively or not breastfed at all, it does not follow that exclusive breastfeeding for a year will further decrease the risk of allergies. Furthermore, there is no study showing an increased risk of allergies in the baby breastfed exclusively only five months, say, compared to one breastfed exclusively six months.

The babies who are very late in starting solid foods are often those from allergic families, and tend to have allergies themselves (although these may not be apparent until they are older). These babies may adamantly refuse food at six months, seven months, eight months or longer. They may be willing to eat only very small amounts of certain foods, even at ten months or a year.

It is also possible that babies may develop deficiencies in iron and zinc if they are exclusively breastfed for nine months or more. Your baby may also have difficulty getting enough calories from just breastmilk. If your baby is still resisting solids at this age, you may want to consider giving him supplements of iron and zinc.

The best policy is to start solids when the baby shows interest in foods and a willingness to eat them. This is usually at around six months. If you keep offering a variety of foods, just making them available, your baby will probably start when the time is right for him.

What if he really wants to eat at 4½ months?

Well, it seems he is ready. Why stop him? I do not believe that if the baby wants to eat, the parents should stop him just to get to a theoretical "best age" to start introducing solids. It is often said that starting solids earlier than about six months of age will result in a decreased milk supply. This is possible, and there are studies that show this, but it usually doesn't matter that much. The baby will still like breastfeeding and get plenty of milk, and eat solids as well.

My baby is four months old and seems hungry (or not gaining well anymore).

The best approach here is not to start formula, as many mothers are tempted to do or are advised to do by their physicians. It would be far more appropriate to start solids (again, not necessarily cereal).

Refer to Chapter 5, Not Enough Milk. Compression may help the baby get more milk (see description in that chapter). If you are on a birth control pill that contains estrogen, stop it. Switch back and forth from breast to breast, as long as the baby is sucking well and clearly getting milk. Try the herbs. Domperidone could also be used.

If none of that works, well, start the solids. I think starting solids a bit early is better than giving the baby a bottle with formula—which, by the way, he may not take anyway. If he does take it, you may find that he will be taking it more and more, until he stops breastfeeding altogether.

Diaper Changes

When your baby begins eating solid foods, you will notice some changes in his bowel movements. Some babies may become constipated if they eat a lot of solids, especially highly processed foods (such as prepared baby cereals) or foods with added iron. Extra breastmilk will usually remedy that.

You might also see a number of foods—corn and raisins, for example—which arrive in the diaper completely undigested, even in an 18-

month-old. This is normal and not a cause for concern.

Some foods will also change the color of your baby's bowel movements—beets, for example, can turn them a dark reddish color. Large amounts of carrots or sweet potato will make them—you guessed it—bright orange. Again, no cause for concern.

When should I give solids, before or after breastfeeding?

Most of the time it does not matter. I think it is best to take a relaxed attitude toward this. After all, what do you do if the baby wants to eat solids because you are sitting at the table? Force him to take the breast on the assumption that he will take more milk if he feeds at the breast first? He probably will, actually, but so what? Breastfeeding, and the baby's and mother's enjoyment of it, almost always suffers when we make rules.

Let the baby eat when you eat. If it turns out that he hasn't nursed first, that's fine. As the baby gets older, there will be times when he will absolutely refuse to take the breast because he wants to eat what you are eating. Eight-month-old babies can be very determined. Other times, he'll be too hungry to mess with solids (which take longer for him to eat because he's still mastering the art of getting food from the high chair tray to his mouth), and he'll insist on nursing first.

On the other hand, sometimes it does matter. One way to get a baby off a lactation aid is to start him eating solids. As he takes more and more solids as food, the mother can usually wean him from the lactation aid. But not always. The reason? Even when he takes a lot of food, he likes the fast flow of milk when he's at the breast. If the milk is flowing quickly, he is usually content. If not, he may not be. A mother who has had a problem with milk supply may not have rapid flow. Even if all the formula has been replaced by an equivalent amount of calories in solid food, the flow of milk from the breast may not be fast enough for the baby, even though the mother is producing enough to make up the difference. The baby does not care what is *in* the breast, though. He cares what he gets. Compression can help, but not always, especially if the baby is very hungry. Thus, a solution to the problem of the baby who is fussy at the breast because of slow flow would be to feed him solids first, and then offer the breast. If the baby is not ravenous and has eaten some food first, he may nurse more calmly.

My 12-month-old (14-month-old, 18-month-old) is not eating and wants only to breastfeed.

It is better not to get into this situation. It is not always easy to deal with. And it is certainly easier to start babies on solids when they are showing signs of readiness. Some babies can maintain their caloric intake with breastmilk alone and gain weight appropriately, and that is good. But the baby will be needing extra iron, probably extra zinc and perhaps other elements as well. Some babies begin to gain poorly past six or seven months if they are only breastfeeding.

Some physicians will tell mothers to stop breastfeeding when the family is in this situation. This is not a good idea. A baby will not necessarily eat food if the breast is withheld. I have seen more than one case in which the child was forcibly weaned, but did not eat more. In one case, a 15-month-old was breastfeeding only, though she would take some Jell-O as well. When she would not eat other food, the mother was urged to wean her. She did, but the baby took only Jell-O, and instead of maintaining her weight as before (not gaining, but not losing), she started to lose weight.

Babies who are not getting adequate calories from breastfeeding alone should want to eat other food as well. But often they don't. They spend so much time at the breast that they refuse other foods. Therefore, one approach is to continue breastfeeding, but to stop each feeding as soon as the baby is not drinking well.

At this point, after the baby comes off the breast, he might take some solids. Anything, even chocolate, might be reasonable, just to get him to eat and get to like eating. Often a baby will take it better off a parent's finger than from a spoon. Banana is an easy food to give, and so is applesauce. Cooked, mashed sweet potato is another food that seems to appeal to many of these "fussy eaters."

It is often useful to take the baby to a parent and child drop-in center, especially around meal or snack times. Children are remarkable in noticing other children and what they do. Even if the other children are much older (say four or five years old), the baby will be fascinated by them, will want to imitate them, and often will copy their eating. Of course, if you have a toddler or older child, having him try to feed your baby may work.

Patience is necessary, for both you and the baby's doctor, who is often pushing to get your baby to take food. It is better not to get into a power struggle with your child. You will almost certainly lose. Put food in front of him, but don't watch him anxiously. He will know what you are doing. If the baby is not eating at 12 months, does it have to be today that he starts? A few weeks won't make any difference, as long as you are making progress. Slowly but surely is fine.

Sometimes what makes mealtimes more pleasant for the baby or toddler—and increases the odds of his eating—is to have him on your lap while you are eating and talking with other people. In that situation, when you are not paying much attention to him but are obviously enjoying the food, many babies will reach out and grab the food from your plate or spoon. I find many of these "noneaters" have either not been part of mealtimes with the family, or have spent the whole meal being coaxed to eat.

I have heard that zinc deficiency may cause a child to reject food.

I doubt this, but anything is possible. If you can get the baby to take zinc in medicinal form, perhaps he will start eating. And zinc deficiency may cause less than optimal growth, so it is a concern.

Ultimately, these children do start eating, but many of them are "picky eaters" all through childhood. As mentioned before, it is better to avoid getting into this situation. Do not delay the introduction of solids if your baby is showing readiness.

My baby won't take a bottle.

So? Babies can learn to drink from a cup, often by four months or younger, though they often resist learning when they are around four months. Once they are about six months of age, it is a good time to start offering a cup—especially since many babies are showing a desire to copy you by between five and six months of age. Start with water, because they are going to spill a lot of whatever is in that cup at first. Spilled water is less of a problem than apple juice, and not as heartbreaking as spilled breastmilk.

Many breastfed babies never drink from a bottle. They begin breastfeeding, start solid foods at around the middle of the first year, begin drinking from a cup soon after, and continue that way until they eventually wean from the breast.

Nutrition

Under most circumstances, babies will eat what they need. Do not try to force them to eat food that is "good for them." If your food is good for you, it will be good for them as well. No food, except breastmilk, is essential. If the baby does not like vegetables, but eats fruit and meat, that's fine. Trying to force him to eat spinach or mashed lima beans will only cause problems. Back in 1929, a study was done that showed if given a choice of a wide variety of foods, babies of about eight months of age will choose a balanced diet, even if on a particular day they eat only bananas and the next day only potatoes. Over a period of time, the diet is balanced.

Let your baby learn the pleasure of eating. Keep mealtimes relaxed. If he is enjoying eating, you don't have to worry about exactly what amounts of foods, and what foods, he gets. Offer a wide variety, and he will have a balanced diet.

By the way, eight-month-old babies make a real show of independence. They will often not want you to put the spoon into their mouths, but will try to grab it out of your hand. If they use the spoon themselves, they often turn it upside down, and the food falls into their laps. Fine. Encourage this independence and desire to do things on their own. Strip the baby down to a diaper and put a plastic cloth—an old shower curtain works well—under the high chair. It all washes off. His table manners will improve in a few years.

If you start adding other foods to your baby's diet when he is showing signs of being ready, and if you take a relaxed attitude about the whole thing, you allow your baby to learn that eating is a pleasant experience.

16

Sleep:
Yours and Your Baby's

Myth: Formula-fed babies sleep better than breastfed babies.

Fact: Even though many breastfeeding promoters say so, this is not really true, or not necessarily true.

Myth: If you bring your baby into your bed at night, you are starting a "bad habit" that will create ongoing sleep problems.

Fact: Babies have slept with their mothers for thousands of generations, and there is absolutely no evidence that this is harmful.

Many breastfeeding mothers find it easy to manage feedings at night if they keep the baby in bed with them, or if the baby sleeps in a bassinet or crib right beside their bed. Then it's a simple matter to just roll over and breastfeed the baby when he wakes in the night, or to pick the baby up and breastfeed. The "family bed" seems to be associated with breastfeeding for a longer period of time.

Does this mean you have to have your baby in bed with you to breastfeed? No, not at all. Each family needs to figure out what works best for them.

But I often hear from mothers who want to keep their babies in their beds, and who have been breastfeeding their babies each time they wake at

night, that they are dealing with a lot of criticism from other people. They are told that having the baby in bed with them and responding when the baby wakes at night will cause "unhealthy sleep habits," and that the baby who wakes at night and is nursed back to sleep has a "sleep problem."

There is a whole group of new pediatric specialists who deal with "sleep problems." These specialists believe that babies should not be breastfed to sleep, and that after a certain age, babies should not be nursed during the night. The old tactic of "letting the baby cry it out" is back in vogue (even though now it may be called "controlled crying" or "learning to self-soothe"). These specialists believe that a baby who wakes during the night after three or four months is not exhibiting "normal" behavior and has a sleep problem. This becomes a new classification of medical problem, and, unfortunately, many of the recommended "treatments" end up interfering with breastfeeding.

Let's consider, first of all, the question of the baby waking at night to feed. Is this normal, or is it a symptom of a sleep problem with potentially harmful long-term consequences?

Our perceptions of sleep have changed considerably over the past century. Here is a quote from a baby book of not too long ago:

"At birth the baby should sleep almost 23 hours out of 24.

He should sleep at least 18 hours a day until six months old.

At least 16 hours until one year old.

At least 14 hours until four years old, part of which should be in the afternoon at a regular hour.

The baby should sleep alone in a room or at least have a crib or a bed to himself. Never rock a baby to sleep. Never put a baby to sleep in your arms; it is a bad habit, tiresome for yourself and unwholesome for the baby."

(*Canada's Baby Book*, 17th edition, Rice Publishers, Montreal, 1928)

Really? He should sleep 18 hours a day until he is six months of age? Whose baby are they talking about? I have never heard of a baby at six months of age sleeping 18 hours a day, unless he was drugged up. Not even at three months. Perhaps some babies sleep a lot in the first two or three days of life, but after that—23 out of 24 hours? That's actually not good if the baby is over a few days old. Think about this in terms of actually looking after the baby, even if the baby is feeding just once every four hours, that means six feedings in 24 hours. He has only an hour, total, of time to get in six feedings, so we're alloting 10 minutes per feeding. Apparently the baby is also expected to sleep through bathtime and diaper changes.

Was this really true in 1928, or was this something that health professionals decided was "best for baby"? Probably it is the latter. And the same is true in this new century, when sleep experts decide at what age babies should sleep through the night and other "rules" for "normal infant sleep."

Let's look back to the time when our ancestors were living in tribal communities. Babies and their mothers slept together, usually with older children and fathers, too. It was safer that way. There was nothing easier for a lion or other carnivore to pick off than a single human sleeping alone. Humans slept together because it was safe, and because they felt secure doing it. Gorillas and other primates sleep this way. And of course, it is still the rule in traditional human societies around the world.

Human milk has adapted to this situation—or perhaps it is the other way around, that humans have adapted to their milk. There is a general relationship between the type of milk a species produces and how often the nursling goes to the breast. For example, rabbits feed only occasionally, and the protein in the mother rabbit's milk is quite high. The same is true for other animals that cannot afford to nurse too often, since, as prey of other animals, they have to be ready to run. Humans belong to another group of mammals that have low concentrations of protein in their milk, keep their young close to the parents, especially the mothers, and feed their young frequently.

In traditional societies, babies sleep next to their mothers and generally feed on and off throughout the night. Our society has changed a lot, and it is not always easy to do things as they were done before. But we should look carefully at any traditional activity we consider discarding. There may be greater consequences than we imagine.

It is quite normal for babies to want and need to feed at night. Most adults are used to sleeping a certain number of hours of uninterrupted sleep. Babies do not have to sleep an uninterrupted number of hours at night, and are usually quite happy and content to wake up frequently.

Just as in the case of colic, which eventually gets better, there will come a time when your child will sleep through the night. There will also be a time when he leaves your bed. You can be sure that when he is 16 years old, those night feedings and night wakings will be a distant memory! I have, in my office, a drawing called "Night Feeding" by a mother who nursed five children. It is obvious that, at least from a distance of several years, this was not a terrible time for her. Indeed, many mothers remember the night feedings as the best time they had with their babies—when it was just the baby and her, away from the rush and hubbub of the day.

Often, once mothers are reassured that night feedings won't lead to "unhealthy sleep habits" or an overly dependent child, or the other problems they've been warned about, they stop being concerned. When the baby sleeps next to his mother, their sleep and wake cycles match, so the mother is never jarred out of a deep sleep. She wakes up as her baby wakes up, they nurse, and they drift back to sleep together.

Be assured of the following:

Nursing your baby to sleep is not harmful

I suppose that it is nice if the baby can also fall asleep without nursing, but he will eventually be able to do that. Guaranteed. Maybe not at six months of age, maybe not at a year, maybe not even at two years, but eventually. Some pediatricians and other physicians view nursing a baby to sleep as being on a level with child abuse, yet are enthusiastic about making a baby cry himself to sleep. Something doesn't fit here.

One of the great pleasures of parenthood, in my opinion, is having a baby fall asleep in your arms. It makes you feel good. It makes you feel competent. *The little guy trusts me so much he will just fall asleep in my arms.* And the heat he gives off when he just falls into sleep—what a pleasure it is to feel that. But too many parents are being advised to make sure this never happens, because this will be spoiling the baby and he will never sleep through the night. It is not true.

Sleeping with your baby is not harmful for your baby, for you or for your partner

On the contrary, it is healthy for everyone. Many mothers and babies prefer sleeping together, and many fathers enjoy it, too. You are much less tired if the baby is sleeping next to you and wakes up for nursing. No need to get up and go for the baby. Yes, you must become very inventive with regard to intimacy—it just adds to the excitement.

Sleeping Arrangements

Parents have come up with many ingenious methods to keep their babies close to them at night. The simplest, of course, is just to bring the baby into your bed. Other strategies parents have used include:

A very young baby can sleep in a bassinet next to the bed.

An adjustable crib can be pushed up against the bed, so that the crib mattress is level with the bed, and the side dropped or removed.

"Side-car" beds are now available that attach to the parents' bed and consist of a small mattress with a railing around the other three sides.

Mattresses on the floor—queen-sized mattress for the parents, plus a single mattress pushed up beside it for the baby and any other children—provide lots of space, and no worries about falls.

A bed in the baby's room has helped some families where the father finds he doesn't sleep well with the baby close by. The baby goes to sleep, and is put in a crib in his room. When he wakes up, Mom feeds him in the bed in the baby's room, and they both spend the rest of the night there.

You will not roll over on your baby

Most parents will wake up when the baby changes his breathing, unless they have had a few drinks too many. How could a mother roll over on her baby and not know it? There is some evidence that crib death is slightly more common in babies who sleep in the same bed as their parents, *if either or both are smokers*, than in babies who sleep in a crib beside their bed. But the rate is still lower than if the baby sleeps in another room. Perhaps smokers should have their babies in a crib next to their bed, but in most cases it is perfectly safe to have the baby in your bed.

The Consumer Product Safety Commission in the United States recently started a campaign against co-sleeping based on a very flawed study. The study used reports of infant deaths—taken from newspapers and other unreliable sources, as well as coroner's reports—and came to the unwarranted conclusion that co-sleeping was unsafe for babies. The study lumped together all babies who died in places other than cribs—including those who died sleeping on couches and left alone in waterbeds. In some cases, the cause of death was unknown and could have been deliberate suffocation by an abusive parent, for example. The Commission also made no comparison to the number of babies who died in cribs. In fact, about 80 babies over 5 years died while in their parents' bed. Apparently 10 babies a day die of SIDS in the United States every day, which means that thousands of babies died while sleeping outside their parents' beds during the same period of time. The Consumer Product Safety Commission should be advocating that babies sleep in their parents' beds, for goodness' sake.

Some recent research from England found that breastfeeding mothers seem to instinctively sleep more safely with their babies. The researchers videotaped mothers and babies in bed together, and found that the breastfeeding mothers slept facing their babies with one arm resting on the bed above the baby's head. It is impossible to roll over on the baby in that position. The baby was also at breast height.

Bottle-feeding mothers, on the other hand, often slept with their backs toward the baby. In this position, the risk of rolling on the baby is somewhat higher (although it is still unlikely). The bottle-fed babies were often placed in the bed with their heads near or on the pillows, increasing the risk of suffocation.

Here is part of an e-mail I received about a 13-month-old baby.

> People comment all the time about how beautiful, sweet, healthy and friendly she is. She is truly a joyous child and is happy 95 percent of the time. She displays very little "separation anxiety," "stranger anxiety," or sleeplessness I read so much about—she has no fear of anyone or anything and happily appeases her curious nature. She is very affectionate and cuddly, yet independent, vastly different from the clingy, anxious, spoiled child I was told she would become if I continued to sleep with her or nurse her past the age of six months.

This mother was told by a psychiatrist "that my feelings of concern and protectiveness were not normal and that I must force myself to put her in her crib at night because that was the 'healthy thing to do.'" This is an incredible statement that the psychiatrist reportedly made. What could be more normal than for a mother to feel concerned and protective about her baby?

Another mother was told that putting the baby in a crib to sleep would help with the baby's verbal development, because when she woke up in the morning and was alone, she would talk to herself. If she kept the baby in her bed, the baby would be deprived of this valuable experience. This is simply not true. The baby who wakes up next to his parents has an actual person to talk to, and can have his babbling and early words responded to—a much better way to encourage language.

> **Research on Long-Term Effects of Co-sleeping**
> (from a paper by Dr. James McKenna)
> Heron found that children who never slept with their parents were less happy and had more temper tantrums than those who occasionally or always slept with their parents. They were also more fearful than those who always slept with their parents.
>
> Lewis and Janda reported that adult college students who had slept with their parents as young children had significantly higher self-esteem and less anxiety than those who had not.
>
> Crawford found that adult women who had slept with their parents as children had higher self-esteem.
>
> A study of children of military families, ages 2 to 13 years, found that co-sleeping children received higher evaluations from their teachers and had lower rates of psychiatric problems than those who had not slept with their parents.
>
> Mosenko studied a number of different ethnic groups, and found that co-sleeping in infancy and early childhood was associated with greater satisfaction in life and a number of other positive traits in adults.

Would my baby sleep longer if he were bottlefed?

This, I believe, is yet another myth that arises from using the bottle-feeding baby as our model

of "normal infant feeding." I believe this based on my understanding of breastfeeding, as well as on the stories of mothers who say that their babies sleep better when fed by bottle. It doesn't matter what is in the bottle. The baby sleeps four hours, for example, after four ounces of formula, but also after four ounces of breastmilk. Yet he will only sleep two hours when breastfed. Why would that be?

The answer goes back to how mothers are taught to breastfeed. When babies go onto the breast, rarely do they latch on in the mechanically most efficient manner for getting milk. This does not always matter, because in the presence of an abundant milk supply, the baby can do fine. However, this often means frequent, long periods on the breast. It also means frequent, long feedings at night. In most traditional societies, this is not a problem. Women in traditional African Bushman society apparently feed as many as four times an hour. If you are walking along, going about the business of the day, and the baby nurses all the while, almost without your noticing it, it is no big deal. If sleeping with your baby and having him nurse all the while is what society sees as normal, it is no big deal.

In North America, though, the baby who does not nurse effectively (for our "lifestyle," since the Bushman baby is nursing quite efficiently for *his* circumstances) will also want more frequent feedings. The baby does not get four ounces as he would from the bottle. The baby may get two ounces or even less, and not surprisingly, sleep only a couple of hours or less. Or he may stay on the breast because he is not satisfied and eventually fall asleep at the breast. The mother eases him off, and a few minutes later he cries.

If you want your baby to sleep longer between feedings, get the best latch possible. Use compression to increase the amount of milk the baby gets at the breast, and try to "finish" the first side before you offer the second. How do you know a baby is finished? Because he no longer actually gets milk (open mouth wide–pause–close mouth type of suck), even with compression. But remember, even when a baby may not be getting milk for a few minutes, there may be another letdown of milk and he will drink plenty. So don't be in a big rush to take him off the breast.

If your baby drinks really well, and gets plenty of the high-fat milk, he will, in fact, go several hours between feedings. As the weeks go by, he may stretch out the feedings at night, and eventually sleep through the night. I usually worry when a two-week-old is sleeping through the night, since this may indicate inadequate intake of milk, but I have seen exclusively breastfed, well-gaining babies who are, in fact, sleeping through the night at two weeks of age. There is nothing about formula that "makes" babies sleep longer. The determining factor is the quantity they get.

I realize that this is different from what you may have read elsewhere about breastmilk emptying out of the stomach faster than formula, or about certain amino acids in artificial milk that make the baby sleepier. There may be something to that, but, essentially, I believe that babies will be hungrier faster if they get less milk at the feeding, whatever that milk is. Overall, the amount the baby gets may be more than enough, but if the baby gets it in little "snacks," he will feed frequently.

So what do I do?

You can work to increase the effectiveness of your baby's latch so that he gets the maximum amount at each feeding, and this may encourage him to sleep longer. You can also continue feeding him at night as long and as often as he needs to with the confidence that this is not harmful or dangerous.

Dr. Spock Was Wrong

This one is our own story, so the names will not be changed to protect the innocent. Our first baby did not sleep through the night until he was four years old. At one point, we had decided it was getting too difficult, and we tried letting him cry it out. This was when he was seven-or-so months old. The first thing we found out was that the baby will cry longer than 20 minutes the first night. Dr. Spock was wrong. Not only will the baby often cry longer than 20 minutes, but even 20 minutes, to the ears of his parents, seems like about two hours. It is awful, and, truthfully, I don't know how some parents can survive it. Perhaps we should have been stronger, but we gave in. I think we were right. But we felt weak.

When our son was over two years of age, we thought we would try it again. (We were slow learners, but our excuse is that we weren't getting much sleep.) We finally gave in, as we heard him cry from his crib, "This is your little boy, Daniel. Why are you doing this?"

We can learn a lot from our children, if we let ourselves. I think we both learned a lot through this issue of sleep. Daniel is 26 years old at this writing. He is a great person (objectively speaking, of course). We survived the four years of sleepless nights. Well, not entirely sleepless—but interrupted. And we are glad we did what we did. It wasn't easy to be awakened every night, night after night. But after all is said and done, it was for the best.

Despite what is said and written about the need to build "healthy sleep habits" by leaving babies to cry themselves to sleep, there is *no* evidence that babies and young children who sleep with their parents, or who are rocked to sleep and responded to at night, grow up to have any more sleep problems than those who are left alone to cry. I always found that my kids were great sleepers—could sleep anywhere, in hotel rooms, other people's houses, tents. And consider this—it is in North America, where crying to sleep has been the approach recommended for babies for some time, that people spend millions on remedies for insomnia and sleep disorders.

A Dog's Life

On more than one occasion, I have seen dogs tied up to bicycle racks or lampposts while their owners are shopping or in the library, or otherwise engaged. The dog whines, cries, and all sorts of people, obviously unknown to the dog, come up, caress and even hug the dog in order to comfort it. Some of the people telling you to let your baby cry it out are probably dog-comforters. Why do people see the dog's crying as a signal that the dog needs comforting and should be responded to, but not have the same response to a baby's crying?

All Wait, No Gain

I have seen babies who stopped gaining weight after being "trained to sleep." The pattern seemed to be that the baby was left to cry, and was perhaps given a pacifier or learned to suck its thumb or two fingers to comfort himself and sleep. This also became common during the day, and the baby would frequently be seen sucking on his thumb or pacifier. The mothers were pleased because despite getting rid of the night feedings, the baby actually seemed to be feeding less often in the day, as well. It was only at the next doctor's visit that they discovered the baby

had gained no weight, or very little weight. And then the mothers called me for help.

Teresa, my co-author, tells me that she spent some time at the home of one of these mothers and it seemed to her that having left the baby to cry had "desensitized" the mother to her baby's cues. This little girl, about five months old, would start to fuss, or even cry, and seem hungry, but her mother would not respond. After a minute or so the child would pop her thumb in her mouth and either just sit in her seat sucking her thumb or actually go to sleep. Teresa spent some time getting the mother to see the child's cues and to offer the breast at those times.

I think that this crying to sleep teaches babies that even if they are hungry, nobody is coming to feed them, and they'd better find some other way to cope with it—and that some of them do the same thing during the day. It also seems to desensitize mothers—if you force yourself to ignore crying at night, I think it's almost inevitable that you become less responsive to your baby's cries in the daytime. And I think that for some babies, the result is that they don't get enough milk, and weight gain becomes a problem.

There are a lot more parents and children sleeping together out there than we know about. Many don't tell. But it's being done—and not only by breastfeeding mothers. Just as a child will eventually stop breastfeeding on his own if you and he allow yourselves the luxury of waiting until you are both ready, so will a child eventually leave your bed, when he's ready and when he's confident enough. When our last child finally left our bed, we were sad. But having children means adjusting to the fact that they will eventually leave you. It seems far off, but it happens much faster than you imagine.

> "The moment she had laid the child to the breast, both became perfectly calm."
>
> —Isak Dinesen, *Ehrengard*

Maybe using a pacifier will help?

In some cases, a pacifier will lengthen the time between feedings, and may result in the baby drinking more effectively. With increased time between feedings, the breast will be fuller, the flow faster, and it is quite possible the baby will drink better and be fuller. It is also quite possible that the baby will be so hungry by the time he gets to the breast that he'll fall asleep before he feeds well, or be too frantic to latch on to the breast well.

Pacifiers can be useful. Some babies drink so much milk so quickly that they are full before they have fulfilled their need for sucking. If they fill up and pull off the breast because they have had enough, but are obviously still needing to suck but fuss when they get more milk, then a pacifier may be the answer. I would suggest, however, trying two or three feedings on each side before resorting to a pacifier. In any case, make sure the baby is breastfeeding well and gaining well before you start the pacifier. Or let the baby suck on one of your fingers. The added benefit of this is that it has to be done with the baby in your arms and getting the same contact he would get if he were still at the breast. A baby with a pacifier can be put down in a crib or a little car seat and left alone, and while he may get the extra sucking he wants, he'll miss out on being held, which is also important.

Will giving cereal in the evening help?

Studies that have looked at this question do not support the notion that giving cereal will help the baby sleep longer. There is actually no reason why they should. If the baby gets enough to drink at the breast, he should not be fuller if given cereal. Some mothers swear that this has helped, though. Perhaps these babies who do sleep better once they get the cereals in the evening are getting much less at their evening feedings. Use of compression, switching back and forth, or herbs may help. If the baby definitely is hungry in the evening, or throughout the day, the milk supply may have decreased. Are you on estrogen-containing medication? Stop the medication if at all possible. Domperidone may help if there has been a significant decrease in milk supply. (For a discussion of increasing milk for the baby, see Chapter 5, Not Enough Milk). It is better to hold off on solids, if possible, because early solids increase the risk of developing allergies, and because the solids—incomplete foods—can replace the complete food, breastmilk. Why start them early? The longer the baby is breast-fed exclusively, up to about the middle of the first year, the better. This is true for formula as well. Avoid it if you can.

To sum all this up, there may be things you can do to encourage your baby to sleep for longer stretches by increasing the amount he gets at each feeding. However, even with these tips, many babies will continue to wake at night to breastfeed. This doesn't mean they have sleep problems. It's normal behavior for human babies. If you find that bringing the baby into bed with you makes it easier to manage night feedings and to get more rest, go ahead. You won't do your baby any harm.

17

Breastfeeding
and Family Relationships

Myth: When a mother breastfeeds, the father is left out of the relationship. He can help if he gives a bottle at night, and this involves him with the baby.

Fact: There is lots the father can do to help with the baby and develop his own relationship with the baby. It is not necessary for him to feed the baby for this to happen.

Fathers and Breastfed Babies

Does breastfeeding mean that the father's relationship with his baby is hindered or diminished? Is it a good idea to give the baby a bottle or two a day from the very beginning so that the father can be involved in feeding? Do the benefits of breastfeeding outweigh the benefits of having both parents share equally in feeding the baby?

All these questions have the same underlying assumption—that feeding a baby is the only way, or the primary way, to develop a close and loving relationship with that baby. The truth is that there are many things to do in caring for a newborn baby that promote that bonding—changing his diapers, bathing him, sleeping with him, carrying him in your arms or in a carrier, singing to the baby, taking him for walks, massaging him, talking to him, burping him, and many, many more. All of these are wonderful ways for fathers (and mothers, grandmothers, siblings, and other family members, too, of course) to interact with the baby without disrupting breastfeeding.

The father who wants to be involved and share in parenting can bring the baby to the mother to nurse, change the baby's diapers, give the baby a bath, and take the baby for a walk afterward. Not only is that baby enjoying time with his father, but he is getting all the benefits of breastfeeding as well. And most fathers who really understand the benefits of breastfeeding want their babies to have "the best."

> "... the idea of bottle feeding just to 'involve the father' is one more instance of preserving the status quo at a price to the baby."
> —Marni Jackson, *The Mother Zone*

Aside from this hands-on involvement, fathers are extremely important in terms of supporting and encouraging their partners in breastfeeding. They can make the difference between forging on through challenging situations, and giving up at the first sign of difficulty.

One mother told me how frustrated she was when her baby was just a few days old. He'd already woken up several times in the night to nurse, and she was tired and worried that she didn't have enough milk. She woke up her husband and asked him to drive to the 24-hour drugstore near their home to buy some formula. Instead, he held her in his arms for a while, told her how much he loved her and their new son and how happy he was that she was breastfeeding. Then he gave her a back rub and brought in some more pillows so that she'd be in a more comfortable position for the next feeding.

That mother says she could feel her milk letting down as her husband rubbed her back. She's convinced that if her husband had brought home the formula, she would have given up on breastfeeding, but his support and encouragement made all the difference that night. This can often be a fine line for fathers to walk, though. It's tough to see your wife struggling with breastfeeding, perhaps crying because her nipples hurt or because she's so frustrated. Formula seems like a quick solution. And maybe that's what she really wants—no father wants to be the "bad guy" who is forcing his partner to keep nursing when she's ready to wean.

But often what women need in this situation is not a solution, but some empathy. Yes, breastfeeding and caring for a newborn is harder than it looked on TV. And boy, you never thought you'd end up with a caesarean, did you? Fathers can also remind their partners of other possible solutions to the problem: calling a lactation consultant or a La Leche League leader, or making an appointment with a breastfeeding clinic. He can remind her of other alternatives—perhaps if she expressed some milk he could feed it to the baby from a cup while she had a little extra time to sleep, go for a walk, read a book, take a long bath, or whatever else she needs.

Many mothers say they rely on their partners to "run interference" for them—to protect and defend them from the criticism of others, including family, friends, and medical professionals. Having to always explain to people that the baby is getting enough to eat, that her breastmilk is good enough and that it's normal for a baby to

eat this frequently can be exhausting for a new mother, especially if this is her first baby and she doesn't have a lot of self-confidence. If the baby's father speaks up and is positive about breastfeeding, it takes some of that burden away from her—and boosts her self-confidence.

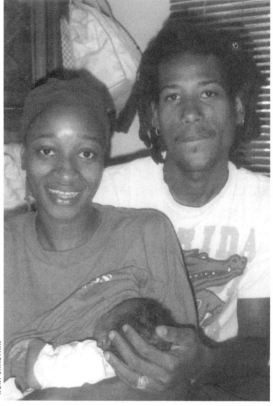

RONI CHASTAIN

Fathers don't have to give bottles in order to get involved with their babies.

Practical help is always appreciated, too. Breastfeeding a baby can take up quite a bit of time, especially in the early weeks while mother and baby are both learning. This is the time to master the art of washing dishes and doing laundry, to arrange for a diaper service or a cleaning lady, to make a nutritious meal (or order in pizza or Chinese food) when supper hasn't made it to the table. In other societies, and in times past, new mothers could often rely on their own mothers or other relatives to take over the house-work and meal preparation during the first weeks and months after a new baby was born. For most North American women, that isn't possible. Their own mothers are probably working full-time. They may live far away from other family members. For them, becoming a mother can be an isolating and overwhelming experience as they try to cope with all the needs of a baby, as well as their other household responsibilities.

Fathers can do a lot to relieve that sense of being overwhelmed, if they recognize that taking the time to get breastfeeding well established is time well-spent.

When Dad's the Best

Mothers are definitely best at breastfeeding. But fathers have their special talents, too:

Dad's deeper voice is more soothing to the baby when he sings or talks to him. Babies seem to really respond and relax when they hear the deep, rumbling sounds of a male voice.

Dad's flatter chest makes a great place for baby to nap. Lie down on the couch, drape the baby over you, and everybody gets a rest.

For the same reason (no breasts to get in the way), Dads can often carry the baby in a sling or soft baby carrier more easily than the baby's mother.

Because men usually have longer arms and larger hands, they are often better at doing some of the "colic holds" described in the colic chapter.

Breastfeeding and Sexual Relationships

One reason fathers are sometimes not as supportive of breastfeeding as they might be is that they see the intimacy of the mother–baby relationship as a threat. *If my wife loves the baby that much*, he may think, *how is she going to have enough time and love for me?*

It may take longer for the new father to take on the role of fatherhood than it does for the mother to take on motherhood. After all, she's had nine months of dramatic and intense physical changes to prepare her. For the father, the baby may not have seemed quite real until it was born. Now he's asking, "Where do I fit in?" His connection to the baby will happen, in time, and he will find his place in the new family he has helped to create.

In some ways, it can seem as though the new, breastfeeding mother is less interested in her husband than she was in those days "before baby." After all, she has a whole new responsibility here. And sex becomes less frequent. Certainly, there is research to show that new mothers have sex with their husbands less often than they did before or during pregnancy, and some studies have found this rate to be lowest for breastfeeding mothers (although others contradict this). Why does this happen? There are several reasons:

- Taking care of a new baby (whether or not you have given birth to the baby and whether or not you are breastfeeding) is tiring. Most people are less interested in sex when they are tired, whatever the cause. (To quote one mother of a six-week-old: "Frankly, I'd rather have a nap than an orgasm.")

- Recovering from pregnancy and birth is also tiring, and the physical changes the mother's body has gone through can certainly decrease interest in sex. The mother may have stitches that make intercourse painful, for example.

- Nursing a baby may meet most of the mother's need for physical contact and affectionate touch. In fact, some mothers describe feeling "touched out"—they've had so much physical stimulation from being in constant contact with their babies that they don't want anyone else to touch them.

- The hormones normally present during breastfeeding can cause the amount of vaginal lubrication produced to be decreased. Even when the woman is sexually aroused, she will have less lubrication, and this may make intercourse uncomfortable or even painful. Using a vaginal lubricant can help.
- The breastfeeding mother's nipples may be tender in the early days, and then become less sensitive to stimulation as breastfeeding continues. If nipple stimulation has been an important part of sexual activity for the couple, this can be a problem.
- Both men and women react differently to full or leaking breasts during sex. Some men like the taste of breastmilk and don't mind a little leaking, while others don't like it at all. Women will sometimes have a strong letdown of milk when they reach orgasm. This bothers some women, and not others. If the milk is a problem, nursing the baby right before sex can help. Putting a towel underneath you helps, too.
- The mother's body is different postpartum. She may be embarrassed by her stretch marks, her blue-veined breasts and her sagging belly. Her husband may not be bothered by this, or he may be turned off by the changes he sees and hope that if she quits breastfeeding she can get her body back into shape more quickly. (In fact, breastfeeding helps the mother's body to return to normal more quickly. Her uterus will contract to its normal size more rapidly, and weight put on during pregnancy is usually lost more easily when the mother breastfeeds.)

- Sex is less spontaneous and more likely to be interrupted now that a baby is in the house.

While some of these factors are directly related to breastfeeding, others are simply part of being new parents. It can be important, though, to recognize that a reduced libido is common and normal during breastfeeding, and that the mother's interest in sex will gradually increase again as her baby grows and as the long weaning process begins.

Intimate relationships are about more than just having sex. During the weeks and months after a baby is born, couples may need to broaden their perspective a bit. If intercourse is uncomfortable, what are the other ways they can express their love for each other and be intimate? This can be a great opportunity to expand your sexual repertoire. If the new mother is feeling "touched out," how can her partner help her feel more comfortable and ready to be close to him? (Hint: a chance to take a long bath, all alone, while Dad takes baby for a walk is usually much appreciated.)

Sex is more enjoyable for breastfeeding mothers if they accept that it will take them longer to become aroused and that vaginal lubrication will be less than normal, and if both partners can accept that they will be interrupted by the baby at least some of the time. Take your time. Enjoy the "warm-up." You can have some touching, fondling, and stimulation, stop for a while to nurse the baby, and then resume what you were doing. (Remember, your baby is only small for a short time, and there will be plenty of opportunities for uninterrupted, leisurely sex in the future.)

Sometimes couples decide to take a weekend away from the baby to be alone together again, hoping this will bring them closer. What usually happens is that the mother spends much of her time calling home to check on the baby and going into the bathroom to pump her milk, only to find that she leaks all over the bed anyway. When they come home, the baby is miserable and clingy and has trouble latching on well after a whole weekend of being fed from a bottle. Mom feels some guilt and regret over leaving her baby, and Dad feels disappointed that the weekend away didn't really recapture the relationship they once had.

The truth is that your relationship will never be exactly the same as it was before you had a baby. The baby has changed your life. Your body is different, your emotions are different, your priorities are different. What you need to do is figure out—and a lot of this will be trial and error—how the two of you can have a close and loving relationship now that you have become a family. This is the "new normal." It can be much better and more satisfying than the relationship you had before the baby arrived—but it will definitely be different.

> "She pictured a child, *her own* . . . at her own breast, with her husband standing by and gazing fondly at her and the child."
> —Leo Tolstoy, *War and Peace*

Often these changes are harder for the father to accept than for the mother. After all, she's been through all kinds of hormonal realignments that encourage falling in love with her new baby. This isn't a rejection of the father, although to some men it feels that way. Dr. Michel Odent, the French obstetrician, shows a series of slides in which a woman gives birth and then sits, holding her baby and gazing into its eyes. She is clearly entranced and falling deeply in love with her child. In the next slide, though, the baby's

father has moved in between the mother and baby in order to kiss her—but Dr. Odent comments that what he is really doing is trying to "break" that intense, loving look between the mother and baby. It's as though he is saying, "Don't forget about me."

Every couple will need to find their own route to keeping their relationship strong while dealing with a new baby and breastfeeding. It may involve some compromise—some nights when she decides to be sexual with her husband even though she isn't feeling "in the mood" because she sees that it's important to him, other nights when he decides to do some laundry and prepare some food for the next day, even though he'd rather be having sex, because he genuinely wants to help his wife get a little extra sleep. It might mean planning ahead rather than being spontaneous, or it might mean taking advantage of whatever moments there are ("Hey! The baby's asleep and just had a good feeding—let's do it!"). It often means doing things with the baby along, rather than just the two of you, but that can work—picnics in the park, going to the drive-in, visiting friends, ordering dinner in instead of going out to a restaurant, renting a movie instead of heading to the theater (although you can certainly take your baby to a restaurant or theater if you want).

The Rest of the Family

Breastfeeding is likely to have an effect on your other family relationships as well. A lot will depend, of course, on their own experiences with breastfeeding and your previous relationships with them.

Often, though, a new mother decides to breastfeed even though her own mother used formula. The new grandmother may feel a bit resentful. Perhaps she thought breastfeeding was a bit "disgusting" or "animalistic," and feels uncomfortable seeing her daughter nurse. She's heard that "breast is best" but can't quite get past feeling that it's somehow "yucky." Or perhaps she wanted to breastfeed, but didn't succeed (thanks to strict schedules and unhelpful advice), and now that old disappointment resurfaces.

As well, she feels cut off from her eagerly awaited grandchild. She had looked forward to taking care of the new baby—perhaps for a nice, long weekend while the new parents went away together—and certainly expected to be able to feed the baby. Now she finds herself having to hand the baby back to the mother every time he fusses. Her helpful advice on feeding schedules, methods of cleaning bottles, and pacifier use is ignored.

Even if the new grandmother did breastfeed, she may have started solid foods very early, fed according to a schedule, and weaned after just a few months. It's hard for her if she feels that her children have decided she did everything "wrong," and she may be concerned that the mother is breastfeeding too often and will damage her breasts or become exhausted, or that the mother's milk will turn "bad" after three months. After all, that's what she was told when her babies were born.

It's a challenge for the new mother, who needs support, encouragement, and practical help at this point in her life, but who may, instead, find herself massaging bruised egos and dealing with unhelpful criticism. Many mothers find it helps to simply say "This is what my doctor advised me to do" when it comes to breastfeeding techniques or timing (even if it hasn't ever been discussed with the doctor). Most people will respect "medical advice." You can also offer books or other materials about breastfeeding, especially those that refute some of the still-prevalent myths. (You could let them read this book, for example.)

18

Breastfeeding and Mother–Baby Separation

Myth: Mothers who work outside the home or go to school can't continue breastfeeding.

Fact: While breastfeeding is obviously easiest when mother and baby are together, many women continue breastfeeding even though they are separated from their babies in order to work, attend school, or because of access visits after a divorce. Not only is it possible, but most mothers feel it is well worth the extra effort.

First, the baby who is separated from his mother will be in the care of another person. Unless this is his father or another person who lives in the home, he is probably being exposed to a variety of germs that he wouldn't encounter if he were at home full-time. If he is being cared for in a day care center, with a large number of other children and several staff people, he's likely to pick up all kinds of viruses and infections. Continued breastfeeding, though, will go a long way to preventing illness and speeding the baby's recovery when he does pick up an infection. Studies have shown that working parents whose small children continue to be breastfed take fewer days off work because their child is sick than those whose children are not breastfed.

Second, breastfeeding is a great way to connect with the baby at the end of a long day of work. When the mother puts her baby to the breast, her body releases the hormone oxytocin, which encourages the milk to flow. Oxytocin and prolactin, another breastfeeding hormone, also have an important side effect—they are natural tranquilizers that help the mother relax. Many women say they can feel all the tension leave their bodies as the baby nurses. They also like the fact that breastfeeding is something only they—and not the babysitter—can do. Employed mothers often find themselves caught in a dilemma: They want their babies to like the caregiver and to be happy while they are at work or school, but they don't want to lose the vital bond and connection between their babies and themselves. They don't want the baby to become more attached to the caregiver than to Mom. Continuing to breastfeed can be very reassuring to mothers with those concerns, because it keeps that special aspect to their relationship. The baby's obvious enthusiasm for nursing lets her know that she is still special to him.

Finally, the long-term benefits of breastfeeding, discussed elsewhere, continue to be important for the baby whose mother is away from him, just as they are to the baby whose mother is with him most of the time.

So how can mothers manage continued breastfeeding, despite separation?

Preparation

Getting breastfeeding well established in the

beginning is especially important for the mother who is anticipating returning to work or being otherwise separated from her baby. Elsewhere we have described the mothers in Africa or other communities who carry their babies with them and nurse several times an hour. When there is that kind of continuous contact and very frequent nursing, it doesn't matter so much if the latch is not as good as it might be, or if the milk supply tends to be a little on the low side. For a mother who will be away from her baby, who will need to pump milk at least some of the time and whose baby may be getting bottles or sucking on a pacifier while at the caregiver's, learning to latch the baby on well and build up a good milk supply are very important. (Of course, if you are returning to school or work outside the home after your baby is six months old, your baby will not need bottles.)

The longer you can be at home with your baby before returning to work or school, the easier it will be to maintain breastfeeding. Not many years ago, women often had to return to work before their babies were six weeks old, and it could be even earlier if the mother had miscalculated her due date and started her maternity leave too early. In Canada today, women can take a full year to be with their new babies, and many companies will extend that with a longer leave (paid or unpaid, depending on the company) if the mother requests it. This allows you to have breastfeeding well established before you must be away. The situation isn't good in the United States (where maternity leaves may be as short as two or three weeks, in some cases) and some other countries, and it is much better in other parts of the world, such as some European countries, where women can take up to three years off work after giving birth.

Of course, even in Canada some mothers must be separated from their babies sooner than six months. Self-employed women, for example, may not be able to stop working for more than a short period of time, and women who are attending school may have to go back to class when the baby is younger than they would like. Also, recent welfare reforms in some places, such as the province of Ontario, require mothers who are receiving welfare to be attending school or actively looking for work by the time the baby is three months old. This is a very short-sighted policy.

During your time at home with your baby, try to resolve any breastfeeding problems you might have. If your supply is low, for example, this is the time to try some of the techniques suggested in Chapter 5, Not Enough Milk. If you let this go on until you are back at work, you may find that your breasts are going without stimulation most of the day, that your baby is getting milk from a faster-flowing bottle, and that your milk supply will gradually decrease until the baby is weaned, long before you had planned.

It is *not* necessary to introduce a bottle early on so that the baby will take a bottle at the sitter's or the day care center. If you take at least six months of maternity leave, your baby will not need a bottle. If your younger baby resists bottles—and some completely breastfed babies do—there are many other ways your caregiver can give him food. She can use a small cup, a spoon, or a syringe (without a needle, of course). If you want the baby to take a bottle, it will probably be easier for the babysitter to introduce it when you aren't around. If you use the gradual introduction to separation suggested later in this chapter, you will give the sitter a good opportunity to try out the bottle. Babies are smart and will often resist taking a bottle when they know you are right there; once they are alone with the sitter and realize that a bottle is the only source of food around, they may take it.

On the other hand, there are many babies who have never taken a bottle and who do just fine with the other methods of feeding when Mom is not around.

Finding the Right Caregiver

Part of your preparation for breastfeeding and working outside the home is finding the right caregiver. Here are some things to consider.

If you find a caregiver close to your work, rather than close to your home, you can minimize the time you are away from your baby. You can nurse the baby when you drop him off, go to work, and then nurse again when you are finished work and before you start for home.

If you are close enough, you may be able to run over to the caregiver's location during your lunch hour, or during breaks, for a nursing session. Or perhaps the caregiver can bring the baby to you during lunch or breaks. Again, discuss with your caregiver to decide how this will work.

Discuss breastfeeding with your caregiver, and ask about any policies that might affect your desire to continue breastfeeding. For example, some day care centers will not allow women to leave breastmilk for their babies, because they consider breastmilk to be a potentially dangerous body fluid. (If you run into this policy, look for another caregiver.) Some centers insist that all babies over a certain age (usually a year) be given regular cow's milk. In this situation, you can keep on breastfeeding at home, but let the baby drink regular milk at day care. Or, the baby can eat other foods during the day and not have any milk while at day care.

Discuss ways of feeding breastmilk without using a bottle, if that is what you want to do to help avoid nipple confusion. You might have to demonstrate how to use the cup or syringe, and see if your sitter is comfortable with this. Or your milk can be mixed with any of the solid foods the baby is eating—there is no reason that liquids need to be taken separately from solids.

Make sure your caregiver knows how breastmilk is supposed to look. Because it is not homogenized—as cow's milk is when we buy it—it will naturally separate into layers when left in the fridge or freezer, with the "cream" on top. Sometimes people assume this means the milk is spoiled, but it isn't. The milk may also be different colors—more bluish or yellowish—at different times. And be sure your caregiver also knows that a breastfed baby's bowel movements are supposed to be yellow in color and very loose.

Talk about how you want the caregiver to deal with the situation when your baby is fussing and you are due back soon. It can be frustrating for the breastfeeding mother to arrive at the day care with full breasts, only to hear that the baby just filled his tummy with milk.

Discuss how you would prefer to handle things if the day care should run out of expressed breastmilk. Do you want to also leave a supply of formula or cow's milk, depending on the baby's age, in case all the breastmilk gets used up, or would you prefer that your sitter give the baby some solid foods, or a little diluted juice, or something else until you get there? The answer, of course, may change with the age of the baby and may depend partly on your baby's temperament. There is no need for a baby older than six months, who is breastfeeding and also eating solid foods, to be given formula—homogenized milk will do just fine. In fact, there is no need for any extra milk to be given in this situation. If you want him to get more calcium (even though he probably doesn't need it), he could be given some cheese or yogurt.

Planning at Work

What are your options at work? Do you have regularly scheduled breaks and lunches that you could use for pumping? Do you have an office with a door that closes (and, ideally, locks), giving you some privacy, or will you need to express in a washroom or the office sickroom or some other location? Are you planning to leave the office and nurse the baby during breaks, or can you arrange to have the baby brought to you?

Women have found various ways to work and still provide milk for their babies. One mother, who managed a golf course, was able to arrange for a sitter to come and care for the baby in her office. Most of the time, she did paperwork in her office while the sitter and baby played nearby. Sometimes the sitter would take the baby out for a walk through the quieter parts of the golf course. When the mother needed to meet with customers or suppliers, she left the baby with the sitter and went to another part of the building. This made it easy to nurse her baby frequently throughout the day.

Another mother arranged with her employer to come in half an hour early each day and stay half an hour later each evening. In exchange, she was given two half-hour breaks—one mid-morning and one mid-afternoon, as well as her normal lunch break. She used those breaks to go over to the day care center, just a block away, and nurse her baby.

The most difficult situations are those in which mothers work long shifts and have no regular breaks. For example, nurses often work 12-hour shifts and may have no breaks if the ward is busy. Flight attendants may also be away from their babies for several days at a time, and while the plane is in flight they don't have many opportunities to express milk or any room to store it. For these mothers, one approach may be to build up a good stock of expressed milk in the freezer while they are on maternity leave. Then, during ordinary bathroom breaks, they can express milk just enough to relieve the fullness.

Incidentally, Canada is a signatory of the International Labor Organization's 1919 paper guaranteeing all nursing mothers two extra 30-minute breaks during the day, either to return home and feed their babies or to express their milk. Of course, just signing a document doesn't mean the provisions will be followed.

Breasts are surprisingly adaptable. Many women have managed to continue breastfeeding or providing milk for their babies despite long separations, irregular schedules, and other challenges. Remember that it is common and typical for mothers who are nursing toddlers or older children to find that they are nursing three times one day, eight times the next day, and four times the day after that. They may find their breasts are slightly fuller on some days, but it all works out.

> **Why your boss should support you breastfeeding**
> • your baby will be sick less often, so you won't need to miss work as much to take care of him
> • your baby's lower prescription costs will mean lower premiums for the employee medical plan
> • you will feel more positive about your work, and will therefore be more productive

Pumping or Expressing Milk

Many mothers who know they will be going back to work begin pumping their milk several months before their maternity leave is over. They store the milk in the freezer, and having this extra supply gives them confidence that even if they can't keep up with pumping all the time once they return to work, there will be milk for their babies.

Others only store a few extra containers of milk, and rely on daily pumping to provide the majority of the milk for the baby's needs while they are away. The method that works best for you will depend a lot on your work and day care situation.

The first step in pumping or extracting milk is to encourage your milk to let down. This is easy if you are pumping at home and have your baby with you, because the baby's suckling will cause the milk to flow. For this reason, some mothers will nurse the baby on one breast and pump the other at the same time. Others will nurse the baby first, and then use the pump. While at first you won't get a lot of milk pumping this way, in time your milk supply will adjust. Even if you just get a couple of ounces, you can save that milk and later mix it with other milk. (Don't add warm milk directly to frozen milk in the storage container, though. Let it chill in the refrigerator first.)

If your baby is not with you, you might need to take some extra steps to get your milk to flow easily. Applying warm, wet washcloths to your breasts can help. Many women find that gentle breast massage helps. Massage from the top of the breasts toward the nipples with gentle strokes. Rubbing the nipple with the palm of your hand held flat can also stimulate the milk to let down, as can rolling the nipples between your finger and thumb. Sometimes looking at a picture of your baby or smelling an undershirt your baby has worn will also help. In time you will figure out what works best for you.

Hand-Expressing

To express your milk by hand, first encourage the milk to let down. Then with one hand, cup the breast on the same side and use the other hand to hold the clean container for storing your milk. Place your thumb near the top of the areola and have your forefinger in about the same position on the bottom of your breast. Now press your thumb and forefinger together, at the same time pushing back toward your ribs. Finally, squeeze forward. You don't need to do this very hard—you shouldn't be leaving bruises—and you shouldn't slide your hand on the skin, which will irritate it. You may get just a drip or two of milk, or you may get a spray. Repeat the pressing movement a few times, and if the flow of milk slows down, move your hand slightly and press again. The milk ducts form a circle around the nipple, so your goal is to keep moving your hand until you have squeezed all of them.

If, after a few minutes of hand-expression, the milk stops flowing or slows down drastically, try expressing from the other breast. Then repeat the breast massage, nipple rubbing, and perhaps smelling your baby's clothes before you go back to the first breast, to encourage another letdown of milk.

This often takes practice, but mothers usually soon learn where their own milk ducts are located and how much pressure to apply to achieve the maximum flow of milk. You can also, with a little practice, express both breasts at the same time. The procedure is the same as with one, but this will take half the time and may produce more milk.

The best things about hand-expression are that it is free and that you can't forget to bring your hands to work! You are also in control of the process, and this makes you less likely to experience bruising or other damage to the breast that can sometimes happen with a pump.

Using a Breast Pump

As interest in breastfeeding has increased, many manufacturers have come out with their own versions of the breast pump. Some are basically useless—in fact, they may be worse than useless because when the mother uses them and discovers she can't get any milk out, she may assume this means her milk supply is low. This is not true. There are women who are never able to use a pump or to hand-express with much success, who nevertheless exclusively breastfeed their babies successfully. A baby who is properly latched on and feeding well is much more efficient at getting milk from the breast than any pump.

The most effective pumps for mothers who are separated from their babies are the high-grade electric models. The best of these are designed to allow the mother to pump from both breasts at the same time, and to allow her to adjust the pressure and speed of the pumping action. Many come with a handy carrying and storage case that the mother can use to bring the pump to work or school, and will convert from electricity to rechargeable battery.

I even knew one mother who would use the pump while driving to and from work. She'd attach the pump under her blouse, let it work away while she navigated through traffic, and then wait until she was stopped before she detached the pump. Since her schedule didn't provide for pumping time during the day, this allowed her to get enough milk for her baby's next day at the sitter's.

Each pump is a little different, just as every woman's breasts are a little different. What you want is a pump that fits your breast, creating a good but comfortable seal, and that produces the right amount of pumping pressure for you. If the first pump you try is not working well for you, don't just assume that means you can't get enough milk this way for your baby. Maybe all you need is a different pump. You can also use breast compression, in the same way you would if the baby were nursing (see Chapter 5, Not Enough Milk), to help the pump get more milk out.

Breast tissue is sensitive and can be easily bruised. The electric pumps have strong suction and can cause sore nipples if the mother does not get her breast centered in the attachment, causing the nipple to rub against the side of the pump. If pumping is hurting, you should stop right away. See if readjusting the position of the pump or decreasing the amount of pressure will help make it more comfortable.

Storing Your Milk

Breastmilk is a "live" fluid and can actually fight off bacteria. Research has shown that even when left at room temperature, breastmilk will kill off any bacteria and remain perfectly safe and healthy for the baby to drink for many hours.

It is important to be sure the containers are clean. The white cells in human milk—an important form of protection against illness—can stick to the side of glass containers, but not to plastic. However, some of the fats in the breastmilk will stick to plastic, but not to glass. The white cells are also destroyed by freezing. There are some special plastic bags designed for storing human milk; these are more durable than the plastic bottle liners many women have used. However, recommendations for the best containers for expressed milk change all the time, and there probably isn't a big difference. Personally, I prefer glass containers because of information that plastic containers may leech toxins into any foods that they are holding.

Expressed breastmilk keeps safely at room temperature for up to about 10 to 12 hours, and can be refrigerated for up to five days. This is good news for mothers who don't have access to a fridge or freezer at work. You can express your milk and simply keep the container in your office or locker until you go home. Then you can either put it in the fridge for use in the next few days, or freeze it. In a deep freeze, expressed milk will keep for six months or longer; in the freezer compartment of a refrigerator, it will keep for two to four months. Be sure to mark the date on each container so you use up the oldest milk first.

The milk can best be thawed by holding the container under warm running water, then shaking well to mix. Check the temperature before giving it to the baby. It is not a good idea to use a microwave to thaw frozen breast-milk, for two reasons. One, some of the anti-bodies in the milk can be destroyed by the microwaves, and two, the microwaves can produce pockets of very hot milk that could burn the baby's mouth.

Common concerns

Mothers frequently mention that they put milk in the refrigerator and two hours later it smells funny and tastes bad. This is not due to spoiling, but is thought to be a situation where the mother has a lot of lipase in her milk. Lipase is an enzyme that breaks down fat, and in this case it is quickly breaking down the fat in the milk. The by-products of the breakdown are what taste unpleasant to adults, but it is not at all harmful to the baby—it is like drinking predigested milk.

This is often a concern of women who have frozen significant quantities of milk, and then notice this change in smell and taste. They worry that they may have to throw all this carefully saved milk away. But the milk can definitely be given to the baby if he'll take it (some older babies will not drink it because of the different taste), or mixed in with his food to mask the flavor.

Scalding the milk before freezing it seems to solve this problem.

If you have had a candida (yeast) infection, you do not need to throw away the milk you collected while you had the infection. Candida is everywhere, you can't get rid of it.

When should I stop pumping?

Some mothers don't pump at all after they return to work. If your baby is six months old or older and already eating solid foods, this approach can work. Plan to have the sitter give the baby solid foods, juice, and water during the day, and then you can nurse frequently during the evening, night, and early morning. Sometimes mothers in this situation will need to pump or express milk for their own comfort, though.

Other women prefer to leave breastmilk for their babies, and will pump for as long as the baby seems to be consuming the milk they leave behind. This would also be important for a baby who is allergic to cow's milk.

As your baby gets older, and the number of feedings at the breast naturally decrease, it becomes easier and easier to manage breastfeeding and working. Your older baby will be able to have a variety of foods and drinks at day care, and yet will still benefit from nursing when you are together.

When You Leave

Your baby's reaction when you go back to work or school may catch you by surprise. Some babies seem almost unconcerned that their mothers are not around. But many breastfeeding babies will protest and cry when they realize you are gone. Even a very good caregiver won't have your smell, your special way of holding the baby, your voice, or your milk—and your baby will miss all those things.

Some mothers leave behind handkerchiefs they have worn in their bras, or T-shirts they have slept in, to provide the baby with that comforting and familiar smell. If you usually use a sling or baby carrier with your baby, see if your caregiver can use it while looking after him—another way to keep the familiar things as part of your baby's day.

You might also be surprised by your baby's reaction when you return. It is not unusual for a baby who has been at day care all day to ignore his mother when she comes to pick him up. Sometimes he will start crying when he sees her—not at all the reaction she was hoping for! Some will refuse to be held or picked up by their mothers, or will react with anger by hitting or kicking her when she does hold them.

This is another demonstration of your baby's intense love for you. He is telling you that he did not want you to leave him. Breastfeeding is one of the best ways to soothe both you and your baby after this kind of tense, stormy reunion. Often you can see your baby's whole body relax as you begin to make the familiar gestures that show him you are preparing to breastfeed: settling him on your lap, unbuttoning your shirt, moving him into the nursing position.

You can sometimes make this transition easier by starting small. First, let the baby spend time with you and the caregiver together, either at your home or the day care. Then leave the baby with the new caregiver for a short period of time—less than one hour, perhaps. Gradually, over a period of two or three weeks, increase the amount of time the baby spends away from you. This will also give you a chance to practice pumping, to see how the baby does with the caregiver, to see if the baby will accept your milk from a cup or bottle, and so on.

When you do go back to work, try to begin not on a Monday but perhaps a Thursday, so that you will have a couple of days of work, followed by a weekend during which everyone can get readjusted, and then five days of work (assuming you are working full-time). Some mothers have found it works for them to adjust their schedules to work longer hours on the other four days of the week, so they can have Wednesdays off.

Often mothers who are separated from their babies during the day find that the babies wake up more at night. They may even refuse most of their daytime feedings of expressed milk and make up for it by nursing very frequently during the evening and night. This can be tiring for the mother who now has no opportunity to catch up with naps during the day. Bringing baby into your bed may be the easiest way to help everyone get the sleep they need. With time, you will learn to latch the baby on and then fall back to sleep while he nurses. Sleeping with Mom also lets your baby enjoy the physical closeness to you that he might be missing during the day.

Your baby's behavior will also change as he goes through different developmental stages. Many babies of six months will not be strongly upset about being left at a sitter's. This can change drastically when the baby is about eight or nine months, and the mother may unexpectedly find herself dealing with a baby who clings to her and screams each morning. Another time of developmental change is around the one-year mark, when the baby becomes more active and mobile. Even when their mothers are home full-time, one-year-olds often skip many daytime feedings and then "crash" at night, wanting to be held and nursed as they recharge themselves after a busy day.

Common Concerns About Breastfeeding and Working

Plugged Ducts

Some women find that because they are missing feedings during the day, they end up with plugged ducts, although this problem is surprisingly uncommon. If you have experienced plugged ducts before, when you were with your baby full-time, you may be more prone to them once you return to work. This problem is more common when mothers don't pump or express milk during the day.

If this is a problem for you, the solution is usually to express milk during your workday, even if you can't store it, to relieve the fullness. If you notice the symptoms of a plugged duct beginning—a sore, tender, and hard area in the breast—try to take a break as soon as possible, apply a hot washcloth, massage the area, and express some milk.

Some women with repeated plugged ducts have found that adding lecithin to their diets has been helpful (see Chapter 7, Sore Breasts).

Decreasing Milk Supply

If your baby is getting bottles of formula or previously pumped and stored breastmilk, he will not be nursing as frequently, and you may find that your milk supply begins to diminish. If you are concerned, you can pump during the day to build your milk production back up.

If your schedule is erratic—for example, if you work three 12-hour shifts, followed by four days at home—you may find that your milk supply is constantly shifting. On your first day at home after the three-day shift, your milk supply

may be low and the baby nursing very frequently. By the fourth day, your milk production will probably have caught up to the baby's needs—but then when you get back to work the next day, your breasts will feel very full.

Some mothers try to balance this out by giving the baby bottles on the days they are at home, just as if they were away at work. This seems a shame, though. Why give the baby second-best when the best is right there? Your body will be able to adjust to this cycle, and your baby will benefit from nursing as much as possible.

Leaking Breasts

Usually leaking breasts are not a problem by the time the baby is six months old. But they are for some mothers, and it is more likely to be a problem if you had to return to work when your baby was still very young. Sometimes just thinking about your baby, or hearing another baby cry, can cause leaking.

Wear good, absorbent breast pads, and bring enough that you can change them frequently (milk-soaked pads against your nipples will cause chafing and soreness). Try to express or pump milk before you get too full. If you do feel the tingling or "filling up" sensations that often signal that leaking is about to happen, try pressing against your breasts with your arms folded across your chest. This will often prevent leaking, and can be done without anyone noticing. Wearing patterned blouses, perhaps with a loose vest over a top, or sweaters with a T-shirt underneath, can help disguise any leaks—a plain silk blouse is not a good choice for the potentially leaky lactating mother at work!

Baby Won't Settle or Sleep for the Caregiver

If you have always nursed your baby to sleep, he may find it difficult to fall asleep for your babysitter, and your babysitter may be used to babies who are just put down in their cribs alone to fall asleep, or who take a pacifier.

Here are some ideas that may help:

- Movement can be very soothing. Have your caregiver try taking the baby for a drive in the car (in his car seat, of course) or pushing him around in a stroller or pram. She can just push the stroller around inside the house, if necessary. Rocking in a rocking chair might also work. If your baby is young enough, she can try a wind-up baby swing.
- Give your caregiver a T-shirt or nightgown that you have slept in, and have her wrap it around the baby while she rocks him to sleep. The familiar smell may do the trick.
- Have the caregiver try walking around with the baby in a sling or baby carrier or back-pack carrier.
- If the baby takes a pacifier or bottle, the caregiver can use it as a substitute for the breast at naptime.
- Sometimes a repetitive noise—such as that of a fan or radio static—will drown out noises that may be distracting the baby and keeping him awake.

Baby Starts to Prefer the Bottle to the Breast

This is more common if your milk supply has begun to diminish, so that the baby finds it easier to get milk from the bottle than from your breast. But older babies sometimes like the bottle because they can carry it around with them, and feel more in control of when they can have it—in contrast to breastfeeding, which is now inaccessible to them for much of each day.

Some mothers don't mind this, since they were not planning to nurse much longer anyway, and they see this as an easy step toward weaning. Others, who wanted to nurse at least into toddlerhood, want to reinterest their babies in breastfeeding.

Avoiding bottles altogether will prevent this problem, and stopping bottles, if possible, will help to solve it.

You can start reducing bottles by asking the sitter to hold your baby for every bottle feeding and not allow him to walk around with a bottle. Then ask her to reduce the number of bottles by offering a cup instead when the baby is thirsty. At the same time, the mother should take steps to increase her milk supply—by expressing or pumping more frequently, or by using herbs or domperidone. This should increase his interest in breastfeeding.

Breastfeeding and Shorter or Irregular Separations

Many women plan occasional times away from their babies—for evenings out with their partners, for vacations, or to attend special events. If the separation will be short—less than two or three hours—they may not need to leave any breastmilk. But women who are planning longer separations may find it helpful to begin expressing in advance so that they have a supply of milk in the freezer for these occasions.

Into the Toddler Years

As your baby gets older, separations become easier to manage. Breastmilk is a smaller part of his daily diet, and your milk supply is well-established and easier to maintain. Many women who work full-time enjoy an ongoing nursing relationship with their children who are toddlers or older. The caregiver may not even know that the child is still nursing, because it may be limited to bedtime and first thing in the morning. Even though there are only one or two nursings a day at this point, both mother and toddler definitely benefit.

Separation from the baby doesn't mean that breastfeeding needs to end. In fact, the benefits of breastfeeding are probably even greater for the baby who spends many hours each day away from his mother than for the baby whose mother is at home with him.

19

Breastfeeding the Toddler

Myth: It is unnatural to breastfeed a child past the age of six months, or past one year.

Fact: It is usual, in nonindustrialized societies, to breastfeed each child for two or more years. It is said that the Inuit (Eskimos) of northern Canada often nursed for up to six years or longer.

As more and more mothers are breastfeeding, many are realizing that breastfeeding is more than just providing milk to the baby. Breastfeeding is a relationship, a give and take between a child and his mother that is special, that allows a close physical connection. Because of this, more mothers are continuing past the four or six months that is considered "usual" in North American society. Indeed, some are continuing breastfeeding for years.

I will say immediately that our oldest son, born in 1976, was nursed until he was about two months shy of four years; that our daughter, born in 1981, was nursed until she was about one month shy of three years; and that our youngest, another son, born in 1984, was nursed until he was a few months over three. None of us—my wife, nor I, nor the children—feel that we have done them any harm.

Teresa, the co-author of this book, has four children. One nursed for two years and a couple of months, one nursed for 3½ years, and the other two nursed for more than 4½ years each.

All four have grown into wonderful teens and young adults.

When our oldest was born, neither my wife nor I ever imagined that he would breastfeed so long. But after a trip to France with him when he was about six months old, he started to wake frequently at night, and breastfeeding was the only way to get him back to sleep. The trip overseas, which lasted almost two months and included frequent traveling and changing hotels, resulted in his sleep pattern being upset. He woke frequently but settled easily with the breast. The night feedings did not disappear when we came home with our now eight-month-old. We tried on occasion to get him to sleep through, but the efforts were futile since we weren't able to let our baby cry—the method everyone suggested to get him to sleep. So he kept breastfeeding, and eventually he stopped. Just like that.

With the second, we were expecting breastfeeding to last for at least a couple of years. But in the end, our daughter was almost three years old when my wife was seven months pregnant and could no longer hold her on her lap to nurse. There passed a couple of very difficult weeks for mother and daughter, as the weaning was rather forced.

By the time our third had been nursing over three years, my wife would ask him gently, from time to time, if he wasn't tired of it, if he wasn't a big boy who didn't need to nurse anymore. At those times he would look up at her, and, without letting go of the breast, would smile at her, and then continue nursing. One day, for no obvious reason that I could ascertain, instead of smiling, he burst into tears and said, "No, not today, tomorrow." And he never nursed again after that day. He did ask from time to time, but it was without conviction, and he didn't insist.

These experiences taught us a lot about the

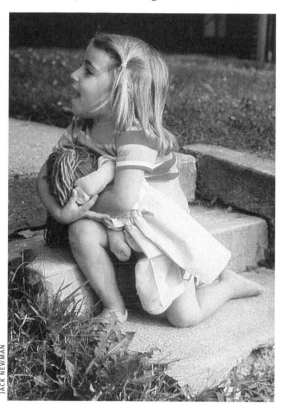

My daughter, Elise, three and a half years old, feeding her doll the only way she knows. She learned about breastfeeding by watching her mother and younger brother.

value of "extended" nursing. Before I go on to discuss the psychological aspects of extended breastfeeding, I would like to put to rest the myth that is repeated by too many health professionals—that there is no nutritional or other value in breastmilk after six months.

Surely, of all the statements generally made about breastmilk and breastfeeding, this one stands head and shoulders above the others in absurdity. One wonders how it is that breastmilk, with all its protein, fat, carbohydrate, trophic factors (those elements in milk that stimulate development of various parts of the body, such as the nervous system and intestines), suddenly, when the baby is six months of age,

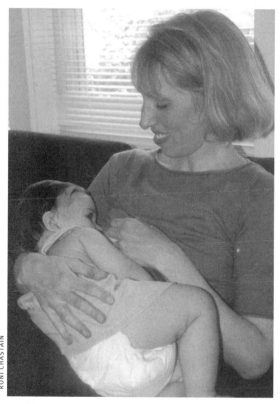

Feeding the older child can be a rewarding experience for both mother and child.

becomes white water with no nutritional value. What happens to all the protein and fat? How does the mother's body do that—turn this nutritious fluid into nothing but water?

To give those health professionals the benefit of the doubt, perhaps what most meant to say

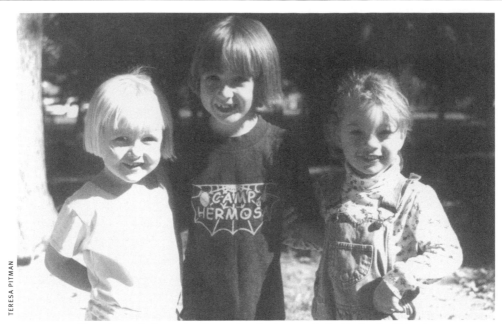

TERESA PITMAN

Three breastfed preschoolers, who also happen to be the best of friends.

was this: Breastmilk is not *necessary* after six months. I suppose that is true, if what they mean is a six-month-old can live without breastmilk. Interestingly, however, in our bottle-feeding society, most health professionals would not say that about formula. They would say that formula is necessary, at least until the baby is nine months of age (some will say 12 months), even though it isn't, actually. That's more formula company marketing. Formula is not necessary after six months of age, as long as the baby is getting a wide variety of solids (including solids rich in iron) in significant quantities, in addition to homogenized milk. This is an illustration of how influential formula company marketing is. Many health professionals are convinced formula (the imitation) is necessary for a baby six months of age or older, whereas breastmilk (the original) is not. In fact, breastmilk is even *more* valuable.

There is more to breastmilk than calories, protein, fat, and carbohydrate, though. The immune factors that protect the three-week-old

are still there. The quantities vary depending on which factor we are talking about, but some factors such as lysozyme, which kill bacteria by breaking up their cell walls, are present in greater quantities at 18 months than they are at six months. The ability of the mother to produce "tailor-made milk" in response to exposure to various bugs and antigens by producing specific secretory IgA and other factors in the milk is still there as well. If the mother gets exposed to a new bacterium, she will start to produce antibodies directed at that very bacterium, and the white cells in her milk will be sensitized to attack and help other immune factors kill any invaders.

So breastmilk is still milk, and still nutritious. Indeed, it is more nutritious than cow's milk, formula, or any other sort of milk. Breastmilk is more than that, though. It also protects babies against infection, helps them to recover from infection, and aids in the development of their bodies. And this continues as long as the baby or child is breastfeeding.

But couldn't this prevent the child from developing his own immunities?

Some physicians and other health professionals argue that if the mother continues breastfeeding, the child will not be able to develop his own immunity. This is so patently absurd, it is difficult to know how to answer it.

Is there a pediatrician who would tell a mother not to immunize her child because if the child is immunized, he would not develop his own immunity? In fact, though immunizations have saved millions of lives, and protected millions from serious illness, there are concerns about some immunizations—that the protection they give is not as good or long-lasting as what the child would get from acquiring the natural disease. Is this a reason not to give the immunizations, given the fact that they have prevented so much disease?

So, does it make any sense to say that the older child who is breastfed will not develop immunities because he is getting protection from his mother's milk? Not at all! Breastfeeding increases the chances that *if* the baby is exposed to an infection, he will become infected but not get sick—or, at the very least, get much less sick than if he weren't breastfeeding. Perfect! This is exactly what we want. He will then become immune without getting sick, and that's the same reason we give babies immunizations.

But that's not all. In fact, breastfeeding and the various immune factors in breastmilk actually stimulate the development of the baby's immune system. This should not be surprising, since breastmilk encourages the development of many of the body's systems, including the digestive system, the brain, and so on. There is some intriguing work to suggest that the breastfed baby's or child's immune system is more mature than that of the artificially fed child. For example, the antibody response of the breastfed baby to certain immunizations is actually greater than that of the baby fed artificially. And if this occurs with immunizations, there is no reason to expect that it would not occur with naturally acquired infections.

Are there other reasons for continuing to breastfeed?

Yes. The special relationship that breastfeeding provides both the mother and the baby is, in my opinion, far more important than the nutritional, immunologic, and developmental value of breastmilk. This is not to say that I feel these factors are unimportant—not at all—but I do feel that the special relationship of the nursing mother and baby is far more important than our society realizes.

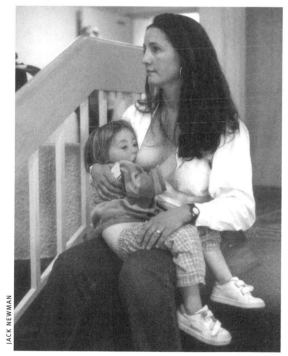

JACK NEWMAN

Mother and toddler able to relax after a long day at a conference.

The act of putting a child to the breast is one of renewal of love. It is a life-affirming act of love. It is a reaffirmation, each time it happens, of a special bond. Older children, especially, get comfort and reassurance and security from the breast. When they fall, they go to the breast to get comfort. When they are frightened, they get reassurance from the breast. When family life is in turmoil, they have security at the breast. A toddler will sometimes spontaneously burst into laughter while nursing, as if his joy knew no bounds. His delight in the breast goes beyond its value as a source of food.

Some argue that this is not good. That children should be able to find comfort and reassurance and security in other ways. They will, they will. No rush to get their thumbs in their mouths, though. Why this worry about getting comfort, reassurance, and security from the breast, as if this were something bad? A child who has a security blanket at age five is not usually scolded for having it or forced to give it up. He needs it. He would be miserable without it. So let him keep his security blanket—everyone knows he will soon give it up. People often think it is kind of cute and charming.

But if the child is getting from the breast what another child might get from a security blanket, the reaction is much more negative. Critics say the child should be able to find another way to get comfort and reassurance. A security blanket, perhaps? A stuffed toy? How can people imagine that this is better than the soft touch and warm milk and loving gazes of his mother?

It is almost impossible to describe the beauty of a three-year-old at the breast (if one is not biased against the idea to begin with). Many paintings from the Middle Ages and Renaissance show Mary breastfeeding Jesus. But more than a casual glance will show that quite often this is not a *baby* Jesus, but rather a *toddler* Jesus. It is obvious that nursing into the second year of life,

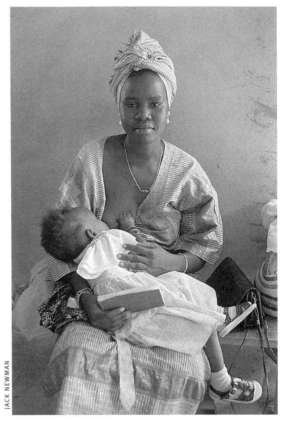

JACK NEWMAN

A mother and child in Burkina Faso. One instance of another culture that accepts and dignifies the breastfeeding relationship even when the child is no longer an infant.

and even longer, was considered normal at that time in Europe.

This has been forgotten in modern industrialized societies. Breastfeeding into the second and third years of life and even longer was considered normal until recently. The Inuit are said to have continued breastfeeding for as long as six years. UNICEF has long stated that babies should be breastfed exclusively for about six months and then given appropriate foods as well as continued breastfeeding to two years and beyond. Fortunately, professional health organizations are now catching up. In December 1997, the American Academy of Pediatrics put out a statement, which, in addition to other positive comments about breastfeeding, encouraged mothers to breastfeed exclusively to about the middle of the first year, and to continue, with the addition of appropriate foods, to a year, and then for as long as the mother and baby desire. No upper limit is mentioned, and this was done deliberately. Even the Canadian Paediatric Society has written in its most recent infant feeding statement that mothers should breastfeed exclusively for six months, and then can continue to two years and beyond, with appropriate addition of solids.

What if I get pregnant again?

While it is very unlikely that you will conceive another baby during the early months, when the baby is breastfeeding exclusively, pregnancy is quite possible if you continue to breastfeed for several years. Some parents decide to wait until their toddler weans before having another baby, but other couples find themselves with a baby on the way and a toddler who is still happily nursing.

Should you wean if you become pregnant? If your previous pregnancies were normal, and this one also seems to be proceeding normally, continuing to breastfeed will not put your expected baby at risk. Sometimes, when mothers have a history of premature labor, or if they are expecting twins or triplets, there is concern that the hormones released during breastfeeding may trigger a premature labor. In those situations, the mother might want to begin a gradual weaning of the older child.

There is some research to show that in a normal pregnancy, breastfeeding does not increase the incidence of premature labor. It does, however, seem to reduce the number of pregnancies that go "post-term"—more than a week past the due date.

There are other things to consider, though. Many women develop sore, tender nipples when they are pregnant, and breastfeeding can become quite uncomfortable. Sometimes this can be improved by reminding your toddler to open wide and latch on well. Other mothers will limit the length of each feeding—counting to 20, for example, and then asking the toddler to stop. The discomfort usually improves after the first three or four months.

Breastfeeding can also cause contractions, and these can get pretty strong toward the end of the pregnancy. Sometimes these contractions are painful enough that the mother needs to end the feeding fairly quickly. It can also be hard to find a comfortable position to nurse in (although determined nursing toddlers will surprise you by their ability to find a way!).

For these reasons, mothers sometimes decide to wean their toddlers or older children when they are pregnant. Also, because the mother's milk supply diminishes rapidly in early pregnancy and then changes to colostrum at the end, many toddlers will wean on their own. They get fed up with the decreasing amount of milk, or they don't like the change in taste, perhaps.

Others don't care that they aren't getting much milk—they want to keep nursing. In this situation, the mother may find herself with a newborn baby and a toddler who still loves to breastfeed. This is called *tandem nursing*—nursing siblings who are not twins.

Some mothers don't want to tandem nurse. They want to focus on the new baby, and find they are resentful of the older child's demands. But others find it helps the older child accept the new baby. It seems to give the message "Yes, we have a new baby, but there is milk for you as well, and you are still welcome at the breast." (Or, you are still welcome in the bosom of the family.)

Won't the toddler take all the milk and not leave enough for the baby?

In the first few days, many mothers will simply make sure that the new baby always nurses first, so that he gets lots of colostrum, and then let the older child nurse afterward. The toddler can also be helpful if the mother experiences any engorgement. As time goes on, the mother's milk supply will adjust to the needs of her two nursing children, just as it would if she had twins or triplets.

> "When she first felt her son's groping mouth attach itself to her breast, a wave of sweet vibration thrilled deep inside and radiated to all parts of her body; it was similar to love, but it went beyond a lover's caress, it brought a great calm happiness, a great happy calm."
>
> —Milan Kundera, *Life Is Elsewhere*

What about the mother?

Well, it is a symptom of how perverse our society has become that I hesitate to write the following. But here goes. If the mother allows herself, she too can get great pleasure and delight from breastfeeding the toddler. Some have suggested that the pleasure mothers get from breastfeeding an older child is perverted, because it is like having sex with children. This is simply bizarre.

I guess it depends on how one defines sexual pleasure. If sexual pleasure means feeling physical pleasure from close contact with someone you love, I guess breastfeeding fits, but then so does almost every other physical contact with those you love: hugging your sister, kissing your friend. To define hugging your sister as sexual pleasure is absurd in the vast majority of cases. Our problem in North America, and much of Europe, is that we cannot understand breasts except in a sexual context. Therefore any plea-

sure while breastfeeding can only be sexual in nature, and sexual pleasure with a three-year-old can only be perverted. It is our society that is perverted.

Some women have, indeed, described erotic thoughts and feelings while breastfeeding. Does this change the equation? Not at all. The mothers who describe these thoughts and feelings do not talk about having sexual feelings for their child, but simply having sexual thoughts and feelings while nursing—just as they might while drifting off to sleep on the couch, just as they might while daydreaming. Breastfeeding an older child allows mothers to relax, and in that state, yes, erotic thoughts and feelings may occur to them. This is as normal as can be and does not mean that breastfeeding is a sexual encounter between a child and his mother. We really do have an uptight society.

Of course, breastfeeding is not always easy or wonderful. Sometimes mothers feel their two-year-old is not asking to nurse at an appropriate time. Sometimes the mother just does not feel like it. But could the same not be said about everything a child wants of us? It may not be appropriate at a given time for the child to have a particular toy, have a particular food, or to go outside without a coat when the temperature is 20 below zero. The parents may not feel like taking time off work or changing their plans for the day when the child is sick, for example—but this is part of parenting. And yet the same child can delight us and make us radiantly happy. No part of parenting is 100 percent aggravation-free, but usually the rewards far outweigh the aggravation. Especially if we take the long view.

Mothers' Stories

The following are word for word what mothers have written to me about breastfeeding their older children. Possible identifying comments have been changed or removed.

LOUISE

I nursed my three children for a total of nine years and yours is the best article I have seen about the warmth and magic ability to comfort a toddler by breastfeeding [referring to some information sheets on the Web]. This is especially true when they are sick. My pediatrician told me to stop nursing on several occasions when my toddlers had the stomach flu (not terrible cases—only mild), recommending . . . instead [an electrolyte solution made by a formula company, naturally]. Now obviously it probably would have been better to keep their stomachs empty, but the stress they would have gone through was not acceptable to me because they obviously wanted to cuddle and nurse. So I let them nurse, figuring if nature intended anything for a sick baby, it would be breastmilk. It allowed them to sleep and rest between the times when they were sick. It gave them liquid so they didn't dehydrate. I don't believe it made things worse. It's funny, but some of my best memories of nursing are those where I was able to take my sick child and hold them and nurse them for hours, giving them the comfort they so desperately needed. To be able to truly help your small, sick child is a feeling I cannot describe and I am certain that I would not have been able to give the same level of comfort if I had only been holding them.

Louise was right about nursing through stomach flu, and the pediatrician was wrong. The pediatrician learned his care of stomach flu from the formula company advertising. You may not be surprised that the formula companies also make special electrolyte solutions for rehydration of

children with diarrhea. They have convinced organizations such as the Canadian Paediatric Society that these solutions are necessary for maintaining hydration when children have gastroenteritis, but in fact they rarely are. It is certainly unnecessary to stop breastfeeding because your baby has the flu. Occasionally adding electrolyte solutions might be useful, but not usually.

Louise understood something that the pediatrician did not—that there is more to taking care of the child than just treating a potential problem. Comforting the child is far more important, especially when comfort is all that is necessary for the majority of illnesses young children have in our society. The mother's relationship with her child takes on a whole new aspect when the child is sick and the mother "nurses" him through the illness. Some of my fondest memories as a child are of the times when I was sick and being coddled—lying on the couch, tucked in under a duvet, being brought drinks, and having cold compresses lovingly applied to my forehead.

> "Rejoice ye with Jerusalem, and be delighted over her, all ye that mourn for her. In order that ye may suck, and be satisfied with the breast of her consolations; in order that ye may sip and find pleasure from the abundance of her glory. For thus hath said the Lord, Behold, I will extend to her peace like a river, and like a rapid stream the glory of nations, that ye may suck; upon the arm shall ye be borne, and upon knees shall ye be dandled."
>
> Isaiah LXVI, 10–13

WENDY

I think that with Jennifer, as with Jane, nursing beyond age two provided a special, intimate emotional bond, that I think is at least if not more important than the nutritional value of nursing at this age. Once she became verbal we could talk about nursing, which provided for many precious moments. She had a nickname for nursing—"at" or "two at" when she wanted to switch. I think we got the idea of using a code word from a La Leche League mother who cited the advantage of privacy. Well, at one point we were at a restaurant with a large group of people I didn't know very well, and Jennifer piped up, "Wanna drink at from Mama's titty!" So much for privacy . . . We also had many private conversations and joked about nursing. Jennifer had had quite the little sense of humor from the start. She'd tell me she wanted to "drink at" from the "squishy one," though it wasn't ever clear which one that was. Or she would say, "Mmm . . . it tastes like candy."

The emotional security provided by nursing became especially valuable and important when I separated from my husband when Jennifer was three. I think it helped her maintain a sense of security during that very difficult time. She also resumed sleeping in bed with me throughout the transition. I was a little uneasy at times about her increased dependency, but kept reminding myself to trust that nurturing her in this way would pay off, which I truly believe it has in terms of her self-esteem and independence (she is now six, in kindergarten). Also in terms of the closeness and trust between us.

Weaning was a very interesting, mutually negotiated process. We discussed it for about a year before it happened. (For about the last year or so, she nursed pretty regularly in the morning and at bedtime, occasionally skipping here and there.) Luckily, Jennifer had a friend in preschool who nursed for as long as she did. She knew when Carmela weaned, and I pointed this out to Jennifer. It gave her an incentive to wean, too.

She pretty much decided which day she would stop, and then never nursed again after that. . . .

She still talks about nursing from time to time, and says she misses it, and sometimes cuddles my breasts as a reminder, but we both feel very good about the way she outgrew it naturally.

ILANA

I have four children. The first three nursed to about 18 months, and weaned themselves (or so it seemed).

My fourth daughter just went on nursing—every day followed the previous one, and there were days when I thought she would nurse forever. She went to the day care from the age of three months, from 7 a.m. to 4 p.m. At first I would come several times a day to nurse, later once a day, and toward her second birthday I stopped visiting her during her stay at the day care. She would nurse when she came home in the afternoon, sometimes every hour till bedtime. She stopped nursing at night around two years, even though she slept with us most of the time. She continued nursing to the age of four and a half years.

As she got older, somehow she nursed less and less—in the morning we were in a hurry, and sometimes she skipped the morning nursing. In the afternoon, she started to be busy—friends, games, etc. We had interesting conversations about nursing. "Mommy, your milk tastes much better than anything else," "When I go to school, I'll stop nursing," and many other things that make nursing an older child a unique experience. Once, when she was around four years old, I asked her if there was still milk coming out when she nursed and she replied, "What do you think? Coca-Cola?"

As she grew older she learned that you can't nurse anywhere, anytime, that when there are visitors it's not always OK to nurse. There started to be days when she wouldn't nurse all day, and other days when she nursed several times. Then there were several days without nursing, and I thought she wouldn't nurse anymore, but she would nurse again. In the end she nursed once every few days, and once, after two or three weeks, when she tried nursing she told me, "There is no more milk! Where did it go?" I explained that because she had been nursing less and less, there is less and less milk. She decided to nurse more, and asked me to remind her to nurse every day when she came home in the afternoon, every evening and morning, but she didn't manage to stick to this plan . . . she was weaned. Nature had taken its course. Babies don't nurse forever.

Nursing an older baby, toddler, or child is a very special experience, and I would recommend it to everyone. Lately more mothers around me have gone on to nurse older babies. I think that seeing me has a lot to do with this.

Ilana is undoubtedly right. Many women do want to breastfeed, and many will breastfeed for years if only people do not tell them it is strange, bizarre, perverted. They need only a role model.

Some mothers are told they are breastfeeding "just for your own gratification." I must say this argument makes me very angry. There are few, if any, women who breastfeed just for their own gratification. This is once again taking breastfeeding as some sort of sexual activity, in a society that does not understand that the primary purpose of breasts is to nurture children. It is difficult in our society to nurse a six-month-old, never mind a toddler. A mother who does so is fighting the tide of general opinion, something that is not easy to do. And it is not possible to force a child who does not want to nurse to continue nursing. They just won't do it.

Mothers nurse past a year or two for several reasons, one of the major ones being that it is easier just to keep going than to try to force a child who does not feel ready to stop breastfeeding. Some continue because the baby is not sleeping through the night, and it is just easier to nurse a child to sleep than to use any other method. But very few who continue into the second and third years later regret that they did it—especially afterward, when they see their happy, confident, independent youngsters. Independent? Really? Yes, really.

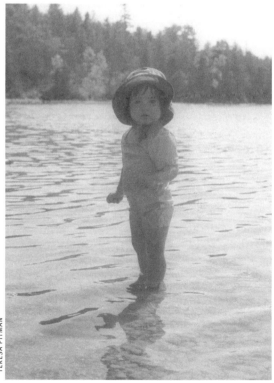

TERESA PITMAN

This nursing toddler is well on her way to being a secure and independent child.

Independence and Extended Breastfeeding

One frequent argument against "extended" nursing (which really should be called "normal duration breastfeeding") is that the child will be overdependent and "sucky" if nursed past a few months. This is yet another example of turning logic upside down.

Are children less independent if they are given security, comfort, and love freely during their first few years? On the contrary, if they are helped to feel secure and loved, they will be independent, not dependent, because they will be secure in that independence and know that they are loved unconditionally. I will admit that you don't need breastfeeding to two years or beyond to give them this, but the argument that continuing breastfeeding to this time causes overdependence is nonsense. It comes from a mistaken notion that nursing past six months or a year is not developmentally appropriate. In fact, it is not "developmentally appropriate" to stop breastfeeding at six months or a year. Of course, it is possible to use breastfeeding to maintain an unnatural dependence, but it is possible to use anything to maintain an unnatural dependence. A mother who uses breastfeeding to control her child would also use toilet training, or food, or bedtimes to do the same thing.

It is possible to force independence, to make a child sleep alone in a dark room at the developmentally inappropriate age of four months. It is possible to make a child accept being left alone with strangers for days at a time. Does this make the child more independent? Not at all. The outward appearance is one of independence, but deep down, the child is not independent—quite the contrary.

Adults often force their own notions of what is appropriate on children. In the 1960s, it was common for children, even young ones, who were admitted to the hospital not to get visits from their parents. Visiting hours were, typically, once a week on Sundays, from 1:00 p.m. to 4:00 p.m. The staff did not like even these occasional visits because the children cried when the parents left. It was generally felt that it was better the children not be visited at all. This was inhuman, and did it serve the interests of the child or parents? Of course not. Just because the child did not cry did not mean all was well. The child simply clammed up, went into depression, and the interpretation of the physicians and nurses was often that the child coped better because he didn't cry. What a disastrous policy! Of course, no one would ever have imagined disallowing visits for an adult in hospital, especially not from his close family.

> **Is there a "natural" age of weaning for humans?**
>
> Anthropologist Kathy Dettwyler has considered this issue by comparing humans to other mammals—and primates in particular. In her book *Breastfeeding: Biocultural Perspectives* she looks at the relationship between the age of weaning and other developmental traits in gorillas, chimpanzees, orangutans, and other primates. For example, in most of the large primates, the number of months of lactation is about six times the length of pregnancy (gestation). As another example, the baby usually weans when it reaches about four times its birthweight. Her conclusion: The natural age of weaning for humans would be somewhere between 2.5 years and 7 years.

You want an independent child? Give him love and security freely. If part of the way you do this is breastfeeding until he is ready to stop, then feel secure yourself that you are doing the right thing. This does not mean letting the child do anything he wants. Children also get security from knowing where their limits are. But forcing independence does not work. How independent do you want your child to be, anyway? Do you want him to leave home at 14? Let him take his steps when he is ready. You will have your independent child.

Extended (Normal Duration) Breastfeeding and Teeth

Dentists these days have made some quite negative comments about breastfeeding longer than a year, especially night nursing. The American Dental Association and the Canadian Dental Association both have policies of discouraging breastfeeding after a year. The reason: Children who are put to sleep *with a bottle* at night often have their teeth destroyed by the sugar in the milk or juice that bathes their teeth.

It is quite right for us to be concerned about babies being put to sleep with a bottle, not only because of their teeth, but also because of possible ear infections and possible aspiration of fluid into their lungs. We should also ask ourselves this: If a child needs something to help him sleep at night, is the bottle the appropriate "something"? To me, the obvious answer is that the child needs the comforting presence of a parent to help him feel relaxed and safe so he can sleep.

Unfortunately, using the bottle to keep the child happy in his crib does result in tooth decay in many cases. Nursing during the night only rarely results in the same sort of damage, and if any damage occurs, it tends to be mild. What dentists don't see is that the majority of children who are nursed during the night do *not* get cavities. Since those who do end up at the dentist's office, he or she often concludes that this is a common problem for children nursing past the first year of life. It isn't. Even if the child is brought to the dentist for a routine check, the dentist will not usually ask about night nursing unless the child has cavities. Most dentists probably have no idea that some or even many of their cavity-free 18-month-old patients are still breastfeeding at night (horrors!).

There is evidence, on the other hand, that nursing past a year helps prevent crooked teeth, and possibly sleep apnea, later in life. Sleep apnea (in which children or adults stop breathing at night for longer than normal periods of time) can cause snoring, tiredness during the day, and even heart problems. Why aren't the dentists concerned about these problems?

But even if night nursing does cause cavities, is this a reason to force an 18-month-old or two-year-old to stop breastfeeding? By the way, this is one issue on which health professionals have no problem making mothers feel guilty: "By nursing your child at night, you have caused him to have cavities." Okay, teeth are important, but they are not *all*-important. The child's psychological state matters as well. To force an 18-month-old to wean when he is not ready is likely to cause a lot more damage than continued nursing at night.

If the child does have cavities, it might be reasonable to attempt to stop the night feedings, but if this is obviously causing distress, the mother should not persist with something that is just not worth it. To stop breastfeeding altogether because of the teeth? What are the dentists thinking about? Like the once-a-week hospital visits we described earlier, this is another example of our causing problems while blithely thinking we are doing the best thing.

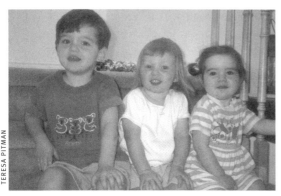

Brother and sister (girl on far right) are tandem breastfeeders. Here they spend time with another breastfed toddler.

Breastfeeding, Parental Separation, and Access

Unfortunately, one problem breastfeeding does not prevent is marriage breakdown. With more mothers breastfeeding for longer periods of time, we see increasing numbers of cases where fathers want access visits with their children while the child is still nursing. Not infrequently, fathers ask for, and unfortunately receive, access that interrupts the breastfeeding relationship. This is short-term gain for long-term pain.

Many toddlers are still nursing at night, and need the breast to fall asleep. Not everyone would agree that this is a good thing, though I certainly think that it is not a bad thing. Even if you don't agree with this as a parenting approach, there is often nothing that can be done about an 18-month-old nursing at night. Some toddlers are feeding frequently through the night. This is a fact. Why would a father insist on overnight access when this is the situation? What is so great about overnight access, anyway? And what if the child cries throughout the night because he cannot have access to the breast? I have, on more than one occasion, heard of the father returning the crying child in the middle of the night because Dad was desperate and unable to handle him. But even if the child does not cry, he will return to the mother, clinging, upset, and wanting to nurse even more than before.

As Wendy mentioned in her story, it was breastfeeding her three-year-old that got Jennifer through the difficult time when the parents' marriage was breaking down. Breastfeeding was a rock on which she could rest when the stress got too much for her. Why would a father who is interested in the welfare of his child insist on yet more stress for the child?

The father can have a considerable amount of time with his child without necessarily interrupting the breastfeeding relationship. There is no need for a father to have alternate weeks with the child. The toddler is not developmentally ready for such a lengthy separation, either from the mother or the father. A few hours at a time, or much of the day—but overnight? Not yet. For the good of the child, it is better to wait until he's older.

Unfortunately, most jurisdictions in North America do not recognize breastfeeding as important, nor do they understand child development. Breastfeeding is seen as expendable. Mothers are often told by judges to give bottles to 18-month-old children who have never taken one—as if the child would listen to the judge!

In the first few years, the mother is more important for the child than the father. That is simply a fact of life. You can argue that it should not be that way, you can argue that it's not fair, but that's the way it is. If the importance of the mother–baby relationship is respected with regard to access, the father's relationship with his child will be better, not worse, in the long run. Most people can be quite inventive about finding a solution without interrupting the breastfeeding relationship, if they want to be. Unfortunately, many do not. They see it as a battle they are determined to win. But no matter which parent wins, the child always loses.

If the child is young (under six months of age), access that results in weaning or unnecessary introduction of formula should not be considered, except in extraordinary situations. The risks of artificial feeding take precedence over the "needs" of the father. Again, arrangements can be made that give the father reasonable access, but not at the risk of the child's health.

Perhaps one day the family court system will understand that bottle-feeding is not, in fact, the normal way of feeding children. Currently, much unnecessary suffering is caused by interruption of the breastfeeding relationship, because we have to consider the father's rights. We should consider them, but let's be creative in finding solutions that do not cause unnecessary weaning.

> "And hence at our maturer years, when any object of vision is presented to us, which by its waving or spiral lines bears any similitude to the form of the female bosom, whether it is found in a landscape with soft gradations of rising and descending surface, or in the forms of some antique vases, or in other works of the pencil or chisel, we feel a general glow of delight, which seems to influence all our senses."
>
> —Erasmus Darwin;
> *Zoonomia*, or *The Laws of Organic Life*. 1794

So, breastfeed a toddler? Of course—why not? Don't worry, he'll stop nursing before he walks down the aisle on his wedding day. You and your child will benefit from it. Go ahead. Let yourself enjoy nursing until you are both ready to wean.

20

Quick Questions and Answers

My mother tried to breastfeed but couldn't. Does this mean I won't be able to?

Of course not. Many women of your mother's generation were getting even worse advice about how to go about breastfeeding than women of this generation. What is actually amazing is that some women who tried to feed by the clock and other "helpful" hints of the day actually managed it quite well. There is no evidence that "insufficient milk supply" is hereditary, even on the off chance that your mother was indeed one of the few women who did not produce enough for their babies (see Chapter 5, Not Enough Milk).

I've heard that there are lots of environmental contaminants in breastmilk, and that if I breastfeed my baby I'll be giving him dangerous chemicals. Is this true, and if so, wouldn't formula be better?

No. It is a measure of how indulgent we are toward formula that we imagine that despite *everything* on our planet being contaminated, somehow formula has escaped contamination. In fact, formula has lots of pollutants—perhaps different ones from those in breastmilk and in different proportions, but nevertheless lots. The concern with contaminants such as PCBs and dioxins in breastmilk is that they diminish the baby's immunity. But babies who are breastfed have *fewer infections* than do artificially fed babies.

Another concern is that these pollutants will increase the chances of the baby getting cancer later on. But the evidence is that breastfed babies have *less* chance of getting certain cancers (see Chapter 1, Why Breastfeeding Is Important).

I was told that you can't eat chocolate or "gassy" foods such as broccoli or spicy foods such as curry when you are breastfeeding, because it will upset the baby. Is this true? What foods should I avoid?

Don't avoid any foods. If you find that certain foods seem to bother the baby, then try avoiding them and see what happens. But don't *expect* that the baby will react to these foods. They don't most of the time (see Chapter 9, Colic).

I'm overweight and have very large breasts. I was told that I probably won't be able to breastfeed because large breasts don't produce enough milk, and also that it's too hard to get the baby positioned on the breast. Is this true?

It is harder to latch a baby on well with large breasts, but it can still be done with good help. Most women with large breasts produce plenty of milk, as do most women with average or tiny breasts (see Chapter 4, Getting Off to the Best Start).

I'm expecting triplets.
Can I breastfeed them?

Of course you can. And with good help and support you may well be able to breastfeed them exclusively. Even if you cannot breastfeed them exclusively, you can still breastfeed. But it is best to supplement at the breast, not use bottles, because breastfeeding continues when you use a nursing supplementer rather than feeding the babies off the breast (see Chapter 5, Not Enough Milk).

I've heard that you shouldn't breastfeed right after you exercise, but instead should pump your milk and throw it away. Will it harm my baby if I nurse him after working out?

Not at all. Maybe after Olympic-type exercise some lactic acid makes the milk taste funny to the baby, but not after normal exercise. Please don't listen to this sort of nonsense. In any case, the lactic acid will not harm the baby. At most, the baby might not like the taste. You don't have to pump the milk even then, since when the lactic acid decreases in your blood it will decrease automatically in the milk.

Won't breastfeeding for a long time—say, more than a year—make your baby too attached and dependent on you?

Attached, yes. Dependent? Well, it depends on how you mean that. Yes, dependent in that he needs you—but isn't that good? That's what love is all about: needing someone. Do you mean that you don't want your baby to need you? Of course you don't. Overly dependent? On the contrary. Babies who get the security they need are more independent (see Chapter 19, Breastfeeding the Toddler).

I'm just seventeen and my baby is due next month. I was told that I'm probably too young to breastfeed because my breasts might not be fully developed. Is this true?

What nonsense. You will probably produce lots and lots of milk. Your breasts have been fully developed for several years. Goodness, if you have what it takes to make a baby, why would your breasts not be up to the task? Nature doesn't goof to that extent.

Breastfeeding was going fine until my baby turned about nine months old. Now he bites me at least once a day while he's nursing—and it hurts! Do I have to wean him? What can I do?

There are a few reasons why babies bite. Sometimes they do so when they have almost finished nursing, are falling asleep at the breast, and suddenly startle. The answer is to ease the baby off the breast when he is falling asleep. Another possibility is that he is playing—trying out his new gums and teeth. This usually occurs after an initial short period of nursing, so the baby isn't terribly hungry or thirsty. The answer is often to bring the baby close to you as when you were feeding him as a newborn. This often works. If not, try not to startle him too much, but just tell him no. Gently but firmly. If he keeps it up, then ease him off the breast, gently, and let him understand that the feeding is over. (Slip your finger into the corner of his mouth so that he doesn't bite down on the nipple to prevent you from removing it!) Just as he can understand that he can't pull hair, he can understand at this age that biting is not acceptable. Usually your baby will stop this behavior after a couple of times of being gently and firmly told it's not okay. Last, babies sometimes bite when milk flow is slow. This may occur quite early in the feeding. Is your milk supply down? Did you go on the birth control pill? Is the baby getting lots of bottles (a nine-month-old does not need bottles)? Correct the problems that might cause a slow flow. Don't stop breastfeeding.

My baby weighed eight pounds at birth and now at four months old he's over 21 pounds. Everyone tells me he's too fat, and I should put him on a diet. Am I overfeeding him? He's had nothing but breastmilk.

Some breastfed babies grow much faster than formula-fed babies. There is no concern—breastfed babies, unlike formula-fed babies, tend to slim down later. How do you put four-month-old babies on a diet? Don't worry, and don't let people worry you (see Chapter 5, Not Enough Milk).

I want to breastfeed but I don't see how I can manage it when I go out. Won't people be offended if they see me nursing?

If they are, that is their problem, isn't it? It's funny that people do not remark on billboards showing 14-year-old girls almost naked selling underwear, but get funny about breastfeeding in public. The good news is that breastfeeding in public is becoming more accepted. If you are really shy, bring a blanket to cover you and your baby. You will get used to nursing in public and you will soon not use the blanket. Why should your baby be hidden if he's nursing? Shouldn't he be able to see you? Make a statement—breastfeed in public. Other women will follow your lead. Many states now have legislation protecting mothers from harassment if they nurse in public. And most provincial human rights commissions will back up a mother's right to nurse in public.

I've tried to quit smoking but I just can't. Would it be better for my baby to get formula than the milk of a mother who is smoking?

No. There is good evidence now that babies whose mothers smoke are healthier if they are breastfeeding than if they are formula-feeding (see Chapter 11, Breastfeeding While on Medication).

My two-month-old is gaining and content, but all his poops are green. Everyone is telling me this is abnormal and the doctor is making me very worried.

If the baby is content and gaining well, ignore the comments from well-meaning friends. Buy yourself a pair of sunglasses so you don't see the color.

Resources
for Good Breastfeeding Help

La Leche League

This is a volunteer organization. Leaders are all mothers who have breastfed at least one baby for at least a year and then had some additional training. They have access to information about many aspects of breastfeeding. Monthly meetings are held in most communities. Dr. Newman is on the Professional Advisory Board of La Leche League International.

LA LECHE LEAGUE INTERNATIONAL
P.O. Box 4079
Schaumburg, IL 60168
Phone: (847) 519-7730
E-mail: LLLHQ@llli.org
Web site: www.lalecheleague.org

To find a La Leche League group or leader in your area:

Phone:(800) LALECHE

Milk Banks in the United States

CALIFORNIA

MOTHERS' MILK BANK
751 South Bascom Avenue
San Jose, CA 95128

Phone: (408) 998-4550
E-mail: mothersmilkbank@hhs.co.santa-clara.ca.us
Web site: www.milkbanksj.org

COLORADO

MOTHERS' MILK BANK AT
PRESBYTERIAN ST. LUKE'S MEDICAL CENTER
1719 E. 19th Avenue
Denver, CO 80218
Phone: (303) 869-1888
E-mail: mmilkbank@health1.org
Web site: http://www.health1.org/milkbank.asp

DELAWARE

MOTHERS' MILK BANK
CHRISTIANA HOSPITAL
4755 Ogletown-Stanton Road
Newark, DE 19718
Phone: (302)733-2340
E-mail: dmore@christianacare.org

INDIANA

INDIANA MOTHERS' MILK BANK, INC.
METHODIST MEDICAL PLAZA II
6820 Parkdale Place, Suite 109
Indianapolis, IN 4654
Phone: (317) 329-7146
E-mail: inmothersmilkbank@clarian.org
Web site: http://www.immilkbank.org/

IOWA

MOTHERS' MILK BANK OF IOWA
DIVISION OF NUTRITION
DEPARTMENT OF PEDIATRICS
CHILDREN'S HOSPITAL OF IOWA
200 Hawkins Drive
Iowa City, IA 52242
Phone: (319) 356-2651
E-mail: Jean-drulis@uiowa.edu or
Janice-jeter@uiowa.edu

MICHIGAN

BRONSON METHODIST HOSPITAL
(DEVELOPING BANK)
601 John Street, Box 306
Kalamazoo, MI 49007
Phone: (269) 341-8849
E-mail: Duffc@bronsonhg.org

NORTH CAROLINA

WAKEMED MOTHERS' MILK BANK AND
LACTATION CENTER
3000 New Bern Avenue
Raleigh, NC 27610
Phone: (919) 350-8599
E-mail: mmould@wakemed.org or
gbuckley@wakemed.org

OHIO

MOTHERS' MILK BANK OF OHIO
GRANT MEDICAL CENTER AT
VICTORIAN VILLAGE HEALTH CENTER
1087 Dennison Avenue
Columbus, OH 43201
Phone: (614) 544-5906
E-mail: gmorrow@ohiohealth.com

TEXAS

MOTHERS' MILK BANK AT AUSTIN
900 E. 30th Street, Suite 214

Austin, TX 78705
Phone: (512) 494-0800
Toll-free: 1 (877) 813-MILK (6455)
E-mail: info@mmbaustin.org
Web site: www.mmbaustin.org

MOTHERS' MILK BANK OF NORTH TEXAS
1300 W. Lancaster, Suite 108
Ft. Worth, TX 76102
Phone: (817) 810-0071
Toll-free: 1 (866) 810-0071
E-mail: mmbnt@hotmail.com
Web site: http://www.mmbnt.org/

CANADA

BC WOMEN'S MILK BANK
C & W LACTATION SERVICES
4500 Oak Street, IU 30
Vancouver, BC V6M 3X4
Phone: (604) 875-2282
E-mail: fjones@cw.bc.ca

Baby-Friendly Hospitals and Birth Centers

For a comprehensive list, please visit
www.babyfriendlyusa.org.

International Lactation Consultants Association (ILCA)

Phone: (919)-861-5577
E-mail: info@ilca.org
Web site: www.ilca.org

Dr. Jack Newman's Breastfeeding Clinics

Phone: (416) 813-5757 (option 3)

General Breastfeeding Information

The Birth Den: www.thebirthden.com/Newman.html
Gentle Mothering: www.gentlemothering.ca

Other Web Sites of Interest

Adopting: www.fourfriends.com/abrw

"Advantages of Formula":
www.cs.colorado.edu/~kolina/advantages-of-formula.html

Baby Milk Action: www.gn.apc.org/babymilk

Bestfed.com: www.bestfed.com

Breastfeeding After Breast Reduction: www.bfar.org

Mothering magazine: www.mothering.com

Breastfeeding.com: www.breastfeeding.com

Compleat Mother: www.compleatmother.com

Drugs and Breastfeeding (Dr. Tom Hale):
http://neonatal.ttuhsc.edu/lact

Famous People Who Have Breastfed:
www.breastfeeding.org/famous_people_who_have_breastfed.htm

International Lactation Consultant Association:
www.ilca.org

Infact Canada: www.infactcanada.ca

International Board of Lactation Consultant Examiners: www.iblce.org

Lactnews: www.jump.net/~bwx/lactnews.html

La Leche League International:
www.lalecheleague.org

Promom: www.promom.org

San Diego County Breastfeeding Coalition:
www.breastfeeding.org

Ted Greiner's Breastfeeding Web site:
www.geocities.com/HotSprings/Spa/3156

UNICEF publications: www.unicef.org/apublic

World Alliance for Breastfeeding Action (WABA):
www.waba.org.br

World Health Organization (WHO) hypoglycemia document: www.who.int/chd/publications/imci/bf/hypoclyc/hypoclyc.htm.

Dutch Web site: www.borstvoeding.com

Italian Web site: http://space.tin.it/salute/uschmid

The La Leche League International Web site also has information in Chinese, Spanish, Italian, and Russian (go to www.lalecheleague.org)

For information in French go to www.allaitement.ca

Acknowledgments

I would like to express my appreciation to La Leche League, to all the women who came to the clinics and helped me learn, and to all those who are dedicated to helping mothers breastfeed. They are the people who taught me what I know about breastfeeding today. Also, special thanks to Ruth Bacon who kept pushing me to write a book, and to Carol Brussel, Yael Wyshogrod, and Kathie Marinelli who read the first drafts and offered comments. Thank you, too, to Nicole Langlois, our editor at Harper Collins, whose enthusiasm and organizational skills have been much appreciated.

Dr. Jack Newman

The authors wish to thank the following mothers and children for allowing their photos to be used in this book:

Susan Bushell and Solana Del Bel Belluz; Karen, Mallachie, and Sadie Campbell; Sherlene Coulanges and Tai-Zel; Victoria DaPonte and Isaac McLellan; Tina and Emily Anne Ditoro; Linda Emanuele; Christine and Brianne Gayfer; Kym Godfrey and Dominic Loss (from Perth, Western Australia); Cleonie Gordon and Kandice Drysdale; Lucy and Lara Hingorani; Tracy and Aaron Kirschner; Hazel Ling and Maren Tracey; Kathleen Ossip; Michele and Cori Sears; Philippa Sheppard and Sophia Oppel; Susan and Austin Speigel; Barbara and Ayden van Koot; Sharon Marie Wheller and Kennedy Elizebeth Marie Wheller; Andrea and Matthew Wronko.

Photographs by Riziero Vertolli and Roni Chastain are used by permission, and with the authors' thanks.

The authors are grateful to the following publishers and authors for the use of excerpts in this book:

Jean Cotterman.

Isak Dinesen (Karen Blixen), *Ehrengard*, London: Penguin Books. Copyright © 1962 by the Curtis Publishing Co; copyright © 1963 by Rungstedlundfonden. Reproduced by permission of Penguin Books Ltd.

Günter Grass, *The Flounder*, Orlando, Fla.: Harcourt, Inc.

Marni Jackson, *The Mother Zone: Love, Sex and Laundry in the Modern Family*, Toronto, Canada: Macfarlane Walter & Ross.

Milan Kundera, *Life Is Elsewhere*, New York: Alfred A. Knopf, Inc.

Ashley Montagu, *Touching: The Human Significance of the Skin*, copyright by Ashley Montagu, New York: HarperCollins Publishers.

Carol Shields, *The Stone Diaries*, Toronto: Random House of Canada. Published in the United States by Viking, and in the United Kingdom by Fourth Estate.

Index

About the Authors

Jack Newman, M.D., is a leading researcher in the field of breastfeeding. The former chief of pediatrics at Doctor's Hospital in Toronto, he is a popular speaker at breastfeeding conferences across North America. He lives in Toronto and is the father of three children, all breastfed.

Teresa Pitman has been a La Leche League leader for more than twenty-five years. She is currently the executive director of La Leche League Canada. The author or coauthor of nine other books on parenting, she is the mother of four breastfed children and lives in Ontario.